Eli Lilly

Lilly's Hand Book of Pharmacy and Therapeutics

Eli Lilly

Lilly's Hand Book of Pharmacy and Therapeutics

ISBN/EAN: 9783742830074

Manufactured in Europe, USA, Canada, Australia, Japa

Cover: Foto ©Lupo / pixelio.de

Manufactured and distributed by brebook publishing software
(www.brebook.com)

Eli Lilly

Lilly's Hand Book of Pharmacy and Therapeutics

LILLY'S

HAND BOOK

OF

PHARMACY

AND

THERAPEUTICS.

FIFTH REVISION. THIRTEENTH EDITION.
ONE HUNDRED AND TWENTY-FIFTH THOUSAND.

PRICE, 25 CENTS.

ELI LILLY & COMPANY,
Pharmaceutical Chemists,
INDIANAPOLIS.
1898

INTRODUCTION

TO THE

FIFTH REVISION.

LILLY'S HAND BOOK OF PHARMACY AND THERAPEUTICS has for years been the standard ready reference in its peculiar field for thousands of Pharmacists and Physicians. The present revision has been most thorough and exhaustive, the work being greatly enlarged both in size and number of pages, introducing many radical changes and improvements, bringing it down to date in every feature.

LILLY'S HAND BOOK furnishes the busy practitioner a reliable means of information, at once concise, systematic and authoritative, to which he may refer with confidence in cases of doubt. Younger members of the profession and medical students will find this little work full of suggestions, which will stimulate them to more extended reading.

The therapeutical notes have been compiled from standard authorites, among which are The United States Dispensatory; The National Dispensatory — Stille & Maisch; The American Dispensatory, with supplement; Hand Book of Therapeutics—Ringer; Materia Medica and Therapeutics—Bartholow; A Treatise on Therapeutics—Trousseau; A Guide to Therapeutics—Farquharson; Modern Materia Medica—Helbing; Materia Medica, Pharmacy and Therapeutics—Potter; Materia Medica, Pharmacology and Therapeutics—Shoemaker.

SPECIAL NOTICE.

LILLY'S HAND BOOK was formerly sent out without charge in paper covers. Copies in leather binding were supplied at 50 cents each. The paper covers however, were not durable and we have discontinued supplying in that way. In substantial muslin binding we now send the HAND BOOK, postage prepaid, on receipt of 25 cents, or in leather binding, 50 cents. These prices barely cover cost of binding and postage, it not being our desire to make a profit on the book. Although an advertisement of our preparations in a way, it also contains such a large fund of collateral information not elsewhere so accessible that we are sure those who desire to to use the Hand Book will not consider the small charge unreasonable.

INDIANAPOLIS, June, 1897.

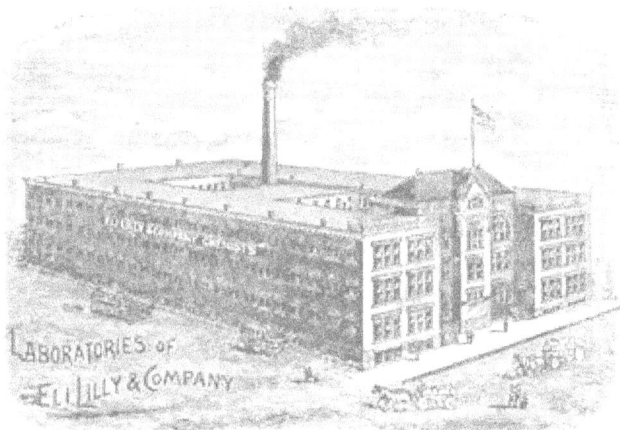

LABORATORIES OF
ELI LILLY & COMPANY

ELI LILLY & COMPANY,

PHARMACEUTICAL CHEMISTS

INDIANAPOLIS, IND., U. S. A.

JOSIAH K. LILLY, PRESIDENT.

JAMES E. LILLY, VICE-PRESIDENT.   EVAN F. LILLY, SECRETARY.

TABLE OF CONTENTS.

For Complete Index see Page 333.

FLUID EXTRACTS.

For nearly a quarter of a century the products of Eli Lilly & Company have borne the highest reputation with the medical and pharmaceutical professions. In no part of their work have they presented greater excellence or demonstrated higher qualities of leadership than in their line of Fluid Extracts.

Having the closest relations with the best sources of foreign crude drugs, with direct surveillance of the collection of indigenous supplies, very largely obtained through their own collectors, the usual course through the markets with consequent uncertainty of quality is avoided.

Not content, however, under any circumstances to accept any drug at its face, it must pass the most rigid examination, botanically in all cases and chemically where practicable, in order that the resulting extract may be of the highest attainable quality. Scientific departments for these purposes were introduced here in advance of any other pharmaceutical laboratory and here were produced the first Fluid Extracts standardized to definite strength.

The natural result of such painstaking care has brought about, in the course of years, a very great preference for the brand of Eli Lilly & Company, a preference it will always be a pleasure to maintain by honest adherence to the methods by which it was originally produced.

All Fluid Extract labels of Eli Lilly & Company carry the most complete information, giving in each case the name of the preparation, dose, botanical name of the drug and authority, natural order, botanical and common synonyms, range, habitat, part used, standard of strength, action and uses, antidotes in case of poisons, formulas for preparing syrups, wines, tinctures, infusions, etc. To insure preservation of Fluid Extracts, they are always sent out in amber glass bottles and it is advised they be kept in a moderately cool situation, as little exposed to variations of temperature as possible.

SPECIAL CAUTION.

The processes and menstrua of other manufacturers being so different, any attempt to apply our formulas to other Fluid Extracts will certainly lead to disappointment. Be careful, therefore, in purchasing always to specify "Lilly's".

ELI LILLY & COMPANY'S
STANDARD FLUID EXTRACTS.
See also Appendix, page 331.

FL. EXT. ABSCESS ROOT.... ....   **Dose 30 to 60 m.**

Polemonium reptans Linn.   **Nat. Ord.** –*Polemoniaceæ*.

Synonyms—American Greek valerian, Jacob's ladder, Blue bells.

Range—United States; from Minnesota east and south.

Habitat—Damp woodlands and shady banks of streams.

Part used—The root.

Standard of strength—That of the U. S. Pharmacopœia, 1890; 1 c.c. representing 1 gram of the drug; or, practically, minim for grain.

Action and uses—Alterative, astringent and diaphoretic. Has been found valuable in scrofula, pleurisy, febrile and inflammatory diseases, and as a gargle in bronchial and laryngeal affections.

PREPARATIONS.

Syrup Abscess Root—Fl. ext. Abscess root, Lilly, 4 fl. ozs.; Syrup, 12 fl. ozs.; Mix—Dose 2 to 4 fl. drs.

Infusion Abscess Root—Fl. ext. Abscess root, Lilly, 2 fl. ozs.; Hot water, 14 fl. ozs.; Mix—Dose ½ to 1 fl. oz. or as a gargle.

FL. EXT. ACONITE LEAVES. .... **Dose 2 to 5 m.**

Aconitum Napellus Linn.   **Nat. Ord.**—*Ranunculaceæ*.

Synonyms—A. vulgare D. C.,—Monkshood, Wolfsbane.

Range—Europe, Asia and Northwestern North America; cultivated.

Habitat—Mountain forests.

Part used—The leaf.

Standard of strength—That of the U. S. Pharmacopœia, 1890; 1 c. c. representing 1 gram of the drug; or, practically, minim for grain.

Aconite leaves have been discarded from the U. S. P., the root alone being official. Fl. Ext. Aconite *root*, Lilly, is standardized to uniform strength and should always be prescribed.

Action and uses—*Aceronarcotic poison*, nerve sedative and antiphlogistic. Antagonizes the fever process. Of greatest value in high resisting pulse, dry hot skin and elevated body temperature. Valuable in acute throat affections and in the onset of inflammations of the respiratory organs, catarrhal croup, acute pleuritis and peritonitis before the stage of effusion; also in simple and eruptive fevers, puerperal and surgical fevers and in the short sharp feverish affections of children. Externally and internally in neuralgia of the fifth nerve.

Antidotes—None reliable. Recumbent posture absolute. **Stomach** pump. Heat to extremities, stimulants, artificial respiration if necessary. Caffeine hypodermically or by the mouth. Atropine, morphine, ammonia, ether and amyl nitrite have been used.

PREPARATION.

Tincture Aconite Leaves—Fl. ext. Aconite leaves, Lilly, 2 fl. ozs.; Alcohol, 1½ fl. ozs.; Water, 2½ fl. ozs.; Mix—Dose 15 to 30 fl. drs.

FL. EXT. ACONITE ROOT, U. S................ .. **Dose 1-2 to 2 m.**

Aconitum Napellus Linn.   **Nat. Ord.** *Ranunculaceæ*.

Synonyms—A. vulgare D. C.,—Aconitum U. S., Monkshood, Wolfsbane.

Range—Europe, Asia and Northwestern North America.

Habitat—Mountain forests.

Part used—The tuber.

Standard of Strength—0.5 per cent. of alkaloid estimated gravimetrically. This preparation will also respond to the following test: 1 minim diluted with water to 10 fluid drams will give from one fluid dram placed in the mouth (previously rinsed with water) and retained for one minute, a distinct tingling sensation, lasting for some minutes.

Note—Fluid extract aconite upon the market **varies greatly in color**. Some makers retaining the menstruum of the **Pharmacopœia of 1880.**

which makes a light colored extract, others, including ourselves, utilize the menstrua of the present pharmacopœia which produces an extract some thicker than the above. Again some employ dilute alcohol which gives to the extract a very dark color.

Action and uses—*Acronarcotic poison*, nerve sedative and antiphlogistic. Antagonizes the fever process. Of greatest value in high resisting pulse, dry hot skin and elevated body temperature. Valuable in acute throat affections and in the onset of inflammations of the respiratory organs, catarrhal croup, acute pleurisy and peritonitis before the stage of effusion; also in simple and eruptive puerperal and surgical fevers and in the short sharp feverish affections of children. Externally and internally in neuralgia of the fifth nerve.

Antidotes—None reliable. Recumbent posture absolute. Stomach pump, stimulants, heat to extremities, artificial respiration if necessary. Give mechypodermically or by the mouth. Atropine, morphine, ammonia, ether and amyl nitrite have been used.

PREPARATION.

Tincture Aconite Root. U. S.—Fl. ext. Aconite root, Lilly, 5½ fl. ozs.; Alcohol, 7¾ fl. ozs.; Water, 2¾ fl. ozs. Mix—Dose 1 to 5 m.

FL. EXT. ADONIS VERNALIS........................ Dose 1 to 2 m.
Adonis vernalis Linn. **Nat. Ord.**—*Ranunculaceæ.*

Synonyms—False hellebore, Birdseye.

Range—Europe, Asia.

Part used—The herb.

Standard of strength—That of the U. S. Pharmacopœia, 1890; 1 c.c. representing 1 gram of the drug or, practically, minim for grain.

Action and uses—*Poisonous.* Reputed valuable as a cardiac stimulant and useful in dropsy and diseases of the heart. Employed in much the same manner as digitalis but is said to be much more prompt and to have no cumulative tendency.

Antidotes—Prompt emetics. Tannic acid is the chemical antidote, but the tannate should be evacuated. Aconite the best antagonist for large doses. Opium to those of long continued use. Recumbent position.

FL. EXT. AGRIMONY. .... Dose 20 to 40 m
Agrimonia Eupatoria Walt. **Nat. Ord.**—*Rosaceæ.*

Synonyms—Agrimonia striata Michx.,—Cocklebur, Sticklewort.

Range—United States; common.

Habitat—Borders of woodlands.

Part used—The herb.

Standard of strength—That of the U. S. Pharmacopœia, 1890; 1 c.c. representing 1 gram of the drug or, practically, minim for grain.

Action and uses—Astringent, stimulant and tonic. Used in popular practice as a gargle for sore throat, wash for ulcers and internally for the cure of bowel complaints, gravel, asthma, coughs and gonorrhea.

PREPARATION.

Infusion Agrimony—Fl. ext. Agrimony, Lilly, 2 fl. ozs.; Hot water, 14 fl. ozs.; Mix—Dose 1 to 2 fl. ozs., or as a gargle or wash for ulcers.

FL. EXT. AILANTHUS .... Dose 15 to 30 m.
Ailanthus glandulosa Desf. **Nat. Ord.**—*Simarubaceæ.*

Synonyms—Tree of Heaven, Chinese sumach.

Range—China; in the U. S. cultivated as a shade tree.

Part used—The bark.

Standard of strength—That of the U. S. Pharmacopœia, 1890; 1 c.c. representing 1 gram of the drug or, practically, minim for grain.

Action and uses—Nervine and antispasmodic. Said to be useful in anorexia, dyspepsia and for the expulsion of tenia.

PREPARATION.

Infusion Ailanthus—Fl. ext. Ailanthus, Lilly, 2 fl. ozs.; Hot water, 14 fl. ozs.; Mix—Dose 2 to 4 fl. drs.

WHEN ORDERING OR PRESCRIBING.

FL. EXT. ALKANET.

Alkanna tinctoria Tausch.   **Nat. Ord.**—*Boraginaceæ.*

Synonym—Anchusa tinctoria Lam.

Range—Western Asia and Southeastern Europe.

Part used—The root.

Standard of strength—That of the U. S. Pharmacopœia, 1890; 1 c.c. representing 1 gram of the drug; or, practically, minim for grain.

Action and uses—Alkanet is not a medical plant, being used as a coloring for oils and pomades, for which purpose this extract is well adapted.

FL. EXT. ALOES .... **Dose 5 to 20 m.**

Aloe Perryi Baker.   **Nat. Ord.**—*Liliaceæ.*

Synonyms—Aloe Socotrina U. S.,—Socotrine aloes.

Range—Shores of Red Sea and Indian Ocean, Southern Africa.

Habitat.—Partial to limestone districts from sea level to an altitude of 3000 feet.

Part used—The inspissated juice of the leaves, purified.

Standard of strength—This preparation though listed as a fluid extract is not properly so called, being made in the proportion of 1 gram purified Socotrine aloes to 2 c.c. of the fluid extract.

Action and uses—Cathartic, emmenagogue, vermifuge and slightly cholagogue.

PREPARATIONS.

Tincture Aloes U. S.—Fl. ext. Aloes, Lilly, 3 fl. ozs.; Fl. ext. Licorice, Lilly, 3 fl. ozs.; Diluted Alcohol, 10 fl. ozs; Mix—Dose as a laxative, 30 to 60 m.; as a purgative 2 to 4 fl. drs.

Wine Aloes, U. S.—Fl. ext. Aloes, Lilly, 2 fl. ozs.; Fl. ext. Cardamom, Lilly, 1 fl. dr.; Fl. ext. Ginger, Lilly, 1 fl. dr.; Stronger white wine, 13¾ fl. ozs.; Mix—Dose as a stomachic, 1 to 2 fl. drs.; as a purgative ½ to 1 fl. oz.

FL. EXT. ARBOR VITÆ, aqueous, see Appendix, page 831.

FL. EXT. ALOES AND MYRRH .... **Dose 10 to 20 m.**

Standard of strength—One pint represents: Purified aloes, Myrrh and Licorice root, of each 5 avd. ounces.

Action and uses—Purgative, tonic and emmenagogue.   Chiefly employed in chlorosis and amenorrhœa when there is constipation.

PREPARATION.

Tincture Aloes and Myrrh, U. S.—Fl. ext. Aloes and Myrrh, Lilly, 4½ fl. ozs.; Alcohol, 5½ fl. ozs.; Water, 2½ fl. ozs., Mix—Dose 1 to 2 fl. drs.

FL. EXT. ALSTONIA CONSTRICTA .... **Dose 5 to 20 m.**

Alstonia constricta F. v. Mueller.   **Nat. Ord.**—*Apocynaceæ.*

Synonym—Australian fever bark.

Range—Warmer parts of East Australia.

Habitat—Dry soil.

Part used—The bark.

Standard of strength—That of the U. S. Pharmacopœia, 1890; 1 c.c. representing 1 gram of the drug; or, practically, minim for grain.

Action and uses—Tonic and antiperiodic.   Said to be used in Central Australia with great success in malarial fevers.

FL. EXT. ALUM ROOT .... **Dose 10 to 60 m.**

Heuchera Americana Linn.   **Nat. Ord.**—*Saxifragaceæ.*

Synonym—American sanicle.

Range—United States; Connecticut to North Carolina, west to Minnesota and Mississippi.

Habitat—Rocky woodlands.

Part used—The root.

Standard of strength—That of the U. S. Pharmacopœia, 1890; 1 c.c. representing 1 gram of the drug; or, practically, minim for grain.

Action and uses—Astringent. Used in domestic medicine as a remedy for diarrhea and menorrhagia; as a mouth wash for aphthæ and as an application to ulcers.

PREPARATION.

Infusion Alum Root—Fl. ext. Alum root, Lilly, 2 fl. ozs.; Hot water, 14 fl. ozs.; Mix—Dose ¼ to 1 fl. oz.

FL. EXT. AMERICAN CENTAURY.................Dose 30 to 60 m.

Sabbatia angularis (Linn.) Pursh.　　**Nat. Ord.**—*Gentianaceæ.*

Synonyms—Chironia angularis Linn.,—Red Centaury.

Range—North America; New York to Ontario and Michigan, south to Florida and Louisiana.

Habitat—Low rich soil.

Part used—The herb.

Standard of strength—That of the U. S. Pharmacopœia, 1890; 1 c.c. representing 1 gram of the drug; or, practically, minim for grain.

Action and uses—Tonic. Used as a prophylactic and remedy in autumnal intermittent and remittent fevers; also useful in dyspepsias and convalescence from fevers.

PREPARATION.

Infusion American Centaury—Fl. ext. American Centaury, Lilly, 1 fl. oz.; Hot water, 15 fl. ozs.; Mix—Dose 1 to 2 fl. ozs.

FL. EXT. AMERICAN COLUMBO..................Dose 20 to 30 m.

Frasera Carolinensis Walt.　　**Nat. Ord.**—*Gentianaceæ.*

Synonyms—F Walteri Michx.,—Yellow gentian, Meadowpride, Indian lettuce.

Range—Western New York to Wisconsin, south to Georgia.

Habitat—Rich, dry soil.

Part used—The root.

Standard of strength—That of the U. S. Pharmacopœia, 1890; 1 c.c. representing 1 gram of the drug; or, practically, minim for grain.

Action and uses—Mild tonic. Purgative and sometimes emetic in overdoses. Valuable in general debility, in atonic dyspepsia and to promote appetite and digestion in convalescence.

PREPARATION.

Infusion American Columbo—Fl. ext. American Columbo, Lilly, 1 fl. oz.; Hot water, 15 fl. ozs.; Mix—Dose ½ to 1 fl oz.

FL. EXT. AMERICAN HEMP..............Dose 5 to 60 m.

Cannabis sativa Linn, var, *Americana.*　　**Nat. Ord.**—*Urticaceæ.*

Synonyms—American cannabis, Common hemp.

Range—Cultivated in the Central United States.

Part used—The inflorescence of the female plant.

Standard of strength—That of the U. S. Pharmacopœia, 1890; 1 c.c. representing 1 gram of the drug; or, practically, minim for grain.

Action and uses—Not poisonous although formerly so regarded; however coma may be produced by excessive doses. Antispasmodic, analgesic, anesthetic, narcotic, aphrodisiac. Its general properties are the same as Cannabis Indica only in lesser degree.

Antidotes—Stomach pump, strychnine and Faradism are antagonistic. Caustic alkalies are incompatible. Stimulants cautiously, artificial respiration.

FL. EXT. AMERICAN IVY........................Dose 30 to 60 m.

Ampelopsis quinquefolia Michx.　　**Nat. Ord.**—*Vitaceæ.*

Synonyms—Parthenocissus quinquefolia (Linn.) Planch, Vitis quinquefolia Lam., Hedera quinquefolia Linn.,—Virginia creeper, Fiveleaved ivy.

Range—Common in the United States; New England, south to Florida, west to Texas and the Dakotas.

Habitat—Low or rich ground along banks of streams; climbing.

Part used—Bark and twigs.

Standard of strength—That of the U. S. Pharmacopœia, 1890; 1 c.c. representing 1 gram of the drug; or, practically, minim for grain.

Action and uses—Alterative, tonic, astringent, expectorant. Useful in scrofula, syphilis, dropsy, bronchitis and pulmonary complaints.

PREPARATIONS.

Syrup American Ivy—Fl. ext. American Ivy, Lilly, 4 fl. ozs.; Syrup, 12 fl. ozs.; Mix—Dose 2 to 4 fl. drs.

Infusion American Ivy—Fl. ext. American Ivy, Lilly, 1 fl. oz. Hot water, 15 fl. ozs.; Mix—Dose 1 to 2 fl. ozs.

FL. EXT. AMERICAN SAFFRON .... Dose 15 to 30 m.
Carthamus tinctorius Willd.   **Nat. Ord.**—*Compositæ.*

Synonyms—Safflower, Dyer's saffron.

Range—India, Levant and Egypt; cultivated in Europe and the United States.

Part used—The florets.

Standard of strength—That of the U. S. Pharmacopœia, 1890; 1 c.c. representing 1 gram of the drug; or, practically, minim for grain.

Action and uses—Stimulant, emmenagogue and diaphoretic. The warm infusion is said to restore the menstrual discharge when recently suppressed by cold; also used as a diaphoretic among children, in measles, scarlet fever and other eruptive diseases.

PREPARATION.

Infusion American Saffron—Fl. ext. American Saffron, Lilly, 1 fl. oz.; Hot water, 15 fl. ozs.; Mix—Dose ½ to 1 fl. oz.

FL. EXT. AMERICAN SARSAPARILLA .... Dose 30 to 60 m.
Aralia nudicaulis Linn.   **Nat. Ord.**—*Araliaceæ.*

Synonym—Small spikenard.

Range—North America; Newfoundland to Rocky Mountains, British Columbia south to New Jersey and Georgia.

Habitat—Moist deep woods and ravines.

Part used—The root.

Standard of strength—That of the U. S. Pharmacopœia, 1890; 1 c.c. representing 1 gram of the drug; or, practically, minim for grain.

Action and uses—Alterative. May be used in the place of Smilax officinalis whenever an alterative is required.

PREPARATIONS.

Syrup American Sarsaparilla—Fl. ext. American Sarsaparilla, Lilly, 4 fl. ozs.; Syrup, 12 fl. ozs.; Mix—Dose 2 to 4 fl. drs.

Infusion American Sarsaparilla—Fl. ext. American Sarsaparilla, Lilly, 1 fl. oz.; Hot water, 15 fl. ozs.; Mix—Dose 1 to 2 fl. ozs.

FL. EXT. AMERICAN WHITE ASH .... Dose 15 to 30 m.
Fraxinus Americana Linn.   **Nat. Ord.**—*Oleaceæ.*

Synonyms—F. alba Marsh,—American ash.

Range—Nova Scotia, west to Minnesota, south to Texas and Florida.

Habitat—Rich woodlands, banks of streams and lakes.

Part used—The bark.

Standard of strength—That of the U. S. Pharmacopœia, 1890; 1 c.c. representing 1 gram of the drug; or, practically, minim for grain.

Action and uses—Tonic and cathartic. Useful in constipation and in

dropsical affections. The wine has been extensively used for the cure of
ague-cake or enlarged spleen.

PREPARATION.

Wine American White Ash—Fl. ext. American White Ash, Lilly,
2 fl. ozs.; Stronger white wine, 14 fl. ozs.; Mix—Dose 1 to 4 fl. drs.

FL. EXT. AMERICAN WORMSEED .... **Dose 30 to 60 m.**
Chenopodium anthelminticum Linn.

Nat. Ord.—*Chenopodiaceæ.*

Synonyms—C. ambrosioides Linn. var. anthelminticum Gray,—Chenopodium U. S.

Range—West Indies and Central America; naturalized in the United
States.

Habitat—In waste places, along roadsides in dry soil.

Part used—The root.

Standard of strength—That of the U. S. Pharmacopœia, 1890; 1 c.c.
representing 1 gram of the drug; or, practically, minim for grain.

Action and uses—An efficient anthelmintic, particularly in the expulsion of round worms in children. It may be given night and morning for
two or three days, followed by a purgative dose of castor oil.

PREPARATIONS.

Syrup American Wormseed—Fl. ext. American Wormseed, Lilly,
4 fl. ozs.; Syrup, 12 fl. ozs.; Mix—Dose 2 to 4 fl. drs.

Infusion American **Wormseed**—Fl. ext. American Wormseed,
Lilly, 1 fl. oz.; Hot water, 15 fl. ozs.; Mix—Dose 1 to 2 fl. ozs.

FL. EXT. ANGELICA ROOT .... **Dose 15 to 30 m.**
Angelica atropurpurea Linn.   **Nat. Ord.**—*Umbelliferæ.*

Synonyms—Archangelica atropurpurea Hoffm.,—High angelica, Dead-
nettle, Purple angelica.

Range—Labrador to Delaware, Illinois and Minnesota.

Habitat—Banks of streams.

Part used—The root.

Standard of strength—That of the U. S. Pharmacopœia, 1890; 1 c.c.
representing 1 gram of the drug; or, practically, minim for grain.

Action and uses—Tonic, stimulant, diuretic and diaphoretic. Used
with some success in chronic bronchitis, chronic rheumatism, gout and
intermittent fever. It is said to promote menstrual discharge. In diseases of the urinary organs, calculi and passive dropsy, it is used in infusion with other diuretics.

PREPARATIONS.

Tincture Angelica Root—Fl. ext. Angelica root, Lilly, 4 fl. ozs.;
Alcohol, 9 fl. ozs.; Water, 3 fl. ozs.; Mix—Dose 1 to 4 fl. drs.

Infusion Angelica Root—Fl. ext. Angelica root, Lilly, 1 fl. oz.;
Hot water, 14 fl. ozs.; Mix—Dose ½ to 1 fl. oz.

Comp. Infusion Angelica Root—Fl. ext. Angelica root, Lilly,
½ fl. oz.; Fl. ext. Gravel plant, Lilly, ½ fl. oz.; Hot water, 15 fl. ozs.;
Mix—Dose ½ to 1 fl. oz.

FL. EXT. ANGELICA SEED. ....**Dose 15 to 30 m.**
Angelica atropurpurea Linn.   Nat. Ord.—*Umbelliferæ.*

Synonyms—Archangelica atropurpurea Hoffm.,—High angelica, Dead-
nettle, Purple angelica.

Range—Labrador to Delaware, west to Illinois and Minnesota.

Habitat—Banks of streams.

Part used—The seed.

Standard of strength—That of the U. S. Pharmacopœia, 1890; 1 c.c.
representing 1 gram of the drug; or, practically, minim for grain.

Action and uses—Tonic, stimulant, diuretic and diaphoretic. Used
with some success in chronic bronchitis, chronic rheumatism, gout and
intermittent fever. Promotes menstrual discharge. In diseases of the

urinary organs, calculi and passive dropsy it is used in infusion with other diuretics.

PREPARATIONS.

Tincture Angelica Seed—Fl. ext. Angelica seed, Lilly, 4 fl. ozs.; Alcohol, 9 fl. ozs.; Water, 3 fl. ozs.; Mix—Dose 1 to 2 fl. drs.

Infusion Angelica Seed—Fl. ext. Angelica seed, Lilly, 1 fl. oz.; Hot water, 15 fl. ozs.; Mix—Dose ½ to 1 fl. oz.

Comp. Infusion Angelica Seed—Fl. ext. Angelica seed, Lilly, ½ fl. oz.; Fl. ext. Gravel plant, Lilly, ½ fl. oz.; Hot water, 15 fl. ozs.; Mix—Dose ½ to 1 fl. oz.

FL. EXT. ANGUSTURA BARK ....Dose 15 to 30 m.

Galipea Cusparia St. Hil.   *Nat. Ord.—Rutaceæ.*

Synonyms—G. officinalis Hancock, Cusparia trifoliata Engler, C. febrifuga Humb. and Bonpland.

Range—Northern Brazil and Venezuela.

Part used—The bark.

Standard of strength—That of the U. S. Pharmacopœia, 1890; 1 c.c. representing 1 gram of the drug; or, practically, minim for grain.

Action and uses—A tonic operating without astringency but with a slight stimulating action. Used in typhoid state of fevers and inflammations especially that of tropical dysentery.

PREPARATION.

Infusion Angustura Bark—Fl. ext. Angustura bark, Lilly, 1 fl. oz.; Hot water, 15 fl. ozs.; Mix—Dose ½ to 1 fl. oz.

FL. EXT. ANISE SEED ....Dose 15 to 30 m.

Pimpinella Anisum Linn.   *Nat. Ord.—Umbelliferæ.*

Synonyms—Anisum, U. S., Common anise.

Range—Western Asia, Egypt, Southeastern Europe; cultivated.

Part used—The fruit.

Standard of strength—That of the U. S. Pharmacopœia, 1890; 1 c.c. representing 1 gram of the drug; or, practically, minim for grain.

Action and uses—Stimulant, carminative, aromatic. Removes flatulent colic of infants, nausea and griping. Is supposed to have the property of increasing the secretion of milk.

PREPARATION.

Infusion Anise Seed—Fl. ext. Anise seed, Lilly, 1 fl. oz.; Hot water, 15 fl. ozs.; Mix—Dose ½ to 1 fl. oz.

FL. EXT. ARALIA COMPOUND ....Dose 15 to 30 m.

Standard of strength—One pint represents American sarsaparilla, Yellow dock, Burdock root, Guaiac wood, of each 2½ troy ounces; Prickly ash bark, Elder flowers and Blue flag, of each 2 troy ounces.

Action and uses—Alterative. Valuable in rheumatism, syphilis, scrofula and cutaneous diseases. It is however very inferior to *Succus Alterans*, Lilly, in those affections.

PREPARATION.

Syrup Aralia Compound—Fl. ext. Aralia compound, Lilly, 4 fl. ozs.; Syrup, 12 fl. ozs.; Mix—Dose 1 to 4 fl. drs.

FL. EXT. BAYBEERRY COMP., see Appendix, page 331.

FL. EXT. ARBOR VITÆ ....Dose 15 to 30 m.

Thuja occidentalis Linn.   *Nat. Ord.—Coniferæ.*

Synonyms—Thuya occidentalis Linn.,- False white cedar.

Range—New Brunswick to Pennsylvania, along mountains to North Carolina, west to Minnesota.

Habitat—Swamps and cool rocky banks.

Part used—Leaves and twigs.

Standard of strength—That of the U. S. Pharmacopœia, 1890; 1 c.c. representing 1 gram of the drug; or, practically, minim for grain.

Action and uses—Tonic, stomachic and febrifuge. Recommended in the treatment of intermittent and remittent fevers, scurvy and rheumatism. As a local remedy, valuable as an application to cancerous ulcerations, and **venereal** excrescences.

PREPARATIONS.

Lotion Arbor Vitæ—Fl. ext. Arbor vitæ, Lilly, 2 fl. ozs.; Water, 14 fl. ozs.; Mix—Saturate cloths and apply frequently.

Syrup Arbor Vitæ—Fl. ext. Arbor vitæ, Lilly, 4 fl. ozs.; Syrup, 12 fl. ozs.; Mix—Dose 1 to 2 fl. drs.

Ointment Arbor Vitæ—Fl. ext. Arbor vitæ, Lilly, 2 fl. ozs.; Lard 4 troy ozs.; Heat the lard and fluid extract together and stir till cold.

FL. EXT. ARECA NUT ....Dose 120 to 180 m.
Areca Catechu Linn.　　　　　　　　Nat. Ord. *Palmeæ.*

Synonym—Betelnut.

Range—Cochin China, Malayan Peninsula and Islands; cultivated.

Part **used**—The seed.

Standard of strength—That of the U. S. Pharmacopœia, 1890; 1 c.c. representing 1 gram of the drug; or, practically, minim for grain.

Action and uses—Astringent, exhilarant and vermifuge, especially for tape worm. The dose is as given above, first cleaning the bowels by fasting and castor oil. It is used in mixtures for bowel complaints, its effect being similar to catechu.

FL. EXT. ARNICA FLOWERS ....Dose 5 to 10 m.
Arnica montana Linn.　　　　　　　**Nat. Ord.—***Compositæ.*

Synonyms— Arnica flores, U. S.,—Mountain tobacco, Leopardsbane.

Range—Europe, Siberia and Northern United States; cultivated.

Habitat—In meadows and plains of cold countries, farther south on mountains.

Part used—The flower heads.

Standard of strength—That of the U. S. Pharmacopœia, 1890; 1 c.c. representing 1 gram of the drug; or, practically, minim for grain.

Action and uses—Stimulant, irritant, depressant, antipyretic, diuretic and vulnerary. In small doses it increases the heart action, raises the arterial tension and stimulates the action of the skin and kidneys. Internally, its effects are uncertain and sometimes dangerous. The tincture is largely used and very valuable, ecchymoses being rapidly dispersed by its administration both internally and externally and in internal bruises from shocks or concussion its internal use is very efficacious. It is a popular remedy for sprains, bruises, local paralysis, etc.

PREPARATIONS.

Tincture Arnica Flowers, U. S.—Fl. ext. Arnica flowers, Lilly, 2 fl. ozs.; Alcohol, 6 fl. ozs.; Water, 6 fl. ozs.; Mix—Dose 15 to 30 m.

Poultice Arnica Flowers—Fl. ext. Arnica flowers, Lilly, 1 fl. oz.; Vinegar 3 fl. ozs.; Mix and add linseed meal to bring to proper consistence.

FL. EXT. ARNICA ROOT, U. S. ....Dose 5 to 10 m.
Arnica montana, Linn.　　　　　　　**Nat. Ord.** *Compositæ.*

Synonyms—Arnicæ radix, U. S.,— Mountain tobacco, Leopardsbane.

Range—Europe, Siberia and Northern United States; cultivated.

Habitat—In meadows and plains of cold countries, farther south on mountains.

Part used—The rhizome and roots.

Standard of strength—That of the U. S. Pharmacopœia, 1890; 1 c.c. representing 1 gram of the drug; or, practically, minim for grain.

Action and uses—Stimulant, irritant, depressant, antipyretic, diuretic and vulnerary. In small doses it increases the heart action, raises the arterial tension and stimulates the action of the skin and kidneys. Internally its effects are uncertain and sometimes dangerous. The tincture is largely used and very valuable, ecchymoses being rapidly dispersed by its administration both internally and externally and in internal bruises from shocks or concussion its internal use is very efficacious. It is a popular remedy for sprains, bruises, local paralysis, etc.

PREPARATION.

Tincture Arnica Root, U. S.—Tincture Arnica root, Lilly, 3¼ fl. ozs.; Diluted alcohol, 28¾ fl. ozs.; Mix—Dose 15 to 30 m.

FL. EXT. AROMATIC, U. S. .... **Dose** 10 to 20 **m.**, diluted with water or dropped **on sugar.**

From Pulvis Aromaticus, U. S.

Standard of strength—One pint represents Cinnamon and Ginger, of each 5¼ troy ounces, Cardamom and Nutmeg, of each 2½ troy ounces.

This extract is prepared by a cold process from the choicest material, is an excellent liquid aromatic and therefore not only useful as an addition to liquids when an aromatic is desired, but also to dry powders as pepsin, bismuth, etc.

Action and uses—Stimulant and carminative.

FL. EXT. ASAFETIDA... .... Dose 5 to 30 m.

Ferula foetida (Bunge) *Regel.*   Nat. Ord. *Umbelliferæ.*

Synonym—Asafetida U. S.

Range—Western Thibet, Persia, Turkestan and Afghanistan.

Habitat—Dry soil in or near deserts.

Part used—The gumresin.

Standard of strength—That of the U. S. Pharmacopœia, 1890; 1 c.c. representing 1 gram of the drug; or, practically, minim for grain.

Action and uses—A powerful antispasmodic, stimulant to the brain and nerves, a stimulating expectorant, emmenagogue, aphrodisiac and anthelmintic. The emulsion is very effective in the flatulent colic of infants and as an enema in infantile convulsions. It has been highly spoken of in the treatment of habitual abortion.

PREPARATIONS.

Tincture Asafetida, U. S.—Fl. ext. Asafetida, Lilly, 3 fl. ozs.; Alcohol, 13 fl. ozs.; Mix—Dose 30 to 60 m.

Syrup Asafetida—Fl. ext. Asafetida, Lilly, 5 fl. drs.; Syrup, 15½ fl. ozs.; Mix—Dose ½ to 1 fl. oz.

Emulsion Asafetida, U. S.—Fl. ext. Asafetida, Lilly, 5 fl. drs.; Alcohol 7 fl. drs.; Water, 14½ fl. ozs. Mix the alcohol and the fluid extract, add to the water, shake well and strain—Dose ½ to 1 fl. ozs.

FL. EXT. ASPARAGUS ROOT.................... Dose 30 to 60 m.

Asparagus officinalis Linn.   Nat. Ord.—*Liliaceæ.*

Synonym—Common asparagus.

Range—Europe; in United States escaped from cultivation.

Part used—The root.

Standard of strength—That of the U. S. Pharmacopœia, 1890; 1 c.c. representing 1 gram of the drug; or, practically, minim for grain.

Action and uses—Diuretic. Said also to be beneficial in repressing undue excitement of the circulatory system, hence, used in enlargement of the heart, dropsy, etc.

FL. EXT. AVENA SATIVA......................... Dose 30 to 60 m.

Avena sativa Linn.   Nat. Ord.—*Gramineæ.*

Synonym—Common oats.

Range—Probably Asia; cultivated.

Part used—The inflorescence.

Standard of strength—That of the U. S. Pharmacopœia, 1890; 1 c.c. representing 1 gram of the drug; or, practically, minim for grain.

Action and uses—Tonic, laxative and nerve stimulant. Said to be specially efficacious in the treatment of chorea, epilepsy, insomnia, nervous exhaustion, alcoholism and the opium habit.

FL. EXT. BALM OF GILEAD............ ...... Dose 30 to 60 m.

Populus balsamifera candicans (Ait.) A. Gray.

Nat. Ord.—Saticacea.

Synonyms—P. candicans Ait.,—Balsam poplar, American balm of Gilead.

Range—Common in cultivation, but rare or unknown in a wild state.

Part used—The buds.

Standard of strength—That of the U. S. Pharmacopœia, 1890; 1 c.c. representing 1 gram of the drug; or, practically, minim for grain.

Action and uses—Stimulant, tonic, diuretic, antiscorbutic. Beneficially employed in affections of the chest, stomach and kidneys and in rheumatism and scurvy.

PREPARATION.

Tincture Balm of Gilead—Fl. ext. Balm of Gilead, Lilly, 4 fl. ozs.; Alcohol, 9 fl. ozs.; Water, 3 fl. ozs.; Mix—Dose 2 to 4 fl. drs.

FL. EXT. BALMONY.. ....Dose 30 to 60 m.

Chelone glabra Linn. **Nat. Ord.—Scrophulariaceæ.**

Synonyms—C. alba Pursh.,—Turtlebloom, Turtlehead, Snakehead.

Range—Newfoundland to Manitoba and Minnesota, south to New Jersey and Florida.

Habitat—Forests; in swamps and marshy places.

Part used—The herb.

Standard of strength—That of the U. S. Pharmacopœia, 1890; 1 c.c. representing 1 gram of the drug; or, practically, minim for grain.

Action and uses—Tonic, cathartic, anthelmintic. Valuable in jaundice and hepatic diseases. Removes worms and excites the digestive organs to action. Used in form of ointment as an application to painful and inflamed tumors, ulcers, breasts, piles, etc.

PREPARATIONS.

Ointment Balmony—Fl. ext. Balmony, Lilly, 2 fl. ozs.; Lard, 7 troy ozs.; Wax, 1 troy oz.; Melt the lard and wax together, add the fluid extract and stir till cold.

Infusion Balmony—Fl. ext. Balmony, Lilly, 1 fl. oz.; Hot water, 15 fl. ozs.; Mix—Dose 1 to 2 fl. ozs.

FL. EXT. BAMBOO BRIER ROOT.............. ....Dose 30 to 60 m.

Smilax lanceolata Linn. **Nat. Ord.—Liliaceæ.**

Synonyms—S. ovata Pursh.,—Southern sarsaparilla.

Range—Virginia to Florida, west to Arkansas and Texas.

Habitat—Rich woods and margins of swamps.

Part used—The rhizome.

Standard of strength—That of the U. S. Pharmacopœia, 1890; 1 c.c. representing 1 gram of the drug; or, practically, minim for grain.

Action and uses—Alterative. It has long been a favorite domestic remedy with the Southern Negroes and the Indians before them. Valuable in the treatment of syphilis, eczema, scrofula and all diseases of the blood. It is an ingredient in SUCCUS ALTERANS, Lilly, and is seldom otherwise used.

FL. EXT. BARBERRY BARK .... Dose 30 to 60 m.

Berberis vulgaris Linn. **Nat. Ord.—Berberidaceæ.**

Range—Europe and Western Asia; naturalized in North America.

Habitat—Thickets and waste ground.

Part used—The bark.

Standard of strength—That of the U. S. Pharmacopœia, 1890; 1 c.c. representing 1 gram of the drug; or, practically, minim for grain.

Action and uses—Tonic, laxative, febrifuge. Used in atonic dyspepsia, chronic diarrhea and dysentery and for enlarged spleen from malarial poisoning.

PREPARATIONS.

Jaundice Bitters—Fl. ext. Barberry bark, Lilly, 2 fl. ozs.; Fl. ext.

Orange peel, bitter, Lilly, 2 fl. ozs.; Fl. ext. Prickly ash bark, Lilly, 2 fl. ozs.; Diluted alcohol, 26 fl. ozs.; Mix—Dose 2 to 4 fl. drs.

Infusion Barberry Bark—Fl. ext. Barberry bark, Lilly, 2 fl. ozs.; Hot water, 14 fl. ozs.; Mix—Dose ½ to 1 fl. oz.

FL. EXT. BAY..For preparing bay rum.

Standard of strength—The finest oils are used in the preparation of this extract and, when it is diluted as per formula below, will yield a spirit comparing most favorably with the best imported bay rum.

PREPARATION.

Bay Rum—Fl. ext. Bay, Lilly, 2 fl. ozs.; Alcohol, 4 pints; Water, 4 pints. Mix the extract with the alcohol, then add the water gradually, with constant stirring. The use of deodorized alcohol adds to the elegance of the spirit.

FL. EXT. BAYBERRY ....Dose 15 to 30 m.

Myrica cerifera Linn.   **Nat. Ord.—***Myricaceæ.*

Synonyms—Waxmyrtle, Waxberry, Candleberry.

Range—Coast, from Nova Scotia to Florida and Alabama, also on Lake Erie.

Habitat—Sandy soil.

Part used—The bark of root and stem.

Standard of strength—That of the U. S. Pharmacopœia, 1890; 1 c.c. representing 1 gram of the drug; or, practically, minim for grain.

Action and uses—Astringent and stimulant. Used with success in diarrhœa, jaundice, canker in the mouth and as a wash for spongy gums.

PREPARATION.

Infusion Bayberry—Fl. ext. Bayberry, Lilly, 1 fl. oz.; Hot water, 15 fl. ozs.; Mix—Use as a gargle.

FL. EXT. BEARSFOOT.............................Dose 5 to 10 m.

Polymnia Uvedalia Linn.   **Nat. Ord.—***Compositæ.*

Synonym—Yellow leaf cup.

Range—Western New York and New Jersey to Missouri and southward.

Habitat—Rich soil.

Part used—The root.

Standard of strength—That of the U. S. Pharmacopœia, 1890; 1 c.c. representing 1 gram of the drug; or, practically, minim for grain.

Action and uses—Tonic and stimulant. The ointment is said to be valuable in lumbago, ague-cake and spinal irritation.

PREPARATION.

Ointment Bearsfoot—Fl. ext. Bearsfoot, Lilly, 4 fl. ozs.; Lard, 8 troy ozs. Heat the lard and the fluid extract together until the alcohol is evaporated and stir till cold.

FL. EXT. BEECH BARK.............................Dose 30 to 60 m.

Fagus atropunicea (Marsh.) Sudw.   **Nat. Ord.—***Fagaceæ.*

Synonyms—F. ferruginea Ait.,—American beechnut.

Range—Nova Scotia to Florida, west to Wisconsin, Eastern Illinois, Missouri and Texas.

Habitat—Rich woodlands.

Part used—The bark.

Standard of strength—That of the U. S. Pharmacopœia, 1890; 1 c.c. representing 1 gram of the drug; or, practically, minim for grain.

Action and uses—Astringent, tonic, antiseptic.

PREPARATION.

Infusion Beech Bark—Fl. ext. Beech bark, Lilly, 1 fl. oz.; Hot water, 15 fl. ozs.; Mix—Dose 1 to 2 fl. ozs.

FL. EXT. BEECH DROPS.................................Dose 10 to 20 m.
Epiphegus Virginiana (Linn.) Bart. **Nat. Ord.**—*Orobanchaceæ.*
Synonyms—Orobanche Virginiana Linn., Epifagus Americana Nutt.,—Cancer root.
Range—New Brunswick to Wisconsin, south to Florida and Arkansas.
Habitat—Common under beech trees, parasitic on their roots.
Part used—The entire plant.
Standard of strength—That of the U. S. Pharmacopœia, 1890; 1 c.c. representing 1 gram of the drug, or, practically, minim for grain.
Action and uses—Astringent. Used in hemorrhage of the bowels and of the uterus and in diarrhœa.

FL. EXT. BELLADONNA LEAVES.....................Dose 1 to 2 m.
Atropa Belladonna Linn. **Nat. Ord.**—*Solanaceæ.*
Synonyms—Belladonnæ folia, U. S.,—Deadly nightshade, Dwale, Black cherry.
Range—Europe, Asia Minor; cultivated.
Habitat—Hedges, waste places, clearings of woods; in England on chalky and limestone soils.
Part used—The leaf.
Standard of strength—0.3 per cent. of alkaloid, estimated by titration with acid.
Action and uses—Poisonous. A powerful narcotic, diaphoretic and diuretic, having a wide range of use. Valuable in checking tendency to nocturnal seminal emissions, nocturnal incontinence of urine in children; for undue sweating as in phthisis and rheumatism. It exerts tonic influence on the bowels and checks excessive salivation.
Antidotes—In poisoning by this drug tannic acid and emetics should be used, then morphine, physostigmine or pilocarpine for the nervous disturbance. Caustic alkalies decompose atropine and are therefore incompatible with preparations of Belladonna.

PREPARATION.

Tincture Belladonna, U. S.—Fl. ext. Belladonna leaves, Lilly, 2½ fl. ozs.; Alcohol, 75 %, 13½ fl. ozs.; Mix—Dose 5 to 15 m.

FL. EXT. BELLADONNA ROOT, U. S................Dose 1 to 2 m.
Atropa Belladonna Linn. **Nat. Ord.**—*Solanaceæ.*
Synonyms—Belladonnæ radix, U. S.,—Deadly nightshade, Dwale, Black cherry.
Range—Europe, Asia Minor; cultivated.
Habitat—Hedges, waste places, clearings of woods; in England on chalky and limestone soils.
Part used—The root.
Standard of strength—0.45 per cent. of alkaloid, estimated by titration with acid.
Action and uses—Poisonous. A powerful narcotic, diaphoretic and diuretic having a wide range of use. Valuable in checking tendency to nocturnal seminal emissions, nocturnal incontinence of urine in children; for undue sweating as in phthisis and rheumatism. It exerts tonic influence on the bowels and checks excessive salivation.
Antidotes—In poisoning by this drug tannic acid and emetics should be used, then morphine, physostigmine or pilocarpine for the nervous disturbance. Caustic alkalies decompose atropine and therefore are incompatible with preparations of Belladonna.

PREPARATIONS.

Tincture Belladonna Root—Fl. ext. Belladonna root, Lilly, 2½ fl. ozs.; Alcohol, 19½ fl. ozs.; Water, 3½ fl. ozs.; Mix—Dose 5 to 15 m.
Liniment Belladonna, U. S.—Fl. ext. Belladonna root, Lilly, 15½ fl. ozs.; Camphor, 354 grains; Dissolve the camphor in the fluid extract.

FL. EXT. BENNE LEAVES..................................Dose 30 to 60 m.

Sesamum Indicum Linn.   **Nat. Ord.**—*Pedaliaceæ.*

Synonyms—S. orientale Linn.,—Sesame, Teal.

Range—Indian Peninsula; cultivated in nearly all parts of the tropical and hot districts of the globe.

Part used—The leaf.

Standard of strength—That of the U. S. Pharmacopœia, 1890; 1 c.c. representing 1 gram of the drug; or, practically, minim for grain.

Action and uses—Demulcent and vulnerary, used in cholera infantum, dysentery, etc.

PREPARATION.

Syrup Benne Leaves—Fl. ext. Benne leaves, Lilly, 4 fl. ozs.; Syrup, 12 fl. ozs.; Mix—Dose 2 to 4 fl. drs.

FL. EXT. BENZOIN..................................Dose 5 to 10 m.

Styrax Benzoin Dryander.   **Nat. Ord.**—*Styraceæ.*

Synonyms—Laurus Benzoin Houtt., Benzoin officinale Hayne,—Benzoinum, U. S.,—Gum benjamin.

Range—Sumatra, Java, Borneo, Laos and Siam; cultivated.

Habitat—Along the coast and hills of the interior.

Part used—The balsamic resin.

Standard of strength—That of the U. S. Pharmacopœia, 1890; 1 c.c. representing 1 gram of the drug; or, practically, minim for grain.

Action and uses—Antiseptic and disinfectant. Employed in chronic mucus profluvia of the bronchial and urinary organs, in chronic diarrhœa and dysentery, by atomizer in chronic laryngeal and bronchial catarrh. Externally for ulcers and wounds, bed sores, sore nipples and chaps.

PREPARATIONS.

Tincture Benzoin, U. S.,—Fl. ext. Benzoin, Lilly, 3¼ fl. ozs.; Alcohol, 12¾ fl. ozs; Mix—Dose 30 to 60 m.

Benzoinated Lard—Fl. ext. Benzoin, Lilly, 2½ fl. drs.; Lard, 1 pound avd.; Melt the lard on a water bath, add the fluid extract, stir until the alcohol is evaporated and strain through muslin. If to be kept in warm weather, replace 5 or 10 per cent. of the lard with white wax.

FL. EXT. BENZOIN COMPOUND..................Dose 5 to 10 m.

For preparing Tr. Benzoin Compound, U. S.

Standard of strength—One pint represents Benzoin, 7½ troy ounces; Purified aloes, 1½ troy ounces; Storax, 4½ troy ounces; Tolu, 2½ troy ounces.

Action and uses—Antiseptic and disinfectant. Employed in chronic mucus profluvia of the bronchial and urinary organs, in chronic laryngeal and bronchial catarrh. Externally for ulcers and wounds, bed sores, sore nipples and chaps.

PREPARATION.

Tincture Benzoin Compound, U. S.—Fl. ext. Benzoin Compound, Lilly, 4 fl. ozs.; Alcohol, 12 fl. ozs.; Mix—Dose 30 to 60 m.

FL. EXT. BERBERIS AQUIFOLIUM...... .... Dose 15 to 30 m.

Berberis aquifolium Pursh.   **Nat. Ord.**—*Berberidaceæ.*

Synonyms—B. nervosa Pursh., B. repens Lindley,—Mountain grape, Mahonia, Hollyleaved barberry, Oregon grape.

Range—Rocky Mountains and westward.

Habitat—Mountainous and hilly districts.

Part used—The rhizome and roots.

Standard of strength—That of the U. S. Pharmacopœia, 1890; 1 c.c. representing 1 gram of the drug; or, practically, minim for grain.

Action and uses—Alterative, tonic, diuretic and diaphoretic. It has been recommended in syphilitic, scrofulous and cancerous affections and in cutaneous diseases.

FL. EXT. BETH ROOT............................. Dose 60 to 120 m.
Trillium erectum Linn. **Nat. Ord.—*Liliaceæ.***

Synonyms—T. rhomboideum Michx.,—Ground lily, Birthroot, Wakerobin.

Range—Nova Scotia to North Carolina, west to Minnesota and Missouri.

Habitat—Rich woods.

Part used—The rhizome.

Standard of strength—That of the U. S. Pharmacopœia, 1890; 1 c.c. representing 1 gram of the drug; or, practically, minim for grain.

Action and uses—Tonic, astringent, antiseptic. Used successfully in spasmodic cough, asthma, also in hemorrhages and to hasten parturition.

PREPARATION.

Infusion Beth Root—Fl. ext. Beth root, Lilly, 1 fl. oz.; Hot water, 15 fl. ozs.; Mix—Dose 2 to 4 fl. ozs.

FL. EXT. BISTORT........................... Dose 30 to 60 m.
Polygonum Bistorta Linn. **Nat. Ord.—*Polygonaceæ*,**

Range—Widely distributed over the Northern Hemisphere, though scarcely common; Northwestern United States.

Habitat—Wet or swampy meadows, borders of damp woods.

Part used—The rhizome.

Standard of strength—That of the U. S. Pharmacopœia, 1890; 1 c.c. representing 1 gram of the drug; or, practically, minim for grain.

Action and uses—Mild astringent. Used in domestic medicine in Europe, in diarrhea, passive hemorrhages, leucorrhœa, relaxations of the throat, anus and vagina.

FL. EXT. BITTER ROOT. Dose, Tonic **4 to 8 m.; Emetic 15 to 30 m.**
Apocynum androsæmifolium Linn. **Nat. Ord.—*Apocynaceæ.***

Synonyms—Catchfly, Dogsbane, Flytrap.

Range—Atlantic to Pacific, New England to British Columbia, south to North Carolina and New Mexico.

Habitat—Borders of woods and thickets, banks of streams.

Part used—The root.

Standard of strength—That of the U. S. Pharmacopœia, 1890; 1 c.c. representing 1 gram of the drug; or, practically, minim for grain.

Action and uses—Tonic, emetic, laxative and diaphoretic. Used in chronic liver complaint, scrofulous affections and low stages of typhoid fever.

PREPARATION.

Infusion Bitter Root—Fl. ext. Bitter root, Lilly, 1 fl. oz.; Hot water, 15 fl. ozs.; Mix—Dose, tonic 1 to 2 fl. drs.; emetic ½ to 1 fl. oz.

FL. EXT. BITTERSWEET, U. S. .... Dose 30 to 60 m.
Solanum Dulcamara Linn. **Nat. Ord.—*Solanaceæ.***

Synonyms—Dulcamara, U. S.,—Woody nightshade, Violetbloom, Scarletberry.

Range—Europe; naturalized in the United States.

Habitat—Moist banks, thickets and hedges; climbing.

Part used—The young branches.

Standard of strength—That of the U. S. Pharmacopœia, 1890; 1 c.c. representing 1 gram of the drug; or, practically, minim for grain.

Action and uses—Narcotic in large doses but generally used as an alterative, diuretic, diaphoretic and discutient. Valuable in scaly eruptions of the skin and in chronic rheumatism and catarrh. Claimed to be aphrodisiac.

PREPARATION.

Syrup Bittersweet—Fl. ext. Bittersweet, Lilly, 4 fl. ozs.; Syrup, 12 fl. ozs.; Mix—Dose 2 to 4 fl. drs.

WHEN ORDERING OR PRESCRIBING.

FL. EXT. BLACK ALDER .... **Dose 60 to 120 m.**

Prinos verticillatus Linn. **Nat. Ord.—***Aquifoliaceæ.*

Synonyms—Ilex verticillata (Linn.) Gray, I. verticillata **tenuifolia** (Torr.) Britton,—Striped alder, False alder, Winterberry.

Range—Nova Scotia to Minnesota, **south to** Florida, west to Arkansas.

Habitat—Low woodlands.

Part used—The **bark.**

Standard of strength—That of the U. S. Pharmacopœia, 1890; 1 c.c. representing 1 gram of the drug; or, practically, minim for grain.

Action and uses—Tonic, alterative and astringent. Successfully **used** in jaundice, diarrhœa and dyspepsia; also locally and internally **in** chronic cutaneous eruptions.

PREPARATION.

Syrup Black Alder—Fl. ext. Black Alder, Lilly, 4 fl. ozs.; Syrup, 12 fl. ozs.; Mix—Dose ½ to 1 fl. oz.

FL. EXT. BLACK ASH BARK .... **Dose 30 to 60 m.**

Fraxinus nigra Marsh. **Nat. Ord.—***Oleaceæ.*

Synonyms—Fraxinus sambucifolia Lam.

Range—Nova Scotia to Minnesota, south to Virginia and Missouri.

Habitat—Rich woods, edges of swamps and banks of streams.

Part used—The bark.

Standard of strength—That of the U. S. Pharmacopœia, 1890; 1 c.c. representing 1 gram of the drug; or, practically, minim for grain.

Action and uses—Tonic and astringent.

PREPARATION.

Infusion Black Ash Bark—Fl. ext. Black Ash bark, Lilly, 2 fl. ozs.; Hot water, 14 fl. ozs.; Mix—Dose ½ to 1 fl. oz.

FL. EXT. BLACKBERRY ROOT, U. S .... **Dose 30 to 60 m.**

From Rubus villosus Aiton, *Rubus Canadensis* Linn. *and Rubus trivalis* Michx. **Nat. Ord.—***Rosaceæ.*

Range—First two species are widely distributed over North America; R. trivalis Michx. is confined to the Southern States.

Habitat—Waste ground, woods and thickets.

Part used—The bark of the root.

Standard of strength—That of the U. S. Pharmacopœia, 1890; 1 c.c. representing 1 gram of the drug; or, practically, minim for grain.

Action and uses—Astringent and tonic. Used in diarrhœa, dysentery, cholera infantum and in relaxed conditions of the intestines in children; also as an injection in gleet, gonorrhœa and prolapsus uteri and ani.

PREPARATION.

Syrup Blackberry Root, U. S.—Fl. ext. Blackberry root, Lilly, 4 fl. ozs.; Syrup, 12 fl. ozs.; Mix—Dose 1 to 2 fl. drs.

FL. EXT. BLACKBERRY COMPOUND. ... **Dose 30 to 60 m.**

Standard of strength—One pint represents Blackberry root, 14 **troy** ounces; Cloves and Cassia, of each 1½ troy ounces.

Action and uses—An excellent combination of the astringent blackberry root and the aromatics, cloves and cassia.

A very agreeable cordial may be made by the following formula:

PREPARATION.

Blackberry Cordial—Fl. ext. Blackberry Compound, Lilly, 1½ fl. ozs.; Brandy, 8 fl. ozs.; Water, 5 fl. ozs.; Sugar, 3 troy ozs.; Mix—Dose 2 to 4 fl. drs.

FL. EXT. BLACK COHOSH, U. S. .... Dose 30 to 60 m.

Cimicifuga racemosa (Linn.) Nutt. **Nat. Ord.**—*Ranunculaceæ.*

Synonyms—Actæa racemosa Linn.,—Black snakeroot, Rattleroot, Squawroot, Bugsbane.

Range—Maine to Wisconsin and Eastern Kansas, south to Florida.

Habitat—Rich woodlands.

Part used—The rhizome.

Standard of strength—That of the U. S. Pharmacopœia, 1890; 1 c.c. representing 1 gram of the drug; or, practically, minim for grain.

Action and uses—Antiperiodic, nervine and antispasmodic. It appears to be a sedative to the nervous and vascular systems and has been used with success in rheumatic chorea, muscular rheumatism, amenorrhœa, dysmenorrhea, leucorrhœa and other uterine diseases. It closely resembles digitalis in action but is safer and should be more frequently used when the latter drug is indicated. It is particularly beneficial in ovarian neuralgia.

PREPARATIONS.

Tincture Black Cohosh, U. S.,—Fl. ext. Black Cohosh, Lilly, 3½ fl. ozs.; Alcohol, 9½ fl. ozs.; Water, 3¼ fl. ozs.; Mix—Dose 2 to 4 fl. drs.

Infusion Black Cohosh—Fl. ext. Black Cohosh, Lilly, 1 fl. oz.; Hot water, 15 fl. ozs.; Mix—Dose 1 to 2 fl. ozs.

FL EXT. BLACK COHOSH COMPOUND ... Dose 30 to 60 m.

Standard of strength—One pint represents Black Cohosh, 6 troy ounces; Bloodroot, 2 troy ounces; Cherry bark and Licorice root, of each 4 troy ounces.

Action and uses—A valuable expectorant.

PREPARATION.

Syrup Black Cohosh Compound—Fl. ext. Black Cohosh Compound, Lilly, 4 fl. ozs.; Syrup, 12 fl. ozs.; Mix—Dose 2 to 4 fl. drs.

FL. EXT. BLACK HAW, U. S. .... Dose 30 to 60 m.

Viburnum prunifolium Linn. **Nat. Ord.**—*Caprifoliaceæ.*

Range—New York to Michigan, Kansas and southward.

Habitat—Dry or moist soil; in thickets.

Part used—The bark of **the root.**

Standard of strength—That of the U. S. Pharmacopœia, 1890; 1 c.c. representing 1 gram of the drug; or, practically, minim for grain.

Action and uses—Considered to be nervine, antispasmodic, astringent, diuretic and tonic. Highly recommended in nervous disorders of pregnancy and to prevent abortion; also in spasmodic dysmenorrhea. It may be combined with cannabis indica, morphine or nerve sedatives. As it sometimes produces nausea when given in large doses it may be combined with simple aromatics.

PREPARATIONS.

Tincture Black Haw—Fl. ext. Black Haw, Lilly, 8 fl. ozs.; Alcohol, 5½ fl. ozs.; Water, 2½ fl. ozs.; Mix—Dose 1 to 2 fl. drs.

Infusion Black Haw—Fl. ext. Black **Haw, Lilly,** 2 fl. ozs.; Hot water, 14 fl. ozs.; Mix—Dose ½ to 1 fl. oz.

FL. EXT. BLACK HELLEBORE .... Dose 10 to 20 m.

Helleborus niger Linn. **Nat. Ord.**—*Ranunculaceæ.*

Synonym—Christmas rose.

Range—Southern and temperate Europe; cultivated.

Habitat—Mountainous regions.

Part used—The rhizome.

Standard of strength—That of the U. S. Pharmacopœia, 1890; 1 c.c. representing 1 gram of the drug; or, practically, minim for grain.

Action and uses—Poisonous in large doses. Drastic, hydragogue cathartic and emmenagogue. Useful in dropsies and as a revulsant in acute cerebral affections.

Antidotes—Stomach pump. Heat to extremities, stimulants, artificial respiration if necessary. Caffeine hypodermically or by the mouth, atropine, morphine, ammonia, amyl nitrite.

PREPARATION.

Tincture Black Hellebore—Fl. ext. Black Hellebore, Lilly, 2 fl. ozs.; Alcohol, 10½ fl. ozs.; Water, 3½ fl. ozs.; Mix—Dose 50 to 60 m.

FL. EXT. BLACK INDIAN HEMP, U. S. .... Dose 5 to 20 m.

Apocynum cannabinum Linn.   Nat. Ord. *Apocynaceæ.*

Synonyms—Canadian Hemp. This should **not** be confounded with Indian cannabis nor with American cannabis.

Range—North America; Atlantic to Pacific coast; Canada to Florida and Southern California.

Habitat—Moist ground, borders of thickets and banks of streams.

Part used—The root.

Standard of strength—That of the U. S. Pharmacopœia, 1890; 1 c.c. representing 1 gram of the drug; or, practically, minim for grain.

Action and uses—Powerfully emetic and cathartic in full doses, also diaphoretic, expectorant and diuretic. It lowers the pulse-rate, produces nausea and drowsiness. Valuable in dropsy and especially the anasarca of Bright's disease and ascites.

PREPARATION.

Infusion Black Indian Hemp—Fl. ext. Black Indian Hemp, Lilly, ½ fl. oz.; Hot water, 15½ fl. ozs.; Mix—Dose ¾ to 1 fl. oz.

FL. EXT. BLACK WALNUT HULLS, green ....**Dose 60** to 120 m.

Juglans nigra Linn.   Nat. Ord. *Juglandaceæ.*

Synonym—Black walnut.

Range—Bolivia, North America; New England, south to mountains of Georgia, west to Minnesota and Eastern Kansas.

Habitat—Rich woodlands.

Part used—Green hulls of the fruit—the fleshy epicarp.

Standard of strength—That of the U. S. Pharmacopœia, 1890; 1 c.c. representing 1 gram of the drug; or, practically, minim for grain.

Action and uses—Recommended in diphtheria. Long used as an application to scrofulous sores, tetter and skin diseases generally and in leucorrhœa. Used also internally in scrofula and is reputed to be vermifuge.

PREPARATIONS.

Syrup Black Walnut Hulls—Fl. ext. Black Walnut hulls, Lilly, 4 fl. oz.; Syrup, 12 fl. ozs.; Mix—Dose ½ to 1 fl. oz.

Lotion Black Walnut Hulls—Fl. ext. Black Walnut hulls, Lilly, 2 fl. ozs.; Hot water, 14 fl. ozs.; Mix—Use locally.

FL. EXT. BLACK WALNUT LEAVES. ....Dose 60 to 120 m.

Juglans nigra Linn.   Nat. Ord. —*Juglandaceæ.*

Synonym—Black walnut.

Range—Bolivia, North America; New England, south to mountains of Georgia, west to Minnesota and Eastern Kansas.

Habitat—Rich woodlands.

Part used—The green leaves.

Standard of strength—That of the U. S. Pharmacopœia, 1890; 1 c.c. representing 1 gram of the drug; or, practically, minim for grain.

Action and uses—Recommended in diphtheria. Long used as an application to scrofulous sores, tetter and skin diseases generally and in leucorrhea. Used also internally in scrofula and is reputed to be vermifuge.

PREPARATIONS.

Syrup Black Walnut Leaves Fl. ext. Black Walnut leaves, Lilly, 4 fl. ozs.; Syrup, 12 fl. ozs.; Mix—Dose ½ to 1 fl. oz.

Lotion Black Walnut Leaves Fl. ext. Black Walnut leaves, Lilly, 2 fl. ozs.; Hot water, 14 fl. ozs.; Mix—Use locally.

FL. EXT. BLACK WILLOW BARK.............Dose 30 to 60 m.
Salix nigra Marsh.   **Nat. Ord.**—*Salicaceæ.*
Synonym—Pussy willow.
Range—Common throughout nearly all parts of the United States.
Habitat—Banks of lakes and streams.
Part used—The bark.
Standard of strength—That of the U. S. Pharmacopœia, 1890; 1 c.c. representing 1 gram of the drug; or, practically, minim for grain.
Action and uses—Antiaphrodisiac. Highly recommended in spermatorrhea. The dose may be largely increased if necessary.

FL. EXT. BLACK WILLOW BUDS.............Dose 30 to 60 m.
Salix nigra Marsh.   **Nat. Ord.**—*Salicaceæ.*
Synonym—Pussy willow.
Range—Common throughout nearly all parts of the United States.
Habitat—Banks of lakes and streams.
Part used—The flower buds.
Standard of strength—That of the U. S. Pharmacopœia, 1890; 1 c.c. representing 1 gram of the drug; or, practically, minim for grain.
Action and uses—Antiaphrodisiac. Highly recommended in spermatorrhea. The dose may be largely increased if necessary.

FL. EXT. BLADDERWRACK.............Dose 30 to 60 m.
Fucus vesiculosus Linn.   **Nat. Ord.**—*Fucaceæ.*
Synonyms—Seawrack, Gulfweed, Seaweed.
Range—North Atlantic Ocean, Baltic and Adriatic seas, and the North American Pacific coast.
Habitat—On rocks and stones, sides of piers along the coast, which are left uncovered at low water.
Part used—Entire plant.
Standard of strength—That of the U. S. Pharmacopœia, 1890; 1 c.c. representing 1 gram of the drug; or, practically, minim for grain.
Action and uses—Alterative and tonic. Employed in goitre, enlargements of the glands and joints, psoriasis, irritable bladder and malnutrition. It reduces obesity by causing absorption of adipose tissue. For this purpose the dose may be gradually increased to ½ a fluid ounce three times a day. It requires to be used several weeks before the effect is observed.

FL. EXT. BLESSED THISTLE.............Dose 15 to 30 m.
Cnicus benedictus Gærtn.   **Nat. Ord.**—*Compositæ.*
Synonyms—Centaurea benedicta Linn.—Holy thistle, Bitter thistle.
Range—Europe; naturalized in the South Atlantic states; rare.
Habitat—Roadsides and waste ground.
Part used—The herb.
Standard of strength—That of the U. S. Pharmacopœia, 1890; 1 c.c. representing 1 gram of the drug; or, practically, minim for grain.
Action and uses—Bitter tonic. Reputed valuable in pulmonary, urinary, hepatic and digestive disorders.

PREPARATION.

Infusion Blessed Thistle—Fl. ext. Blessed Thistle, Lilly, 2 fl. ozs.; Hot water, 14 fl. ozs.; Mix—Dose 2 to 4 fl. drs.

FL. EXT. BLOOD ROOT, U. S.................................**Dose 3 to 5 m.**
Sanguinaria Canadensis Linn.   **Nat. Ord.—***Papaveraceæ.*
Synonyms—Sanguinaria, U. S.,—Red puccoon, Indian paint.
Range—Nova Scotia to Manitoba and North Dakota, south to Florida and Arkansas; common.
Habitat—Rich soil in open woodlands.
Part used—The rhizome.
Standard of Strength—1 per cent. of alkaloid.
Action and uses—ACRONARCOTIC POISON. Sialagogue, expectorant and emmenagogue. A systemic emetic, a cardiac paralyzer and an alterative. It is a tonic to the stomach and stimulates the liver. Especially valuable in chronic nasal catarrh, asthma and chronic bronchitis. Its largest use is as an addition to cough syrups for its expectorant qualities.
Antidotes—Its poisonous action is antagonized by opium, amyl nitrite, atropine, etc. Alkalies, tannin and most of the metallic salts are incompatible.

PREPARATION.

Tincture Blood Root, U. S.—Fl. ext. Blood root, Lilly, 2½ fl. ozs.; Alcohol, 13½ fl. ozs.; Mix—Dose 15 to 30 m.

FL. EXT. BLUE COHOSH....................................**Dose 10 to 20 m.**
Caulophyllum thalictroides (Linn.) Michx.
   Nat. Ord.—*Berberidaceæ.*
Synonyms—Leontice thalictroides Linn.,—Caulophyllum, U. S.,—Squaw root, Pappoose root.
Range—Japan and Manchuria. North America; New Brunswick to Minnesota, south to Nebraska and South Carolina.
Habitat—In rich soils in deep woodlands, along streams and lakes.
Part used—Rhizome and rootlets.
Standard of strength—That of the U. S. Pharmacopœia, 1890; 1 c.c. representing 1 gram of the drug; or, practically, minim for grain.
Action and uses—Sedative, antispasmodic, oxytocic and parturient. A favorite remedy in chronic uterine diseases and as a preparatory medicine for labor.

PREPARATIONS.

Tincture Blue Cohosh—Fl. ext. Blue cohosh, Lilly, 4 fl. ozs.; Diluted alcohol, 12 fl. ozs.; Mix—Dose 30 to 60 m.

Syrup Blue Cohosh—Fl. ext. Blue cohosh, Lilly, 2 fl. ozs.; Syrup, 14 fl. ozs.; Mix—Dose 60 to 120 m.

FL. EXT. BLUE COHOSH COMP.............................**Dose 5 to 10 m.**
Standard of strength—One pint represents Blue cohosh, 8 troy ounces; Ergot and Waterpepper, of each, 4 troy ounces; Oil savin, 2 fl. ounces.
Action and uses—Emmenagogue. Very useful in amenorrhea, dysmenorrhea and other uterine disorders.

PREPARATION.

Tincture Blue Cohosh Comp.—Fl. ext. Blue cohosh comp., Lilly, 3 fl. ozs.; Alcohol, 9½ fl. ozs.; Water, 3½ fl. ozs.; Mix—Dose 30 to 60 m.

FL. EXT. BLUE FLAG, U. S................................**Dose 5 to 10 m.**
Iris versicolor Linn.   **Nat. Ord.—***Iridaceæ.*
Synonyms—Iris, U. S.,—Flaglily, Liverlily, Waterflag.
Range—New Foundland to Florida, west to Minnesota and Arkansas.
Habitat—Wet meadows and along the edges of streams and swamps.
Part used—The rhizome and rootlets.
Standard of strength—That of the U. S. Pharmacopœia, 1890; 1 c.c. representing 1 gram of the drug; or, practically, minim for grain.
Action and uses—Cathartic, alterative, sialagogue and diuretic. Very serviceable in duodenal catarrh with obstruction of the bile ducts and con-

sequent jaundice; also in malarial poisoning and bilious remittents. Recently demonstrated of greatest value in hepatic disorders as a cholagogue and purgative. It is one of the principal constituents of ELIXIR PURGANS, Lilly.

PREPARATION.

Syrup Blue Flag—Fl. ext. Blue flag, Lilly, 4 fl. ozs.; Syrup, 12 fl. ozs.; Mix—Dose 20 to 40 m.

FL. EXT. BLUE GENTIAN ....Dose 10 to 30 m.
Gentiana puberula Michx.   **Nat. Ord.**—*Gentianaceæ.*
Synonym—American Gentian.
Range—Western New York to Minnesota, south to Kansas and Kentucky.
Habitat—Dry prairies and barrens.
Part used—The root.
Standard of strength—That of the U. S. Pharmacopœia, 1890; 1 c.c. representing 1 gram of the drug; or, practically, minim for grain.
Action and uses—Tonic, stomachic and antibilious. Valuable in atonic dyspepsia and where a pure simple bitter is indicated.

PREPARATION.

Infusion Blue Gentian—Fl. ext. Blue gentian, Lilly, 1 fl. oz.; Hot water, 15 fl. ozs.; Mix—Dose ½ to 1 fl. oz.

FL. EXT. BOLDO LEAVES.....................Dose 5 to 15 m.
Peumus Boldus Molina.   **Nat. Ord.**—*Monimiaceæ.*
Synonyms—P. fragrans Pers., Boldoa fragrans Ruiz et Pavon.
Range—Chili; cultivated.
Habitat—Sunny hillsides.
Part used—The leaves.
Standard of strength—That of the U. S. Pharmacopœia, 1890; 1 c.c. representing 1 gram of the drug; or, practically, minim for grain.
Action and uses—Tonic and in large doses narcotic. Used in anemia, rheumatism, dyspepsia and general debility; also in catarrhal affections of the urinary passages and as a substitute for quinine. Reputed valuable in chronic torpor of the liver and in South America is much used in gonorrhea and chronic cystitis.

PREPARATIONS.

Tincture Boldo Leaves—Fl. ext. Boldo leaves, Lilly, 2 fl. ozs.; Alcohol, 10½ fl. ozs.; Water, 3½ fl. ozs.; Mix—Dose 40 to 120 m.

Syrup Boldo Leaves—Fl. ext. Boldo leaves, Lilly, 4 fl. ozs.; Syrup, 12 fl. ozs.; Mix—Dose 20 to 60 m.

FL. EXT. BONESET. U. S.....................Dose 20 to 60 m.
Eupatorium perfoliatum Linn.   **Nat. Ord.**—*Compositæ.*
Synonyms—Eupatorium, U. S.,—Thoroughwort, Joepye weed, Indian sage.
Range—Nova Scotia to Minnesota, south to Louisiana and Arkansas; common.
Habitat—Low grounds.
Part used—The herb.
Standard of strength—That of the U. S. Pharmacopœia, 1890; 1 c.c. representing 1 gram of the drug; or, practically, minim for grain.
Action and uses—Tonic, diaphoretic, emetic, laxative. Excellent to abort a general cold; also in fevers, dyspepsia, jaundice and general debility.

PREPARATIONS.

Syrup Boneset—Fl. ext. Boneset, Lilly, 4 fl. ozs.; Syrup, 12 fl. ozs.; Mix—Dose 2 to 4 fl. drs.

Infusion Boneset—Fl. ext. Boneset, Lilly, 2 fl. ozs.; Hot water, 14 fl. ozs.; Mix—Dose ½ to 1 fl. oz.

FL. EXT. BROOM CORN SEED............. ....**Dose 30 to 60 m.**

Sorghum saccharatum Person.　　　　**Nat. Ord.—** *Gramineæ.*

Synonyms—Andropogon saccharatus Roxb.,—Broom corn grass.

Range—Tropical Asia; cultivated in the United States.

Part used—The seeds.

Standard of strength—That of the U. S. Pharmacopeia, 1890; 1 c.c. representing 1 gram of the drug; or, practically, minim for grain.

Action and uses—Diuretic, sedative, demulcent and soothing to the irritated urinary organs in vesical catarrh, cystitis and irritable bladder. Produces great relief in the aged who are compelled to urinate frequently at night.

PREPARATION.

Infusion Broom Corn Seed—Fl. ext. Broom corn seed, Lilly, 2 fl. ozs.; Hot water, 14 fl. ozs.; Mix—Dose ½ to 1 fl. oz.

FL. EXT. BROOM TOPS, U. S......................**Dose 20 to 40 m.**

Cystisus scoparius (Linn.) Link.　　　　**Nat. Ord.—** *Leguminosæ.*

Synonyms—Sarothamnus scoparius Koch., S. vulgaris Wimm.,—Scoparius, U. S.,—Broom, Broomflowers.

Range—Western Asia, Southwestern Europe; cultivated in gardens in the United States.

Habitat—Sandy thickets and uncultivated grounds.

Part used—Twigs and inflorescence.

Standard of strength—That of the U. S. Pharmacopeia, 1890; 1 c.c. representing 1 gram of the drug; or, practically, minim for grain.

Action and uses—Diuretic, cathartic and in large doses emetic. Has been employed with great advantage in dropsy.

PREPARATION.

Infusion Broom Tops—Fl. ext. Broom tops, Lilly, 1 fl. oz.; Hot water, 15 fl. ozs.; Mix—Dose 1 to 2 fl. ozs.

FL. EXT. BUCHU, U. S............. ....**Dose 30 to 60 m.**

Barosma betulina (Thunb.) Bartling and Wendland *and B. crenulata* (Linn.) Hooker.　　　　**Nat. Ord.—** *Rutaceæ.*

Range—South Africa, north of Cape Town and other parts of the West of Cape Colony.

Habitat—Mountainous districts.

Part used—The leaves.

Standard of strength—That of the U. S. Pharmacopeia, 1890; 1 c.c. representing 1 gram of the drug; or, practically, minim for grain.

Action and uses—Useful in chronic catarrh of the bladder and **all** mucous discharges of the genital and urinary organs depending on a relaxed condition of the affected parts. Largely employed in subacute and chronic gonorrhea and in incontinence or retention of urine from deficient tone of the bladder.

PREPARATION.

Syrup Buchu—Fl. ext. Buchu, Lilly, 2 fl. ozs.; **Syrup, 14 fl. ozs.; Mix**—Dose ½ to 1 fl. oz.

Tincture Buchu—Fl. ext. Buchu, Lilly, 2 fl. ozs.; Alcohol, 10 fl. ozs.; Water, 4 fl. ozs.; Mix—Dose 1 to 2 fl. drs.

FL. EXT. BUCHU COMP., Formula A ....**Dose 30 to 60 m.**

Standard of strength—One pint represents Buchu, 8 troy ounces; Juniper berries, 4 troy ounces; Pareira brava, 3 troy ounces; Cubeb, 1 troy ounce; Cardamom, ¼ troy ounce.

Action and uses—Diuretic and stimulant.

PREPARATION.

Tincture Buchu Comp.—Fl. ext. Buchu comp., Lilly, 4 fl. ozs.; Alcohol, 9 fl. ozs.; Water, 3 fl. ozs. Mix the alcohol with the water and add the fluid extract.—Dose 2 to 4 fl. drs.

FL. EXT. BUCHU COMP., Formula B, see Appendix, page 331.

FL. EXT. BUCHU, JUNIPER AND POTASSIUM ACETATE.
Dose 20 to **40 m.**
Standard of strength—One pint represents Buchu, 12 troy ounces; Juniper berries, 3 troy ounces; Potassium acetate, 1 troy ounce.

Action and uses—Valuable in the treatment of diseases of the bladder, affections of the genito-urinary mucous membrane, inflammation of the kidneys, etc.

PREPARATION.

Elixir Buchu, Juniper and Potassium Acetate—Fl. ext. Buchu, Juniper and Potassium acetate, Lilly, 2 fl. ozs.; Alcohol, 1 fl. oz.; Simple elixir, 13 fl. ozs.; Mix the alcohol and simple elixir then add the fluid extract—Dose ¼ to 1 fl. oz.

FL. EXT. BUCHU AND PAREIRA BRAVA...........Dose 30 to 60 m.
Standard of strength—One pint represents Buchu, Pareira brava, of each 8 troy ounces.

Action and uses—Very useful in chronic diseases of the urinary passages, kidneys and bladder.

FL. EXT. BUCKBEAN LEAVES............ ....Dose 30 to 60 m.
Menyanthes trifoliata Linn. **Nat. Ord.**—*Gentianaceæ.*
Synonyms—Brookbean, Boybean, Marsh clover.
Range—Europe, Asia, North America; Greenland, Labrador to Alaska, south to New Jersey, Indiana and Central California.
Habitat—Moist places, bogs and wet woodlands.
Part used—The leaves.
Standard of strength—That of the U. S. Pharmacopœia, 1890; 1 c.c. representing 1 gram of the drug; or, practically, minim for grain.
Action and uses—Bitter tonic. Reputed antiscorbutic, emmenagogue and vermifuge.

FL. EXT. BUCKTHORN BARK, U. S............. .....Dose 15 to 30 m.
Rhamnus Frangula Linn. **Nat. Ord.**—*Rhamnaceæ.*
Synonyms—Frangula vulgaris Reich.,—Frangula, U. S.,—Alder buckthorn.
Range—Europe and Russian Asia, except in the far north.
Habitat—Hedges and thickets.
Part used—The bark.
Standard of strength—That of the U. S. Pharmacopœia, 1890; 1 c.c. representing 1 gram of the drug; or, practically, minim for grain.
Action and uses—A safe purgative without irritating qualities, often used in constipation of pregnancy. In this, however, it is quite inferior to ELIXIR PURGANS, Lilly.

PREPARATIONS.

Syrup Buckthorn Bark—Fl. ext. Buckthorn bark, Lilly, 4 fl. ozs.; Syrup, 12 fl. ozs.; Mix—Dose 1 to 2 fl. drs.

Infusion Buckthorn Bark—Fl. ext. Buckthorn bark, Lilly, 1 fl. oz.; Hot water, 15 fl. ozs.; Mix—Dose ½ to 1 fl. oz.

FL. EXT. BUCKTHORN BERRIES. ....Dose 60 to 120 m.
Rhamnus cathartica Linn. **Nat. Ord.**—*Rhamnaceæ.*
Synonyms—Cervispina cathartica Mœnch.
Range—Europe and Russian Asia, except in the extreme north, Northern Africa; cultivated in the United States.
Habitat—Chalky districts, thickets and hedges.
Part used—The fruit.
Standard of strength—That of the U. S. Pharmacopœia, 1890; 1 c.c. representing 1 gram of the drug; or, practically, minim for grain.
Action and uses—Hydragogue cathartic and alterative.

PREPARATION.

Syrup Buckthorn Berries—Fl. ext. Buckthorn berries, Lilly, 4 fl. ozs.; Syrup, 12 fl. ozs.; Mix—Dose ½ to 1 fl. oz.

FL. EXT. BUGLEWEED.......................................Dose 30 to 60 m.

Lycopus Virginicus Linn.   **Nat. Ord.—***Labiatæ.*

Synonym—Paul's betony.

Range—Labrador to Florida, Missouri and northwestward across the continent.

Habitat—Shady moist places.

Part used—The herb.

Standard of strength—That of the U. S. Pharmacopœia, 1890; 1 c.c. representing 1 gram of the drug; or, practically, minim for grain.

Action and uses—A mild narcotic, tonic, astringent and sedative. Used in phthisis, hemorrhage of the lungs, diabetes and chronic diarrhea.

PREPARATIONS.

Syrup Bugleweed—Fl. ext. Bugleweed, Lilly, 4 fl. ozs.; Syrup, 12 fl. ozs.; Mix—Dose 2 to 4 fl. drs.

Infusion Bugleweed—Fl. ext. Bugleweed, Lilly, 1 fl. oz.; Hot water, 15 fl. ozs.; Mix—Dose 1 to 2 fl. ozs.

FL. EXT. BURDOCK ROOT, U. S........................Dose 30 to 60 m.

Arctium Lappa Linn, *and some other species of Arctium.*
           Nat. Ord.—*Compositæ.*

Synonyms—A. majus Schkuhr, Lappa major Gærtn., L. minor D. C., L. officinalis Allioni,—Lappa, U. S.

Range—Asia and Europe; naturalized in North America.

Habitat—Waste places.

Part used—The root.

Standard of strength—That of the U. S. Pharmacopœia, 1890; 1 c.c. representing 1 gram of the drug; or, practically, minim for grain.

Action and uses—Aperient, alterative, diuretic and diaphoretic. Used in scorbutic, syphilitic and scrofulous diseases. The cultivated root is used in the green state by Eli Lilly & Company in the preparation of SUCCUS ALTERANS, Lilly, of which it is a **very** valuable constituent.

PREPARATIONS.

Syrup Burdock Root—Fl. ext. Burdock root, Lilly, 4 fl. ozs.; Syrup, 12 fl. ozs.; Mix—Dose 2 to 4 fl. drs.

Infusion Burdock Root—Fl. ext. Burdock root, Lilly, 1 fl. oz.; Hot water, 15 fl. ozs.; Mix—Dose 1 to 2 fl. ozs.

FL. EXT. BURDOCK SEED..............................Dose 30 to 60 m.

Arctium Lappa Linn, *and some other species of Arctium.*
           Nat. Ord.—*Compositæ.*

Synonyms—A. majus Schkuhr, Lappa major Gærtn., L. minor D. C., L. officinalis Allioni, Lappa, U. S.

Range—Asia and Europe; naturalized in North America.

Habitat—Waste places.

Part used—The seed.

Standard of strength—That of the U. S. Pharmacopœia, 1890; 1 c.c. representing 1 gram of the drug; or, practically, minim for grain.

Action and uses—Aperient, alterative, diuretic and diaphoretic. Used in scorbutic, syphilitic and scrofulous diseases.

PREPARATIONS.

Syrup Burdock Seed—Fl. ext. Burdock seed, Lilly, 4 fl. ozs.; Syrup, 12 fl. ozs.; Mix—Dose 2 to 4 fl. drs.

Infusion Burdock Seed—Fl. ext. Burdock seed, Lilly, 1 fl. oz.; Hot water, 15 fl. ozs.; Mix—Dose 1 to 2 fl. ozs.

FL. EXT. BUTTERNUT, BARK OF ROOT.........**Dose 60 to 120 m.**
Juglans cinerea Linn.　　　　**Nat. Ord.—***Juglandaceæ.*
Synonym—White walnut.
Range—New Brunswick to the mountains of Georgia, west to Minnesota, Eastern Kansas and Arkansas.
Habitat—Rich woodlands and in upper bottom lands.
Part used—The bark of the root.
Standard of strength—That of the U. S. Pharmacopœia, 1890; 1 c.c. representing 1 gram of the drug; or, practically, minim for grain.
Action and uses—A mild and efficient cathartic, evacuating without debilitating the bowels.

PREPARATIONS.

Syrup Butternut, Bark of Root—Fl. ext. Butternut, bark of root, Lilly, 4 fl. ozs.; Fl. ext. Calamus, Lilly, Fl. ext. Rhubarb, Lilly, of each 1 fl. oz.; Syrup, 10 fl. ozs., Mix—Dose 1 to 4 fl. drs.

Cathartic Syrup—Fl. ext. Butternut, bark of root, Lilly, 2 fl. ozs.; Fl. ext. Senna, Lilly, Fl. ext. Calamus, Lilly, of each 1 fl. oz., Fl. ext. Jalap, Lilly, Fl. ext. Ginger, Lilly, of each ½ fl. oz., Syrup, 11 fl. ozs.; Mix—Dose 1 to 4 fl. drs.

FL. EXT. BUTTONSNAKEROOT ....**Dose** 60 to 120 m.
Lacinaria spicata (Linn.) Kuntze.　　**Nat. Ord.** *Compositæ.*
Synonyms—Liatris spicata Willd., Serratula spicata Linn.,—Gay-feather, Devilsbit, Roughroot, Throatwort.
Range—Ontario to New York and Massachusetts, south to Florida, west to Minnesota and Arkansas.
Habitat—Moist soil, low prairies or meadows.
Part used—The tuber.
Standard of strength—That of the U. S. Pharmacopœia, 1890; 1 c.c. representing 1 gram of the drug; or, practically, minim for grain.
Action and uses—Diuretic, tonic and stimulant. Said to be useful in gonorrhœa and sore throat, being employed internally in the former and as a gargle in the latter complaint.

PREPARATION.

Infusion Buttonsnakeroot—Fl. ext. Buttonsnakeroot, Lilly, 1 fl. oz.; Hot water, 15 fl. ozs.; Mix—Dose 2 to 4 fl. ozs.

FL. EXT. CACTUS GRANDIFLORUS................**Dose 5 to 10 m.**
Cactus grandiflorus Linn.　　　　**Nat. Ord.—***Cactaceæ.*
Synonyms—Cereus grandiflorus Miller,—Nightblooming cereus.
Range—Tropical America; cultivated.
Part used—The succulent branches.
Standard of strength—That of the U. S. Pharmacopœia, 1890; 1 c.c. representing 1 gram of the drug or, practically, minim for grain.
Action and uses—Not known to be poisonous. Sedative and diuretic. Highly recommended for functional and organic diseases of the heart, mental derangements and renal congestion. Advantageously used in functional palpitation of the heart, Rubini, 1866, confirmed by N. S. Davis, 1879. In 1883 Dr. Bird reports that it palliates the abnormal action and the pain in rheumatic disorders of the heart and was even beneficial to the rheumatism itself. Dr. Cullen, 1882, claims for it even more remarkable powers in functional heart disease, when lips and fingers are almost stagnant with blood, after failure of the usual remedies, digitalis and bromide potassium. Dr. O'Hara finds cactus grand. peculiarly efficacious in removing the effects of degenerative lesions of the heart, including dropsy, angina, etc. It may be given in water the dose gradually increased.

PREPARATION.

Tincture Cactus Grandiflorus—Fl. ext. Cactus grandiflorus, Lilly, 8 fl. ozs.; Alcohol, 8 fl. ozs.; Mix—Dose 10 to 20 m.

WHEN ORDERING OR PRESCRIBING.

FL. EXT. CALABAR BEAN.................. ....Dose 1 to 3 m.
  Physostigma venenosum Balfour.   **Nat. Ord.—*Leguminosæ.***

Synonyms—Physostigma, U. S.,—Ordeal bean.

Range—Tropical Western Africa, near the mouths of the Niger and Old Calabar rivers, along the Gulf of Guinea.

Habitat Wooded banks of streams.

Part used—The seed.

Standard of Strength—0.2 per cent. of ether soluble alkaloid (Physostigmine).

Action and uses—Poisonous. Calabar bean has a powerful sedative influence upon the spine, and is indicated in all cases of abnormal excitement, or irritation of the spinal marrow, especially in tetanus and the poisonous effects of strychnine. It contracts the pupil of the eye. As a local application to the eye, moisten a small piece of soft paper with the *tincture*, dry it by exposure to the air and place it within the lower lid.

Antidotes—(1) Atropine, which directly antagonizes the respiratory depression; (2) Strychnine, which stimulates the cord.

PREPARATION.

Tincture Calabar Bean. U. S.—Fl. ext. Calabar bean, Lilly, 2½ fl. ozs.; Alcohol, 10¼ fl. ozs.; Water, 3½ fl. ozs.; Mix—Dose 5 to 15 m.

FL. EXT. CALAMUS, U. S. ....Dose 5 to 15 m.
  Acorus Calamus Linn.   **Nat. Ord**—*Aroideæ.*

Synonyms—Sweetflag, Myrtleflag, Sweetrush.

Range—Europe, North America; Nova Scotia to Minnesota, southward to Florida.

Habitat—Margins of streams and swamps.

Part used—The rhizome.

Standard of strength—That of the U. S. Pharmacopœia, 1890; 1 c.c. representing 1 gram of the drug; or, practically, minim for grain.

Action and uses—An aromatic stimulant, tonic and carminative. Used in flatulent colic, dyspepsia and feeble digestion.

PREPARATIONS.

Syrup Calamus—Fl. ext. Calamus, Lilly, 4 fl. ozs.; Syrup, 12 fl. ozs.; Mix—Dose ½ to 1 fl. dr.

Infusion Calamus—Fl. ext. Calamus, Lilly, 1 fl. oz.; Hot water, 15 fl. ozs.; Mix—Dose ½ to 1 fl. oz.

FL. EXT. CALENDULA FLOWERS......... .... Dose 30 to 60 m.
  Calendula officinalis Linn.   **Nat. Ord.—*Compositæ.***

Synonyms—Calendula, U. S.,—Marigold.

Range—Levant and Southern Europe; cultivated.

Part used—The florets.

Standard of strength—That of the U. S. Pharmacopœia, 1890; 1 c.c. representing 1 gram of the drug; or, practically, minim for grain.

Action and uses—Used as a dressing for lacerated wounds; applied on lint it prevents suppuration and causes healing by first intent. Said to be an excellent application to cancerous and other ulcers. Internally it is diaphoretic and stimulant, being useful in spasmodic affections and suppressed menstruation.

PREPARATIONS.

Tincture Calendula Flowers. U. S.—Fl. ext. Calendula flowers, Lilly, 3½ fl. ozs.; Alcohol, 9⅝ fl. ozs.; Water, 3¼ fl. ozs.; Mix—Dose 2 to 4 fl. drs.

Ointment Calendula Flowers—Fl. ext. Calendula flowers, Lilly, 4 fl. ozs.; Ointment, U. S., 4 avd. ozs.; Evaporate the fluid extract to a soft extract and incorporate with the ointment.

Lotion Calendula Flowers—Fl. ext. Calendula flowers, Lilly, 4 fl. ozs.; Water, 12 fl. ozs.; Mix—For external use.

FL. EXT. CALENDULA FLOWERS, NONALCOHOLIC.
Dose 30 to 60 m.

Calendula officinalis Linn.   **Nat. Ord.—***Compositæ.*

Synonyms—Calendula, U. S.,—Marigold.

Range—Levant and Southern Europe; cultivated.

Part used—The florets.

Standard of strength—That of the U. S. Pharmacopœia, 1890; 1 c.c. representing 1 gram of the drug; or, practically, minim for gram.

Action and uses—Preferred to the alcoholic preparation for external use. It may also be used internally. Used as a dressing for lacerated wounds, applied so that it prevents suppuration and causes healing by first intention. It is said to be an excellent application to cancerous and other ulcers. Useful in spasmodic affections and suppressed menstruation.

PREPARATION.

Lotion Calendula Flowers, Nonalcoholic—Fl. ext. Calendula flowers, nonalcoholic, Lilly, 4 fl. ozs.; Hot water, 12 fl. ozs.; Mix—For external use.

FL. EXT. CALENDULA HERB..................... Dose 30 to 60 m.

Calendula officinalis Linn.   **Nat. Ord.—***Compositæ.*

Synonym—Marigold.

Range—Levant and Southern Europe; cultivated.

Part used—The herb.

Standard of strength—That of the U. S. Pharmacopœia, 1890; 1 c.c. representing 1 gram of the drug; or, practically, minim for gram.

Action and uses—Reputed antispasmodic, sudorific, deobstruent and emmenagogue.

PREPARATION.

Tincture Calendula Herb—Fl. ext. Calendula herb, Lilly, 3½ fl. ozs.; Diluted alcohol, 12½ fl. ozs.; Mix—Dose 1 to 4 fl. drs.

FL. EXT. CANADA SNAKEROOT........ ... ... Dose 30 to 120 m.

Asarum Canadense Linn.   **Nat. Ord.—***Aristolochiaceæ.*

Synonyms—Wild ginger, Indian ginger.

Range—New Brunswick to Manitoba and Dakota, south to North Carolina.

Habitat—Shaded river banks and moist woodlands.

Part used—The rhizome.

Standard of strength—That of the U. S. Pharmacopœia, 1890; 1 c.c. representing 1 gram of the drug; or, practically, minim for gram.

Action and uses—Aromatic, stimulant, tonic and diaphoretic. Promotes expectoration and is an excellent carminative.

PREPARATION.

Infusion Canada Snakeroot—Fl. ext. Canada snakeroot, Lilly, 1 fl. oz.; Hot water, 15 fl. ozs.; Mix—Dose 1 to 4 fl. ozs.

FL. EXT. CANADA THISTLE ... . Dose 15 to 30 m.

Carduus arvensis (Linn.) Robs.   **Nat. Ord.—***Compositæ.*

Synonyms—Cirsium arvense Scop., Cnicus arvensis Hoffm.,—Cursed thistle.

Range—Europe; naturalized in the United States.

Habitat—Cultivated fields, pastures and roadsides.

Part used—The root.

Standard of strength—That of the U. S. Pharmacopœia, 1890; 1 c.c. representing 1 gram of the drug; or, practically, minim for gram.

Action and uses—Tonic and astringent. Used principally in diarrhœa and dysentery.

PREPARATION.

Infusion Canada Thistle—Fl. ext. Canada thistle, Lilly, 2 fl. ozs.; Hot water, 14 fl. ozs.; Mix—Dose 2 to 4 fl. drs.

FL. EXT. CANNABIS INDICA .... **Dose 5 to 60 m.**

Cannabis sativa Linn. *var. indica,*   **Nat. Ord.**— *Urticaceæ.*

Synonyms—Cannabis sativa Linn.,—Indian cannabis, U. S.,—Foreign indian hemp, Gunjah, Hashish, Churrus, Bhang, Subjer.

Range—Caucasus, Persia, Northern India; cultivated in Europe, Asia and the United States.

Habitat—Rich moist soil of mountain slopes and banks of streams.

Part used—The inflorescence of the female plant.

Standard of Strength—100 c.c. contain 13 gm. extractive.

Action and uses—Nor poisonous according to best authorities, though formerly so regarded. Antispasmodic, analgesic, anesthetic, narcotic, aphrodisiac. Specially recommended in spasmodic and painful affections; for preventing rather than arresting migraine; almost a specific in that form of insanity peculiar to women, caused by mental worry or moral shock. It is the best hypnotic in delirium tremens. Its anodyne power is marked in chronic metritis and dysmenorrhea. Used with excellent results in habitues of opium, chloral or cocaine. In hysterical cases not calmed by chloral or opium it acts especially well.

PREPARATION.

Tincture Cannabis Indica, U. S.—Fl. ext. Cannabis Indica, Lilly, 2½ fl. ozs.; Alcohol, 13½ fl. ozs.; Mix—Dose 5 minims increased till its effects are experienced.

FL. EXT. CANTHARIDES .... **Dose, diluted, 1-2 to 1 m.**

Cantharis vesicatoria De Geer.

                    Class—*Insecta;* **Ord.**—*Coleoptera.*

Synonyms—Cantharis U. S.,—Spanish fly.

Range—Southern and Central Europe.

Habitat—Upon Oleaceæ and Caprifoliaceæ.

Part used—The dried bodies of the insect.

Standard of strength—That of the U. S. Pharmacopœia, 1890; 1 c.c. representing 1 gram of the drug; or, practically, minim for gram.

Action and uses—IRRITANT POISON in overdoses. A powerful stimulant with a peculiar direction to the urinary and genital organs. In moderate doses it is diuretic. Recommended in low forms of fever, dropsy and chronic bronchitis. In scaly diseases of the skin it has cured where arsenic and the application of tar has failed. In various forms of debility of the bladder, such as produce incontinence of urine in children, and dysuria in old men, it has often been efficient. It is valuable in chronic vesical catarrh and diabetes insipidus has been cured by it.

Antidotes—Evacuation of the stomach, mucilaginous drinks freely, opium for the gastro-enteritis are the best measures. There is **no** chemical or physiological antagonist.

PREPARATIONS.

Tincture Cantharides, U. S.—Fl. ext. Cantharides, Lilly, 1¼ fl. ozs.; Alcohol, 30½ fl. ozs.; Mix—Dose 5 to 10 drops repeated three or four times a day.

Cerate Ext. Cantharides—Fl. ext. Cantharides, Lilly, 5¼ fl. ozs.; Resin, 3 avd. ozs.; Yellow wax, lard, of each 7 avd. ozs.; Evaporate the fluid extract on a water bath until it weighs 3 avd. ozs.; add the remaining ingredients previously melted together and keep at a temperature of 100° C. for 15 minutes. Strain through muslin and stir till cold.

Acetic Cantharidal Vesicant—Fl. ext. Cantharides, Lilly, 9 fl. drs.; Alcohol, 2 fl. drs.; Acetic ether, 4 fl. drs.; Acetic acid 1 fl. dr.; Mix the alcohol, acetic ether and acetic acid, then add the fluid extract. Paint the parts to be blistered several times and cover with oiled silk or rubber.

FL. EXT. CAPSICUM U. S.   Dose, diluted, 1-2 to 1 m.
Capsicum fastigiatum Blume. Nat. Ord.—*Solanaceæ.*
Synonym—Red pepper, Cayenne pepper, Bird pepper.
Range—Southern India; extensively cultivated in tropical America and Africa.
Habitat—Waste places.
Part used—The fruit.
Standard of strength—That of the U. S. Pharmacopœia, 1890; 1 c.c. representing 1 gram of the drug; or, practically, minim for grain.
Action and uses—A topical stimulant to the mucous surfaces—exciting the appetite in small doses, but in larger doses causing gastro-enteritis. In some forms of sore throat, as in the early stages of tonsilitis, the infusion forms a valuable addition to a gargle. Dr. Lyons, of Dublin, has praised it highly for the relief of nausea, depression and drinkcraving of the dipsomaniac, giving 10 minim doses of the tincture before meals.

PREPARATION.

Tincture Capsicum, U. S.—Fl. ext. Capsicum, Lilly, 6 fl. drs.; Alcohol, 15¼ fl. ozs.; Mix—Dose 30 to 60 m., diluted.

FL. EXT. CARAWAY SEED........................Dose 60 to 120 m.
Carum Carvi Linn. Nat. Ord.—*Umbelliferæ.*
Synonym—C. Carvi Linn.
Range—Europe, Central and Western Asia, also extends into the Arctic Circle.
Habitat—In moist meadows and pastures; cultivated.
Part used—The fruit.
Standard of strength—That of the U. S. Pharmacopœia, 1890; 1 c.c. representing 1 gram of the drug; or, practically, minim for grain.
Action and uses—Stomachic and carminative. Used in flatulent colic and as an adjuvant or corrective to other medicines.

FL. EXT. CARDAMOM........................Dose 5 to 10 m.
Elettaria repens (Sonnerat) Baillon. Nat. Ord.—*Scitamineæ.*
Synonyms—Amomum repens Sonnerat,—Cardamomum, U. S.
Range—Malabar; cultivated in India and Ceylon.
Habitat—Newly cleared mountain slopes, in moist soil.
Part used—The fruit.
Standard of strength—That of the U. S. Pharmacopœia, 1890; 1 c.c. representing 1 gram of the drug; or, practically, minim for grain.
Action and uses—Aromatic and carminative.

PREPARATION.

Tincture Cardamom, U. S.—Fl. ext. Cardamom, Lilly, 1½ fl. ozs.; Alcohol, 10¼ fl. ozs.; Water, 6½ fl. ozs.; Mix—Dose 30 to 60 m.

FL. EXT. CARDAMOM COMP........................Dose 15 to 30 m.
Standard of strength—One pint represents Cardamom, Cinnamon, of each, 2½ troy ounces; Caraway, 1¼ troy ounces; Cochineal, ⅝ troy ounce.
Action and uses—An elegant aromatic adjuvant especially intended for the preparation of the U. S. tincture. Its concentrated form commends it as a corrigent, stomachic or carminative.

PREPARATION.

Tincture Cardamom Comp., U. S.—Fl. ext. Cardamom comp., Lilly, 2 fl. ozs.; Diluted alcohol, 14 fl. ozs., Mix—Dose 2 to 4 fl. drs.

FL. EXT. **CAROBA LEAVES**...................... Dose 15 to 30 m.

Jacaranda procera Sprengel.   Nat. Ord.—*Bignoniaceæ.*

Synonyms—Bignonia Copaia Aublet, B. Caroba Vellos.

Range—Guiana and Brazil.

Part used—The leaves.

Standard of strength—That of the U. S. Pharmacopœia, 1890; 1 c.c. representing 1 gram of the drug; or, practically, minim for grain.

Action and uses—Alterative, diuretic and sudorific. This drug has been employed in gonorrhea and in vesical affections attended with purulent and mucopurulent urine. In its native country it is used as a remedy in all venereal diseases.

FL. EXT. **CASCARA AMARGA**........ ....Dose 30 to 60 m.

Picramnia sp.?   **Nat. Ord.**—*Simarubaceæ.*

Synonyms—Honduras bark.

Range—Central America and Mexico.

Part used—The bark. It is from an undetermined species of Picramnia.

Standard of strength—That of the U. S. Pharmacopœia, 1890; 1 c.c. representing 1 gram of the drug; or, practically, minim for grain.

Action and uses—Reputed alterative and tonic. Is asserted to be valuable in syphilis, chronic liver complaints, chronic eczema, chronic nasal catarrh and psoriasis.

FL. EXT. **CASCARA SAGRADA, U. S.**

Dose—As a LAXATIVE, 5 to 15 m. three times a day; as a CATHARTIC, 20 to 60 m. morning and evening; as a STOMACHIC, 4 to 10 m. three times a day.

Rhamnus Purshiana D. C.   **Nat. Ord.**—*Rhamnaceæ.*

Synonym—Chittem bark.

Range—Northern California, Idaho, Washington, Oregon and British Columbia.

Habitat—Sides and bottoms of canyons in coniferous forests.

Part used—The bark.

Standard of strength—That of the U. S. Pharmacopœia, 1890; 1 c.c. representing 1 gram of the drug; or, practically, minim for grain.

Action and uses—Tonic, febrifuge and cathartic. It is recommended in the treatment of habitual constipation, and is especially indicated in those affections in which atony of the stomach and bowels are a feature. In the treatment of constipation, the dose should be regulated so as to fall short of a cathartic effect; one fluid ounce of the fluid extract mixed with two fluid ounces of syrup, and given in doses of a teaspoonful three or four times a day, will generally prove sufficient.

FL. EXT. **CASCARA AROMATIC.**

Dose—As a LAXATIVE, 5 to 15 m. three times a day; as a CATHARTIC, 20 to 60 m. morning and evening; as a STOMACHIC, 4 to 10 m. three times a day.

Rhamnus Purshiana D. C.   **Nat. Ord.**—*Rhamnaceæ.*

Synonyms—Chittem bark.

Range—Northern California, Idaho, Washington, Oregon and British Columbia.

Habitat—Sides and bottoms of canyons in coniferous forests.

Part used—The bark.

Standard of strength—That of the U. S. Pharmacopœia, 1890; 1 c.c. representing 1 gram of the drug; or, practically, minim for grain.

NOTE—An efficient and palatable preparation of Cascara sagrada from which the bitter principle has been removed.

Action and uses—Tonic, febrifuge and cathartic. It is recommended in the treatment of habitual constipation, and is especially indicated in those affections in which atony of the stomach and bowels are a feature. In the treatment of constipation, the dose should be regulated so as to fall short of a cathartic effect; one fluid ounce of the fluid extract mixed with two fluid ounces of syrup, and given in doses of a teaspoonful three or four times a day, will generally prove sufficient.

FL. EXT. CASCARA SAGRADA COMP ....**Dose 15 to 60 m.**

Standard of strength—Each fluid dram represents Cascara sagrada, 40 grs.; Senna, purified, 25 grs.; Alom, c. p., 1-12 gr.

Action and uses—Tonic, laxative and cathartic. Useful in habitual constipation, and valuable in all affections where a tonic effect on the stomach and bowels is needed.

FL. EXT. CASCARA, BITTERLESS.

Dose—As a LAXATIVE, 5 to 15 m. three times a day; as a CATHARTIC, 20 to 60 m. morning and evening; as a STOMACHIC, 1 to 10 m. three times a day.

Rhamnus Purshiana D. C.   Nat. Ord.—*Rhamnaceæ.*

Synonyms—Chittem bark.

Range—Northern California, Idaho, Washington, Oregon and British Columbia.

Habitat—Sides and bottoms of canyons in coniferous forests.

Part used—The bark.

Standard of strength—That of the U. S. Pharmacopœia, 1890; 1 c.c. representing 1 gram of the drug; or, practically, minim for grain.

Action and uses—Tonic, febrifuge and cathartic. It is recommended in the treatment of habitual constipation, and is especially indicated in those affections in which atony of the stomach and bowels are a feature. In the treatment of constipation, the dose should be regulated so as to fall short of a cathartic effect; one fluid ounce of the fluid extract mixed with two fluid ounces of syrup, and given in doses of a teaspoonful three or four times a day, will generally prove sufficient.

FL. EXT. CASCARILLA ....**Dose 20 to 30 m.**

Croton Eluteria Bennett.   Nat. Ord.—*Euphorbiaceæ.*

Range—Bahamas and Cuba.

Habitat—On low hills.

Part used—The bark.

Standard of strength—That of the U. S. Pharmacopœia, 1890; 1 c.c. representing 1 gram of the drug; or, practically, minim for grain.

Action and uses—Aromatic, tonic and stimulant.

PREPARATION.

Infusion Cascarilla—Fl. ext. Cascarilla, Lilly, 1 fl. oz.; Hot water, 15 fl. ozs.; Mix—Dose ½ to 1 fl. oz.

FL. EXT. CASSIA BUDS .... Dose 15 to 30 m.

From one or more *undetermined* species of *Cinnamomum* grown in China.   Nat. Ord.—*Laurineæ.*

Synonyms—Has been attributed to C. Cassia Blume, C. aromaticum Nees, Laurus Cassia Ait.

Range—Southeastern China.

Part used—The small unripe fruit.

Standard of strength—That of the U. S. Pharmacopœia, 1890; 1 c.c. representing 1 gram of the drug; or, practically, minim for grain.

Action and uses—Aromatic, stimulant and carminative.

PREPARATION.

Tincture Cassia Buds—Fl. ext. Cassia buds, Lilly, 4 fl. ozs.; Alcohol, 4½ fl. ozs.; Water, 4½ fl. ozs.; Mix the alcohol and the water, and add the fluid extract—Dose 60 to 120 m.

FL. EXT. CASTOR BEAN .... Dose 30 to 60 m.

Ricinus communis Linn.   Nat. Ord.—*Euphorbiaceæ.*

Range—India and Africa; naturalized and cultivated in most temperate and tropical countries.

Part used—The seed.

Standard of strength—That of the U. S. Pharmacopœia, 1890; 1 c.c. representing 1 gram of the drug; or, practically, minim for grain.

Action and uses—Cathartic. This preparation is thought by some practitioners to operate in much smaller doses than the oil with less tendency to irritate the bowels or cause nausea or vomiting.

WHEN ORDERING OR PRESCRIBING.

FL. EXT. CASTOR LEAVES.

Ricinus communis Linn.   **Nat. Ord.**—*Euphorbiaceæ.*

Range—India and Africa; naturalized and cultivated in most temperate and tropical countries.

Part used—The leaves.

Standard of strength—That of the U. S. Pharmacopœia, 1890; 1 c. c. representing 1 gram of the drug; or, practically, minim for grain.

Action and uses—Galactagogue. Used locally to excite the flow of milk. The fluid extract may be painted over the breasts or may be made into a poultice and applied.

EL. EXT. CATECHU .... Dose 10 to 30 m.

Acacia Catechu (Linn.) Willd.   **Nat. Ord.**—*Leguminosæ.*

Synonyms—Mimosa Catechu Linn.,—Cutch, Terra japonica.

Range—India and East Indies.

Habitat—Dry forests.

Part used—An extract prepared from the wood.

Standard of strength—One pint of this fluid extract represents 8 troy ounces of Catechu.

Action and uses—Powerful astringent and mild tonic.

PREPARATIONS.

Tincture Catechu Comp., U. S.—Fl. ext. Catechu, Lilly, 3½ fl. ozs.; Fl. ext. Cassia, Lilly, 6 fl. drs.; Alcohol, 7½ fl. ozs.; Water, 4½ fl. ozs.; Mix the alcohol and water and add the fluid extracts—Dose 60 to 120 m.

Infusion Catechu, Br.—Fl. ext. Catechu, Lilly, 5 fl. drs.; Fl. ext. Cassia, Lilly, ½ fl. dr.; Hot water, 10 fl. ozs.; Mix—Dose 1 to 3 fl. ozs.

FL. EXT. CATECHU COMP. .... Dose 10 to 40 m.

Standard of strength—One pint represents Catechu, 10½ troy ounces; Cinnamon, 5½ troy ounces.

Action and uses—An excellent astringent.

PREPARATION.

Tincture Catechu Comp., U. S.—Fl. ext. Catechu comp., Lilly, 2½ fl. ozs.; Alcohol, 8½ fl. ozs.; Water, 5½ fl. ozs.; Mix the alcohol and water and add the fluid extract—Dose 1 to 3 fl. drs.

FL. EXT. CATNEP .... Dose 30 to 60 m.

Nepeta Cataria Linn.   **Nat. Ord.**—*Labiatæ.*

Synonyms—Catsmint, Catswort, Fieldbalm.

Range—Asia, Europe; naturalized in the United States.

Habitat—Around dwellings, along fences, etc.

Part used—The herb.

Standard of strength—That of the U. S. Pharmacopœia, 1890; 1 c.c. representing 1 gram of the drug; or, practically, minim for grain.

Action and uses—Carminative, diaphoretic, tonic and antispasmodic. Useful in febrile, nervous and infantile diseases and to restore the menstrual secretions.

PREPARATIONS.

Catnep Mixture—Fl. ext. Catnep, Lilly, 1½ fl. ozs.; Fl. ext. Valerian, Lilly, Scullcap, Lilly, of each 1 fl. oz.; Mix—Dose 15 to 20 m.

Infusion Catnep—Fl. ext. Catnep, Lilly, 1 fl. oz.; Hot water, 15 fl. ozs.; Mix—Dose 1 to 2 fl. ozs.

FL. EXT. CEDRON SEED .... Dose 15 to 30 m.

Simaba Cedron Planch.   **Nat. Ord.**—*Simarubaceæ.*

Range—New Granada and Central America.

Part used—The seed.

Standard of strength—That of the U. S. Pharmacopœia, 1890; 1 c.c. representing 1 gram of the drug; or, practically, minim for grain.

Action and uses—Tonic, antispasmodic and antiperiodic.

FL. EXT. CELERY SEED...................................Dose 30 to 60 m.

Apium graveolens Linn.　　　　　　　　**Nat. Ord.**—*Umbelliferæ.*

Range—Levant and Southern Europe; cultivated in the United States extensively.

Part used—The fruit.

Standard of strength—That of the U. S. Pharmacopœia, 1890; 1 c.c. representing 1 gram of the drug; or, practically, minim for grain.

Action and uses—Said to be diuretic, sudorific and nervine and claimed to be a remedy for sick headache and nervous prostration.

PREPARATIONS.

Syrup Celery Seed—Fl. ext. Celery seed, Lilly, 4 fl. ozs.; Syrup, 12 fl. ozs.; Mix—Dose 2 to 4 fl. drs.

Infusion Celery Seed—Fl. ext. Celery seed, Lilly, 1 fl. oz.; Hot water, 15 fl. ozs.; Mix—Dose 1 to 2 fl. ozs.

FL. EXT. CEVADILLA SEED.

Schoenocaulon officinale Gray　　　　　　**Nat. Ord.**—*Liliaceæ.*

Synonyms—Veratrum Sabadilla Schlecht., Asagræa officinalis Lindl.

Range—Mexico, Guatemala and Venezuela.

Habitat—Grassy places on open hills.

Part used—The seed.

Standard of strength—That of the U. S. Pharmacopœia, 1890; 1 c.c. representing 1 gram of the drug; or, practically, minim for grain.

Action and uses—Poisonous. Acrid, insecticide, rarely used internally. Mostly used externally in destroying vermin in the hair.

PREPARATION.

Tincture Cevadilla Seed—Fl. ext. Cevadilla seed, Lilly, 1 fl. oz.; Alcohol, 15 fl. ozs.

FL. EXT. CHAMOMILE...................................Dose 30 to 60 m.

Anthemis nobilis Linn.　　　　　　　　**Nat. Ord.**—*Compositæ.*

Synonym—Roman chamomile.

Range—Southern and Western Europe; introduced into the United States, cultivated.

Habitat—Gravelly heaths, waste places, etc.

Part used—The flower heads.

Standard of strength—That of the U. S. Pharmacopœia, 1890; 1 c.c. representing 1 gram of the drug; or, practically, minim for grain.

Action and uses—A mild tonic. In large doses emetic. Especially valuable in general debility when accompanied by languid appetite often attending convalescence from idiopathic fevers.

PREPARATION.

Infusion Chamomile—Fl. ext. Chamomile, Lilly, 1 fl. oz.; Hot water, 15 fl. ozs.; Mix—Dose 1 to 2 fl. ozs.

FL. EXT. CHERRY BARK, U. S....................................Dose 30 to 60 m.

Prunus serotina Ehrb.　　　　　　　　**Nat. Ord.**—*Rosaceæ.*

Synonyms—P. Virginiana Linn., Cerasus serotina Loiseleur.—Wild cherry.

Range—North America; Nova Scotia to Florida, west to Minnesota, Eastern Nebraska and Louisiana.

Habitat—Rich woodlands.

Part used—The bark deprived of the corky layer.

Standard of strength—That of the U. S. Pharmacopœia, 1890; 1 c.c. representing 1 gram of the drug; or, practically, minim for grain.

Action and uses—Tonic and sedative. From its pleasant flavor it is much used in cough syrups.

PREPARATION.

Infusion Cherry Bark, U. S.—Fl. ext. Cherry bark, Lilly, 5½ fl. drs.; Water, q.s. to make 16 fl. ozs.; Mix—Dose 2 to 3 fl. ozs.

NOTE—For making Syrup Cherry bark use Fl. Ext. Cherry bark, for Syrup, Lilly.

FL. EXT. CHERRY BARK, for Syrup, Proctor's formula.
Dose 60 to 120 m.

Prunus serotina Ehrh.   Nat. Ord.—*Rosaceæ.*

Synonyms—P. Virginiana Linn., Cerasus serotina Loiseleur,—Wild cherry.

Range—North America; Nova Scotia to Florida, west to Minnesota, Eastern Nebraska and Louisiana.

Habitat—Rich woodlands.

Part used—The bark deprived of the corky layer.

Standard of strength—That of the U. S. Pharmacopœia, 1890; 1 c.c. representing 1 gram of the drug or, practically, minim for grain.

Action and uses—Tonic and sedative.

PREPARATION.

Syrup Cherry Bark, (Proctor)—Fl. ext. Cherry bark, for syrup, Lilly, 5 fl. ozs.; Syrup, 12 fl. ozs.; Mix—Dose 1 to 4 fl. drs. This is not intended to duplicate the official preparation.

FL. EXT. CHERRY BARK COMP. .... Dose 30 to 60 m.

Standard of strength—One pint represents Cherry bark, 12½ troy ounces; Bloodroot, Ipecac, Opium, of each, 1½ troy ounces.

Action and uses—Expectorant and sedative. Principally used to prepare the compound syrup of cherry bark.

PREPARATION.

Syrup Cherry Bark Comp.—Fl. ext. Cherry bark comp., Lilly, 4 fl. ozs.; Syrup, 12 fl. ozs.; Mix—Dose 2 to 4 fl. drs.

FL. EXT. CHERRY BARK, DETANNATED .... Dose 30 to 60 m.

Prunus serotina Ehrh.   Nat. Ord.—*Rosaceæ.*

Synonyms—P. Virginiana Linn., Cerasus serotina Loiseleur,—Wild cherry.

Range—North America; Nova Scotia to Florida, west to Minnesota, Eastern Nebraska and Louisiana.

Habitat—Rich woodlands.

Part used—The bark deprived of the corky layer.

Standard of strength—That of the U. S. Pharmacopœia, 1890; 1 c.c. representing 1 gram of the drug; or, practically, minim for grain.

Action and uses—The process of detannating Cherry bark deprives it largely of its tonic properties but its sedative quality is fully preserved in this preparation and it will be found an excellent addition to cough syrups and especially adapted when it is desired to combine with any of the preparations of Iron.

PREPARATION.

Syrup Cherry Bark, Detannated—Fl. ext. Cherry bark, detannated, Lilly, 4 fl. ozs.; Syrup, 12 fl. ozs.; Mix—Dose 2 to 4 fl. drs.

FL. EXT. CHESTNUT LEAVES, U. S. .... Dose 60 to 120 m.

Castanea dentata Marsh.; Sudworth.   Nat. Ord.—*Cupuliferæ.*

Synonyms—C. sativa var. Americana Watson and Coulter, C. vesca Gaertn.

Range—North America; Ontario, south to Florida, west to Arkansas and Michigan.

Habitat—Dry hills.

Part used—The leaves.

Standard of strength—That of the U. S. Pharmacopœia, 1890; 1 c.c. representing 1 gram of the drug; or, practically, minim for grain.

Action and uses—Tonic, astringent and antispasmodic. It has the reputation of being very efficacious in whooping cough.

PREPARATIONS.

Syrup Chestnut Leaves—Fl. ext. Chestnut leaves, Lilly, 4 fl. ozs.; Syrup, 12 fl. ozs.; Mix—Dose, for a child, 15 to 60 m., six or eight times a day.

Infusion Chestnut Leaves—Fl. ext. Chestnut leaves, Lilly, 1 fl. oz.; Hot water, 15 fl. ozs.; Sugar, 2 troy ozs.; Mix—Dose, for a child, 2 to 4 fl. drs., six or eight times a day.

FL. EXT. CHIRATA, U. S. ....Dose 20 to 30 m.
Swertia Chirata Hamilton. **Nat. Ord.**—*Gentianaceæ.*

Synonyms—Ophelia Chirata Grisebach,—Bitterstick, East India balmony.

Range—Northern India.

Habitat—Mountain slopes, from 5000 to 9000 feet above sea level.

Part used—The entire plant.

Standard of strength—That of the U. S. Pharmacopœia, 1890; 1 c.c. representing 1 gram of the drug; or, practically, minim for grain.

Action and uses—Pure bitter tonic, resembling gentian in its effects. In India it has been successfully used in intermittent and remittent fevers. Overdoses are inclined to nauseate. Particularly useful in the dyspepsia of gouty subjects.

PREPARATIONS.

Tincture Chirata, U. S.—Fl. ext. Chirata, Lilly, 1⅝ fl. ozs.; Alcohol, 7¼ fl. ozs.; Water, 7¼ fl. ozs.; Mix—Dose 2 to 4 fl. drs.

Infusion Chirata—Fl. ext. Chirata, Lilly, 1 fl. oz.; Hot water, 15 fl. ozs.; Mix—Dose ½ to 1 fl. oz.

FL. EXT. CINCHONA AROMATIC .... Dose 10 to 60 m.
Standard of strength—One pint represents Calisaya bark, 12 troy ounces; Sweet orange peel, 2 troy ounces; Fl. Ext. Cardamom comp., 2 fluid ounces. The Calisaya bark used in this preparation conforms to the U. S. standard and contains not less than 5 per cent. of total alkaloids and at least 2½ per cent. of quinine.

Action and uses—Stomachic, cordial, tonic and febrifuge.

FL. EXT. CINCHONA CALISAYA, **U. S.** ....**Dose 10 to 60 m.**
Cinchona Calisaya Weddell. **Nat. Ord.**—*Rubiaceæ.*

Synonyms—Cinchona, U. S.,—Yellow cinchona, Peruvian bark, Jesuit's bark.

Range—Mountainous districts of South America between 10° south latitude and 10° north latitude; cultivated in South America and in the mountains of Java, India and Jamaica.

Habitat—Mountain slopes, moist atmospheres, 3000 to 8000 feet above sea level.

Part used—The bark.

Standard of strength—That of the U. S. Pharmacopœia, 1890. From bark containing not less than 5 per cent. total alkaloids and at least 2.5 per cent. of quinine.

Action and uses—Tonic, febrifuge and antiperiodic.

PREPARATIONS.

Tincture Cinchona Calisaya, U. S.—Fl. ext. Cinchona calisaya, Lilly, 3¼ fl. ozs.; Alcohol, 10 fl. ozs.; Glycerin, ½ fl. oz.; Water, 2 fl. ozs.; Mix the alcohol, glycerin and water and add the fluid extract—Dose 1 to 2 fl. drs.

Infusion Cinchona Calisaya, U. S.—Fl. ext. Cinchona calisaya, Lilly, 1 fl. oz.; Aromatic sulphuric acid, 80 m.; Water, q.s. to make 16 fl. ozs.; Mix—Dose 1 to 2 fl. ozs.

FL. EXT. CINCHONA COMP. .... Dose 10 to **60 m.**
Standard of strength—One pint represents Calisaya bark, 8 troy ounces; Bitter orange peel, 6 troy ounces; Serpentaria 1½ troy ounces. The calisaya bark used in this preparation conforms to the U. S. standard and contains not less than 5 per cent. of total alkaloids and at least 2½ per cent. of quinine.

Action and uses—Stomachic, cordial and tonic. Its principal use is for preparing Huxham's Tincture of Barks.

PREPARATION.

Huxham's Tincture of Barks—Fl. ext. Cinchona comp., Lilly, 3¼ fl. ozs.; Alcohol, 10¼ fl. ozs.; Glycerin, 1½ fl. ozs.; Water, 1¼ fl. ozs.; Mix the alcohol, glycerin and water and add the fluid extract—Dose 1 to 2 fl. drs.

WHEN ORDERING OR PRESCRIBING.

FL. EXT. CINCHONA COMP., DETANNATED ... Dose 10 to 60 m.

Standard of strength—One pint represents Red cinchona bark, 8 troy ounces; Bitter orange peel, 6 troy ounces; Serpentaria, 1½ troy ounces. The red bark used in this preparation contains not less than 5 per cent. of total alkaloids.

Action and uses—Stomachic, cordial and tonic. This extract is especially designed for the preparation of a tincture with which iron salts may be combined without forming an inky precipitate.

PREPARATION.

Tincture Cinchona Comp., Detannated—Fl. ext. Cinchona comp., detannated, Lilly, 5¼ fl. ozs.; Alcohol, 10½ fl. ozs.; Glycerin, 1¾ fl. ozs.; Water, 1¾ fl. ozs.; Mix the alcohol, glycerin and water and add the fluid extract—Dose 1 to 2 fl. drs.

FL. EXT. CINCHONA, DETANNATED .... Dose 10 to 60 m.
Cinchona Calisaya Weddell. **Nat. Ord**—*Rubiaceæ.*

Synonyms—Yellow Cinchona, Peruvian bark, Jesuit's bark.

Range—Mountainous districts of South America between 19° south latitude and 10° north latitude; cultivated in South America and in the mountains of Java, India and Jamaica.

Habitat—Mountain slopes in moist atmospheres, 3000 to 8000 feet above sea level.

Part used—The bark.

Standard of strength—That of the U. S. Pharmacopœia, 1890. From bark containing not less than 5 per cent. total alkaloids and at least 2½ per cent. of quinine.

Action and uses—Tonic, febrifuge and antiperiodic. This extract is especially designed for the preparation of the various cinchona compounds and for mixtures containing iron salts, with which it does not form an inky precipitate.

PREPARATION.

Tincture Cinchona, Detannated—Fl. ext. Cinchona, detannated, Lilly, 3½ fl. ozs.; Alcohol, 9½ fl. ozs.; Water, 3¼ fl. ozs.; Mix—Dose 1 to 2 fl. drs.

FL. EXT. CINCHONA, PALE .... Dose 10 to 60 m.
Cinchona officinalis Linn. **Nat. Ord.**—*Rubiaceæ.*

Synonyms—Peruvian bark, Jesuit's bark.

Range—Mountainous districts of South America between 19° south latitude and 10° north latitude; cultivated in South America and the mountains of Java, India and Jamaica.

Habitat—Mountain slopes in moist atmospheres, 3000 to 8000 feet above sea level.

Part used—The bark.

Standard of strength—That of the U. S. Pharmacopœia, 1890; i.e., representing 1 gram of the drug or, practically, minim for grain. From pale bark containing not less than 5 per cent. of total alkaloids.

Action and uses—Tonic, febrifuge and antiperiodic.

PREPARATIONS.

Tincture Cinchona, Pale—Fl. ext. Cinchona, pale, Lilly, 3½ fl. ozs.; Alcohol, 7 fl. ozs.; Glycerin, ½ fl. oz.; Water, 5 fl. ozs.; Mix the alcohol, glycerin and water and add the fluid extract—Dose 1 to 2 fl. drs.

Infusion Cinchona, Pale—Fl. ext. Cinchona, pale, Lilly, 1 fl. oz.; Hot water, 15 fl. ozs.; Mix—Dose 1 to 2 fl. ozs.

FL. EXT. CINCHONA, RED .... Dose 10 to 60 m.
Cinchona succirubra Pavon. **Nat. Ord.**—*Rubiaceæ.*

Synonyms—Peruvian bark, Jesuit's bark.

Range—Mountainous districts of South America between 19° south latitude and 10° north latitude; cultivated in South America and the mountains of Java, India and Jamaica.

Habitat—Mountain slopes in moist atmospheres, 3000 to 8000 feet above sea level.

Part used—The bark.

Standard of strength—That of the U. S. Pharmacopœia, 1890; 1 c.c. representing 1 gram of the drug; or, practically, minim for grain. From bark containing not less than 5 per cent. of total alkaloids.
Action and uses—Tonic, febrifuge and antiperiodic.

FL. EXT. CINCHONA, RED, **COMP**................**Dose 10 to 60 m.**

For making Tincture, U. S.

Standard of strength—One pint represents Red cinchona bark, 8 troy ounces; Bitter orange peel, 6 troy ounces; Serpentaria, 1½ troy ounces. The red bark used in this preparation contains not less than 5 per cent. total alkaloids.
Action and uses—Stomachic, cordial and tonic.

PREPARATION.

Tincture Cinchona, Red, Comp., U. S.—Fl. ext. Cinchona, red, comp., Lilly, 5¾ fl. ozs.; Alcohol, 16⅛ fl. ozs.; Glycerin, 1¼ fl. ozs.; Water, 1½ fl. ozs.; Mix the alcohol, glycerin and water and add the fluid extract—Dose 1 to 2 fl. drs.

FL. EXT. CINNAMON, CEYLON.....................Dose 10 to 30 m.

Cinnamomum zeylanicum Breyne.   **Nat. Ord.**—*Laurineœ.*

Synonyms—Laurus Cinnamomum Linn.
Range—Ceylon and other islands of the East Indies; cultivated in Cayenne, Tropical Africa, America and Asia.
Habitat—Ascending wooded mountain slopes to altitudes of 3000 feet.
Part used—The inner bark of the shoots.
Standard of strength—That of the U. S. Pharmacopœia, 1890; 1 c.c. representing 1 gram of the drug; or, practically, minim for grain.
Action and uses—Aromatic, stimulant, carminative and mildly astringent.

PREPARATION.

Tincture **Cinnamon, Ceylon, U. S.**—Fl. ext. Cinnamon, Ceylon, Lilly, 1½ fl. ozs.; Alcohol, 12 fl. ozs.; Water, 2⅜ fl. ozs.; Mix the alcohol and water then add the fluid extract—Dose 60 to 120 m.

FL. EXT. **CLEAVERS**...........................**Dose 30 to 60 m.**

Galium Aparine Linn.   **Nat. Ord.**—*Rubiaceœ.*

Synonyms—Goosegrass, Bedstraw, Catchweed.
Range—Europe, Asia, North America; throughout the continent.
Habitat—Moist woods and copses.
Part used—The herb.
Standard of strength—That of the U. S. Pharmacopœia, 1890; 1 c.c. representing 1 gram of the drug; or, practically, minim for grain.
Action and uses—Aperient, antispasmodic and diuretic. Valuable in suppression of urine and in inflammation of the kidneys and bladder.

PREPARATION.

Infusion Cleavers—Fl. ext. Cleavers, Lilly, 2 fl. ozs.; Hot water, 14 fl. ozs.; Mix—Dose 1 to 2 fl. ozs.

FL. EXT. CLOVES.........................Dose 5 to 20 m.

Eugenia aromatica (Linn.) Kuntze.   **Nat. Ord.**—*Myrtaceœ.*

Synonyms—E. caryophyllata Thunb., Caryophyllus aromaticus Linn.
Range—Molucca Islands; cultivated in tropical countries.
Part used—The unexpanded flowers.
Standard of strength—That of the U. S. Pharmacopœia, 1890; 1 c.c. representing 1 gram of the drug; or, practically, minim for grain.
Action and uses—Aromatic and stimulant.

PREPARATIONS.

Tincture Cloves—Fl. ext. Cloves, Lilly, 3 fl. oz.; Alcohol, 13 fl. ozs.; Mix—Dose 1 to 2 fl. drs.

Infusion Cloves—Fl. ext. Cloves, Lilly, ½ fl. oz.; Hot water, 15½ fl. ozs.; Mix—Dose ½ to 1 fl. oz.

WHEN ORDERING OR PRESCRIBING.

FL. EXT. CLOVER TOPS . . . .**Dose 30 to 60 m.**
Trifolium pratense Linn. **Nat. Ord.**—*Leguminosæ.*
Synonym—Red clover.
Range—Europe; naturalized in the United States, cultivated extensively.
Habitat—Fields and meadows; common.
Part used—The inflorescence.
Standard of strength—That of the U. S. Pharmacopœia, 1890; 1 c.c. representing 1 gram of the drug; or, practically, minim for grain.
Action and uses—Recommended as an application for ill conditioned ulcers and burns; soothing and promoting healthy granulation. Also used in whooping cough. Has been extolled as an alterative but its value in this direction is very doubtful.

PREPARATIONS.

Syrup Clover Tops—Fl. ext. Clover tops, Lilly, 4 fl. ozs.; Syrup, 12 fl. ozs.; Mix—Dose, for children, 1 to 2 fl. drs. three or four times a day.

Ointment Clover Tops—Fl. ext. Clover tops, Lilly, 4 fl. ozs.; Lard, 8 troy ounces; Heat the fluid extract on a water bath until the alcohol is dissipated, add the lard, previously melted, and stir till cold.

FL. EXT. COCA LEAVES, U. S. . . . .**Dose 20 to 60 m.**
Erythroxylon Coca Linn. **Nat. Ord.**—*Lineæ.*
Range—Peru, Bolivia; cultivated in Ceylon, Java and British India.
Habitat—On mountain slopes to an altitude of 8000 feet.
Part used—The leaves.
Standard of strength—0.5 per cent. cocaine.
Action and uses—Poisonous. Anodyne and antispasmodic. It is a powerful nervous stimulant and increases the power of the muscular system to sustain fatigue. It contributes to mental cheerfulness and has been used in the treatment of opium habit in which, however, it has no value except to antagonize certain heart symptoms. It should, in such cases, never be used as a regular remedy.
Antidotes—Alcohol and opium as stimulants to the heart, artificial respiration. Chloral is the most direct antagonist.

PREPARATION.

Tincture Coca Leaves—Fl. ext. Coca leaves, Lilly, 4 fl. ozs.; Diluted alcohol, 12 fl. ozs.; Mix—Dose 1 to 4 fl. drs.

FL. EXT. COCCULUS INDICUS.
Anamirta paniculata Colebrook. **Nat. Ord.**—*Menispermaceæ.*
Synonyms—A. Cocculus Wight et Arnott, Menispermum Cocculus Linn.,—Fishberry.
Range—The Eastern side of the Indian Peninsula and the East Indian Islands.
Part used—The fruit.
Standard of strength—That of the U. S. Pharmacopœia, 1890; 1 c.c. representing 1 gram of the drug; or, practically, minim for grain.
Action and uses—Poison. Seldom used internally. Resembles nux vomica in its action, producing convulsions. Said to be used successfully as a local application in obstinate cutaneous diseases, as scald head, itch, etc. and to destroy vermin in the hair. It should never be used where the surface is abraded.
Antidotes—Chloral hydrate is said to be antagonistic. Emetics, stomach pump, stimulants, artificial respiration. Theoretically, morphine has been suggested.

PREPARATIONS.

Tincture Cocculus Indicus—Fl. ext. Cocculus indicus, Lilly, 2 fl. ozs.; Alcohol, 9 fl. ozs.; Water, 5 fl. ozs.; Mix the alcohol and water and add the fluid extract.

Ointment Cocculus Indicus—Fl. ext. Cocculus indicus, Lilly, ½ fl. oz.; Lard, 4 troy ozs.; Melt the lard, add the fluid extract and stir till cold.

FL. EXT. COFFEE, **the green berry**........ ....**Dose 30 to 60 m.**
Coffea Arabica Linn.   **Nat. Ord.**—*Rubiaceæ.*

Range—Southern Arabia and Tropical Africa; cultivated in Tropical America and the East Indies.

Habitat—Hilly woodlands at an elevation of 1000 to 2000 feet above the sea.

Part used—The seed.

Standard of strength—That of the U. S. Pharmacopœia, 1890; 1 c.c. representing 1 gram of the drug; or, practically, minim for gram.

Action and uses—Astringent, stimulant and stomachic. Substitutes guarana. Valuable in nervous headache and the cephalalgia sometimes following menstruation and that following dissipation. Contraindicated in neuralgia, chronic headache and when it is desirable not to excite the heart.

FL. EXT. COFFEE, **the roasted berry**........... ....**Dose 30 to 60 m.**
Coffea Arabica Linn.   **Nat. Ord.**—*Rubiaceæ.*

Range—Southern Arabia and Tropical Africa; cultivated in Tropical America and the East Indies.

Habitat—Hilly woodlands at an elevation of 1000 to 2000 feet above the sea.

Part used—The seed.

Standard of strength—That of the U. S. Pharmacopœia, 1890; 1 c.c. representing 1 gram of the drug; or, practically, minim for gram.

Action and uses—Principally used for preparing syrup of coffee for flavoring soda water syrups. Valuable in opium poisoning. In asthma, if not habitually used, coffee is useful in the paroxysm.

PREPARATION.

Syrup Coffee—Fl. ext. Coffee, the roasted berry, Lilly, 2 fl. ozs.; Syrup, 14 fl. ozs.

FL. EXT. COLCHICUM ROOT, U. S.... ....**Dose 2 to 8 m.**
Colchicum autumnale Linn.   **Nat. Ord.**—*Liliaceæ.*

Synonyms—Meadow saffron, Naked ladies.

Range—Southern Europe and Northern Africa.

Habitat—Moist pastures and meadows.

Part used—The tuber.

Standard of strength—0.5 per cent. of alkaloid, estimated gravimetrically.

Action and uses—ACRID NARCOTIC POISON. Diaphoretic, diuretic, cathartic, anodyne and sedative. Valuable in the treatment of rheumatism and gout. In acute gout it should be given with an alkali and kept short of emetocatharsis.

Antidotes—Tannic acid to delay absorption. Emetics, cathartics, warm demulcent drinks freely. Morphine hypodermically.

PREPARATIONS.

Tincture Colchicum Root—Fl. ext. Colchicum root, Lilly, 2⅝ fl. ozs.; Alcohol, 11 fl. ozs.; Water, 2⅝ fl. ozs.; Mix the alcohol and water and add the fluid extract—Dose 10 to 30 m.

Wine Colchicum Root, U. S.—Fl. ext. Colchicum root, Lilly, 6⅜ fl. ozs.; Stronger white wine, 93⅝ fl. ozs.; Mix—Dose 10 to 15 m.

FL. EXT. COLCHICUM SEED, U. S...................**Dose 2 to 8 m.**
Colchicum autumnale Linn.   **Nat. Ord.**—*Liliaceæ.*

Synonyms—Meadow saffron, Naked ladies.

Range—Southern Europe and Northern Africa.

Habitat—Moist pastures and meadows.

Part used—The seed.

Standard of strength—0.5 per cent. of alkaloid, estimated gravimetrically.

Action and uses—ACRID NARCOTIC POISON. Diaphoretic, diuretic,

cathartic, anodyne **and sedative**. Valuable in the treatment of rheumatism and gout. In acute **gout it** should be given with an alkali and kept
short of emetocatharsis.

Antidotes—Tannic acid to **delay absorption.** Emetics, cathartics,
warm demulcent drinks freely. Morphine hypodermically.

PREPARATIONS.

Tincture Colchicum Seed, U. S.—Fl. ext. Colchicum seed, Lilly,
2¾ fl. ozs.; Alcohol, 10½ fl. ozs.; Water, 3½ fl. ozs.; Mix—Dose 10 to 30 m.
Wine Colchicum Seed, U. S.—Fl. ext. Colchicum seed, Lilly,
2⅝ fl. ozs.; Stronger white wine, 13½ fl. ozs.; Mix—Dose 10 to 30 m.

FL. EXT. COLOCYNTH .... **Dose 5 to 10 m.**
Citrullus Colocynthis Schrader. **Nat. Ord.**—*Cucurbitaceæ.*
Synonyms—Cucumis Colocynthis Linn.,—Bitter apple, Bitter cu-
cumber.
Range—Turkey and the Archipelago, Africa, Asia; cultivated in Spain.
Habitat—Sandy soil along the coast.
Part used—The fruit deprived of its rind.
Standard of strength—That of the U. S. Pharmacopœia, 1890; 1 c.c.
representing 1 gram of the drug; or, practically, minim for grain.
Action and uses—A powerful drastic hydragogue cathartic and stim-
ulant also of the hepatic secretion and intestinal glands.

PREPARATION.

Tincture Colocynth—Fl. ext. Colocynth, Lilly, 2 fl. ozs.; Alcohol, 5
fl. ozs.; Water, 9 fl. ozs.; Mix the alcohol and water, and add the fluid extract—Dose ½ to 1 fl. dr.

FL. EXT. COLUMBO, U. S. .... **Dose 15 to 30 m.**
Jateorhiza Palmata (Lam.) Miers. **Nat. Ord.**—*Menispermaceæ.*
Synonyms—J. Calumba Miers, Cocculus palmatus D. C.,—Calumba,
U. S.
Range—Eastern Africa; cultivated in parts of East Indies.
Habitat—In forests and underbrush.
Part used—The root.
Standard of strength—That of the U. S. Pharmacopœia, 1890; 1 c.c.
representing 1 gram of the drug; or, practically, minim for grain.
Action and uses—A valuable tonic in deficient appetite from indi-
gestion or simple want of tone. As it contains no tannin it may be used
in combination with iron. It is also given with alkalies and combined
with other tonics.

PREPARATIONS.

Tincture Columbo, U. S.—Fl. ext. Columbo, Lilly, 1⅞ fl. ozs.; Alcohol, 10¼ fl. ozs.; Glycerin, 3¾ fl. ozs.; Mix the alcohol with the glycerin
and add the fluid extract—Dose 1 to 2 fl. drs.
Infusion Columbo—Fl. ext. Columbo, Lilly, 1 fl. oz.; Hot water, 15
fl. ozs.; Mix—Dose ½ to 1 fl. oz.

FL. EXT. COLTSFOOT .... **Dose 60 to 120 m.**
Tussilago Farfara Linn. **Nat. Ord.**—*Compositæ.*
Synonyms—Bullsfoot, Flower velure.
Range—Northern Asia and Europe; naturalized in the United States;
New England, New York and Pennsylvania.
Habitat—Wet places and along brooks.
Part used—The leaves.
Standard of strength—That of the U. S. Pharmacopœia, 1890; 1 c.c.
representing 1 gram of the drug; or, practically, minim for grain.
Action and uses—Demulcent and tonic. Used in coughs and pulmon-
ary complaints, scrofula, scrofulous tumors, etc.

PREPARATIONS.

Syrup Coltsfoot—Fl. ext. Coltsfoot, Lilly, 4 fl. ozs.; Syrup, 12 fl. ozs.;
Mix—Dose ½ to 1 fl. oz.
Infusion Coltsfoot—Fl. ext. Coltsfoot, Lilly, 4 fl. ozs.; Hot water, 12
fl. ozs.; Mix—Dose ½ to 1 fl. oz.

FL. EXT. COMFREY ....Dose 60 to 120 m.
Symphytum officinale Linn.   **Nat. Ord.**—*Boraginaceæ.*
Range—Europe; naturalized in the United States; New England.
Habitat—Moist grounds.
Part used—The root.
Standard of strength—That of the U. S. Pharmacopœia, 1890; 1 c.c.
representing 1 gram of the drug; or, practically, minim for grain.
Action and uses—Demulcent and tonic. Used in pulmonary affections.

PREPARATION.

Compound Wine of Comfrey or Restorative Wine Bitters—Fl. exts. Comfrey, Solomon's seal, Unicorn root, Lilly, of each, 1
fl. oz.; Fl. exts. Chamomile, Gentian comp., Cardamom, Sassafras, Lilly,
of each, ½ fl. oz.; Alcohol, 4 fl. ozs.; Sherry wine, q.s. ad., 4 pints; Mix—
Dose ½ to 1 fl. oz.

FL. EXT. CONDURANGO.......................Dose 30 to 60 m.
Gonolobus Condurango Triana.   **Nat. Ord.**—*Asclepiadaceæ.*
Range—Ecuador.
Part used—The bark.
Standard of strength—That of the U. S. Pharmacopœia, 1890; 1 c.c.
representing 1 gram of the drug; or, practically, minim for grain.
Action and uses—Aromatic tonic. Reputed at one time to be a cure
for cancer but this has proven untrue.

FL. EXT. CONIUM LEAVES......................Dose 5 to 10 m.
Conium maculatum Linn.   **Nat. Ord.**—*Umbelliferæ.*
Synonym—Poison hemlock.
Range—Europe and Asia; naturalized in the United States.
Habitat—Waste places.
Part used—The leaves.
Standard of strength—That of the U. S. Pharmacopœia, 1890; 1 c. c.
representing 1 gram of the drug; or, practically, minim for grain.
Action and uses—Poisonous. Narcotic and sedative. Considered
of value in chorea, in the convulsions of children; said to have remarkable power in effecting muscular relaxation, thus making it beneficial in
laryngismus stridulus, spasmodic wry neck and spasmodic stricture.
Note—Conium and its preparations are contraindicated in cases of great
exhaustion and debility. Diseases interfering with the rhythm of the
heart suggest a cautious use of the medicine.
Antidotes—Nux vomica and its alkaloids are antagonistic. Tannic acid
and caustic alkalies are chemically incompatible.

PREPARATION.

Tincture Conium Leaves—Fl. ext. Conium leaves, Lilly, 2 fl. ozs.;
Alcohol, 10½ fl. ozs.; Water, 3½ fl. ozs.; Mix—Dose 30 to 60 m. increased
gradually as found necessary.

FL. EXT. CONIUM FRUIT, U. S..................Dose 1 to 5 m.
Conium maculatum Linn.   **Nat. Ord.**—*Umbelliferæ.*
Synonym—Poison hemlock.
Range—Europe and Asia; naturalized in the United States.
Habitat—Waste places.
Part used—The full grown fruit.
Standard of Strength—0.5 per cent. of coniine weighed as
hydrochloride.
Action and uses—Poisonous. Narcotic and sedative. Considered of
value in chorea, in the convulsions of children; said to have remarkable
power in effecting muscular relaxation, thus making it beneficial in
laryngismus stridulus, spasmodic wry neck and spasmodic stricture.
Note—Conium and its preparations are contraindicated in cases of great
exhaustion and debility. Diseases interfering with the rhythm of the
heart suggest a cautious use of the medicine.

Antidotes—Nux vomica and its alkaloids are antagonistic. Tannic acid and caustic alkalies are chemically incompatable.

PREPARATION.

Tincture Conium Fruit—Fl. ext. Conium fruit, Lilly, 2½ fl. ozs.; Alcohol, 6¼ fl. ozs.; Water, 6⅓ fl. ozs.; Mix—Dose 5 to 20 m. Increased gradually as found necessary.

FL. EXT. COOLWORT .... Dose 30 to 60 m.
Mitella nuda Linn.   **Nat. Ord.**—*Saxifragaceæ*.

Synonyms—Mitrewort, Gem fruit.

Range—New England to New York, Michigan, Minnesota and northward.

Habitat—Deep moist woods in moss.

Standard of strength—That of the U. S. Pharmacopœia, 1890; 1 c.c. representing 1 gram of the drug; or, practically, minim for grain.

Action and uses—Diuretic. Used in strangury.

FL. EXT. CORIANDER SEED .... Dose 30 to 60 m.
Coriandrum sativum Linn.   **Nat. Ord.**—*Umbelliferæ*.

Range—Mediterranean and Caucasian regions; cultivated.

Habitat—In cultivated ground as a weed.

Part used—The fruit.

Standard of strength—That of the U. S. Pharmacopœia, 1890; 1 c.c. representing 1 gram of the drug; or, practically, minim for grain.

Action and uses—Aromatic and carminative.

PREPARATION.

Infusion Coriander Seed—Fl. ext. Coriander seed, Lilly, 2 fl. ozs.; Hot water, 14 fl. ozs.; Mix—Dose ½ to 1 fl. oz.

FL. EXT. CORN SILK, from green silk .... DOse 60 to 120 m.
Zea Mays Linn.   **Nat. Ord.**—*Gramineæ*.

Synonyms—Silk of Indian corn, Zea.

Range—Tropical and Temperate America; cultivated.

Part used—The styles and stigmas.

Standard of strength—That of the U. S. Pharmacopœia, 1890; 1 c.c. representing 1 gram of the drug; or, practically, minim for grain.

Action and uses—Demulcent, diuretic and anodyne. Recommended in treatment of diseases of the bladder and kidneys and irritation of urine. A certain but mild diuretic when given in full doses at short intervals. Beneficial in vesical catarrh, dysuria, cystitis and uric lithiasis, producing discharges of small calculi. In cases of decomposition of mucoid secretions, accompanied with ammoniacal odor it is especially useful.

PREPARATION.

Syrup Corn Silk—Fl. ext. Corn silk, Lilly, 6 fl. ozs.; Syrup, 10 fl. ozs.; Mix—Dose 2 to 4 fl. drs.

FL. EXT. COTO BARK .... Dose 5 to 20 m.
Para Coto. **Nat. Ord.**—*Probably Laurineæ or Anacardiaceæ*.

NOTE—COTO and PARA COTO are two distinct kinds of Bolivian barks, the botanical origin of which is not known. Their therapeutic properties are similar, and as PARA COTO is generally preferred it is invariably supplied when COTO bark is ordered.

Range—Bolivia.

Part used—The bark.

Standard of strength—That of the U. S. Pharmacopœia, 1890; 1 c.c. representing 1 gram of the drug; or, practically, minim for grain.

Action and uses—Astringent. Said to be a specific for diarrhœa and is recommended in the treatment of dysentery, colic, cholera, cholera morbus, gastric catarrh, night sweats, rheumatism and gout. For internal use it should be diluted with water or disguised in some pleasant vehicle.

FL. EXT. COTTON ROOT BARK, U. S. .... Dose 30 to 60 m.
Gossypium herbaceum Linn. *and other species of Gossypium.*
Nat. Ord.—*Malvaceæ.*

Range—Tropical Asia and Africa; cultivated in the Southern United States.

Part used—The bark of the root.

Standard of strength—That of the U. S. Pharmacopœia, 1890; 1 c.c. representing 1 gram of the drug; or, practically, minim for grain.

Action and uses—Emmenagogue and oxytocic. It appears to act very much like ergot on the uterus and is particularly valuable in dysmenorrhœa and scanty menstruation and especially in suppressed menstruation produced by cold.

PREPARATION.

Infusion Cotton Root Bark—Fl. ext. Cotton root bark, Lilly, 2 fl. ozs.; Hot water, 14 fl. ozs.; Mix—Dose ½ to 1 fl. oz.

FL. EXT. COTTON ROOT BARK, green .... Dose 30 to 60 m.
Gossypium herbaceum Linn., *and other species of Gossypium.*
Nat. Ord.—*Malvaceæ.*

Range—Tropical Asia and Africa; cultivated in the Southern United States.

Part used—The fresh bark of the root. Supposed by some to be more active than the U. S. preparation.

Standard of strength—That of the U. S. Pharmacopœia, 1890; 1 c.c. representing 1 gram of the drug; or, practically, minim for grain.

Action and uses—Emmenagogue and oxytocic. It appears to act very much like ergot on the uterus and is particularly valuable in dysmenorrhœa and scanty menstruation and especially in suppressed menstruation produced by cold.

PREPARATION.

Infusion Cotton Root Bark, green—Fl. ext. Cotton root bark, green, Lilly, 2 fl. ozs.; Hot water, 14 fl. ozs.; Mix—Dose ½ to 1 fl. oz.

FL. EXT. COUCH GRASS, U. S. .... Dose 3 to 6 fl. drs.
Agropyrum repens (Linn.) Beauvois. **Nat. Ord.**—*Gramineæ.*

Synonyms—*Triticum repens* Linn.,—Triticum, U. S.,—Doggrass, Knotgrass, Quickens.

Range—Europe and America.

Habitat—In cultivated fields and in sandy soil and along lakes and water courses.

Part used—The rhizome.

Standard of strength—That of the U. S. Pharmacopœia, 1890; 1 c.c. representing 1 gram of the drug; or, practically, minim for grain.

Action and uses—Diuretic and slightly aperient. Used principally in irritation of the bladder and urinary passages.

PREPARATION.

Infusion Couch Grass—Fl. ext. Couch grass, Lilly, 2 fl. ozs.; Hot water, 14 fl. ozs.; Mix—Dose 2 to 6 fl. ozs.

FL. EXT. CRAMP BARK, U. S. .... Dose 30 to 60 m.
Viburnum Opulus Linn. **Nat. Ord.**—*Caprifoliaceæ.*

Synonyms—High cranberry, Squawbush.

Range—New Brunswick and far westward, south to Pennsylvania.

Habitat—Low grounds along streams.

Part used—The bark.

Standard of strength—That of the U. S. Pharmacopœia, 1890; 1 c.c. representing 1 gram of the drug; or, practically, minim for grain.

Action and uses—A powerful antispasmodic. Effective in relaxing cramps of all kinds as in asthma, hysteria, cramps of the limbs and other parts especially in pregnant women.

PREPARATION.

Infusion Cramp Bark—Fl. ext. Cramp bark, Lilly, 2 fl. ozs.; Hot water, 14 fl. ozs.; Mix—Dose ½ to 1 fl. oz. or, may be used as a gargle.

FL. EXT. CRANESBILL, U. S. ....**Dose 30 to 60 m.**
Geranium maculatum Linn.   **Nat. Ord.**—*Geraniaceæ.*
Synonyms—Geranium, U. S.,—Astringent root, Crowfoot.
Range—Common throughout the United States.
Habitat—Moist woods, thickets, low grounds.
Part used—The rhizome.
Standard of strength—That of the U. S. Pharmacopœia, 1890; 1 c.c.
representing 1 gram of the drug; or, practically, minim for grain.
Action and uses—A powerful astringent, pleasant to the taste. Used
in second stages of dysentery, diarrhea and cholera infantum; in infu-
sion, both internally and externally, whenever astringents are indicated:
as a gargle in sore throat, hemorrhages, troublesome epistaxis, bleeding
from small wounds; as an injection in leucorrhea, gleet, etc.

PREPARATIONS.

Tincture Cranesbill—Fl. ext. Cranesbill, Lilly, 2 fl. ozs.; Diluted
alcohol, 14 fl. ozs.; Mix—Dose 2 to 4 fl. drs.

Infusion Cranesbill—Fl. ext. Cranesbill, Lilly, 2 fl. ozs.; Hot water,
14 fl. ozs.; Mix—Dose ½ to 1 fl. oz.

FL. EXT. CRAWLEY ROOT ....**Dose 15 to 30 m.**
Corallorhiza odontorhiza (Willd.) Nutt. **Nat. Ord.**—*Orchidaceæ.*
Synonyms—Cymbidium Odontorhizon Willd.,—Chickentoe, Coralroot.
Range—Eastern Massachusetts and Vermont to Florida, west to Michi-
gan and Missouri.
Habitat—Rich woods.
Part used—The rootstock.
Standard of strength—That of the U. S. Pharmacopœia, 1890; 1 c.c.
representing 1 gram of the drug; or, practically, minim for grain.
Action and uses—Diaphoretic, sudorific, sedative and febrifuge.

FL. EXT. CUBEB, U. S. ....**Dose 10 to 40 m.**
Piper Cubeba Linn. f.   **Nat. Ord.**—*Piperaceæ.*
Synonyms—Cubeba officinalis Miquel.
Range—Java; cultivated.
Habitat—Chiefly cultivated in coffee plantations.
Part used—The unripe fruit.
Standard of strength—That of the U. S. Pharmacopœia, 1890; 1 c.c.
representing 1 gram of the drug; or, practically, minim for grain.
Action and uses—Stimulant with special direction to the urinary
organs. A most valuable remedy in acute gonorrhea.

PREPARATION.

Tincture Cubeb, U. S.—Fl. ext. Cubeb, Lilly, 3¼ fl. ozs.; Alcohol,
12¾ fl. ozs.; Mix—Dose 1 to 2 fl. drs.

FL. EXT. CUCUMBER TREE BARK ....**Dose 30 to 60 m.**
Magnolia acuminata Linn.   **Nat. Ord.**—*Magnoliaceæ.*
Synonyms—M. Virginiana var. acuminata L.
Range—Western New York to Illinois and southward.
Habitat—Rich woodlands.
Part used—The bark.
Standard of strength—That of the U. S. Pharmacopœia, 1890; 1 c.c.
representing 1 gram of the drug; or, practically, minim for grain.
Action and uses—Bitter tonic and aromatic. Used principally in
hot decoction to produce diaphoresis in fevers, bronchial catarrh, rheu-
matism and gout and for the cure of intermittent fevers.

FL. EXT. CULVER'S ROOT, U. S............ ....**Dose 20 to 60 m.**
Leptandra Virginica (Linn.) Nutt. **Nat. Ord.—***Scrophulariaceæ.*
Synonyms—Veronica Virginica Linn.—Leptandra, U. S.,—Culver's physic, Black root.
Range—Vermont to Minnesota and southward.
Habitat—Rich woodlands.
Part used—The rhizome and roots.
Standard of strength—That of the U. S. Pharmacopœia, 1890; 1 c.c. representing 1 gram of the drug; or, practically, minim for grain.
Action and uses—Laxative, cholagogue and tonic. Employed successfully in all hepatic affections, causing the liver to act with great energy without active cathasis. It is an excellent laxative in all febrile diseases, peculiarly applicable to typhoid and bilious fevers.

PREPARATIONS.

Tincture Culver's Root—Fl. ext. Culver's root, Lilly, 2 fl. ozs.; Alcohol, 10½ fl. ozs.; Water, 3½ fl. ozs.; Mix—Dose 3 to 6 fl. drs.

Syrup Culver's Root—Fl. ext. Culver's root, Lilly, 4 fl. ozs.; Syrup, 12 fl. ozs.; Mix—Dose 1 to 4 fl. drs.

FL. EXT. DAMIANA................................**Dose 30 to 60 m.**
Turnera diffusa Willd. *var. aphrodisiaca* (Ward) Urban.
                                      Nat. Ord.—*Turneraceæ.*
Synonyms—T. aphrodisiaca Ward.
Range—Mexico and Lower California.
Part used—The leaves.
Standard of strength That of the U. S. Pharmacopœia, 1890; 1 c.c. representing 1 gram of the drug; or, practically, minim for grain.
Action and uses—Damiana increases peristalsis and is effective in constipation of neurotic subjects, especially those whose sexual powers are at low ebb. Increased diuresis follows its use and cases of irritable bladder and urethra are greatly benefited. It is also a tonic sedative to the heart. It is therefore plain why Damiana is so useful in cases of nerve exhaustion resulting from sexual excesses and why, far from being a direct stimulant of erotic desires, it has been found to act as a sedative to abnormal sexual appetite. Everything depends however on the use of the true *Turnera diffusa var. aphrodisiaca* every lot of which is inspected and identified in our botanical department, which amongst botanists everywhere is regarded special authority on this drug. It is the principal ingredient in Pil. Aphrodisiaca, (Lilly,) a most effective remedy. Send for booklet "Demonstration of the true Damiana" to Eli Lilly & Company.

FL. EXT. DANDELION, U. S.......................**Dose 60 to 180 m.**
Taraxacum officinale Weber   **Nat. Ord.—***Compositæ.*
Synonyms—T. Taraxacum (L.) Karst., T. Dens-leonis Desf.
Range—Europe; naturalized in North America.
Habitat—Grassy places near roadsides, etc.
Part used—The root.
Standard of strength—That of the U. S. Pharmacopœia, 1890; 1 c.c. representing 1 gram of the drug; or, practically, minim for grain.
Action and uses—Tonic, diuretic, aperient and alterative. Of special value in torpor and chronic engorgement of the liver.

PREPARATION.

Infusion Dandelion—Fl. ext. Dandelion, Lilly, 2 fl. ozs.; Hot water, 14 fl. ozs.; Mix—Dose 1 to 3 fl. ozs.

FL. EXT. DANDELION COMP......... ....**Dose 30 to 60 m.**
Standard of strength One pint represents Dandelion, 8 troy ounces; Pipsissewa, 4 troy ounces; Uva ursi, Angelica root, of each, 2 troy ounces.
Action and uses—An excellent tonic and diuretic.

PREPARATION.

Syrup Dandelion Comp.—Fl. ext. Dandelion comp., Lilly, 6 fl. ozs.; Syrup, 10 fl. ozs.; Mix—Dose 2 to 4 fl. drs.

FL. EXT. DANDELION AND SENNA..............**Dose 60 to 120 m.**

Standard of strength—One pint represents Dandelion and Senna, of each, 8 troy ounces.

Action and uses—Tonic and laxative.

PREPARATION.

Syrup Dandelion and Senna—Fl. ext. Dandelion and Senna, Lilly, 4 fl. ozs.; Syrup, 12 fl. ozs.; Mix—Dose ½ to 1 fl. oz.

FL. EXT. DIGITALIS, U. S..........................**Dose 1 to 2 m.**

Digitalis purpurea Linn.　　　　**Nat. Ord.**—*Scrophulariaceæ.*

Synonym—Foxglove.

Range—Europe, temperate zone; cultivated in Europe and the United States.

Habitat—In sandy soil along the borders of thickets and woods.

Part used—The leaves.

Standard of Strength—100 c.c. contain 25 gm. extractive.

Action and uses—IRRITANT POISON. Valuable in palpitation and irregular action of the heart, whether depending on organic disease or not. In mitral disease, when the cardiac action is feeble, when lividity and dropsy are setting in, the lungs becoming engorged and the right heart oppressed, here it does good service in small doses, combined with a little iron; it is also considered the best remedy for aneurism, given in increasing doses.

Antidotes—Strong emetics followed by stimulants internally and externally. Tannic acid is the chemical antidote but the tannate is not inert and the stomach should be evacuated. Aconite is the best antagonist to large doses and opium in cases of its long continued use. Cinchona and iron sulphate decompose the active principles of digitalis.

PREPARATIONS.

Tincture Digitalis, U. S.—Fl. ext. Digitalis, Lilly, 2½ fl. ozs.; Alcohol, 9½ fl. ozs.; Water, 4½ fl. ozs.; Mix—Dose 5 to 10 m.

Infusion Digitalis, U. S.—Fl. ext. Digitalis, Lilly, 2 fl. drs.; Cinnamon water, 2½ fl. ozs.; Alcohol, 12 fl. drs.; Water, q.s. to make 16 fl. ozs.; Mix the fluid extract, cinnamon water and water and add the alcohol—Dose 2 to 4 fl. drs.

FL. EXT. DILL................................**Dose 15 to 60 m.**

Anethum graveolens Linn.　　　　**Nat. Ord.**—*Umbelliferæ.*

Synonyms—Peucedanum graveolens Hiern.,—Dill fruit, Garden dill, Dilly.

Range—Levant and Southern Europe; cultivated.

Part used—The fruit.

Standard of strength—That of the U. S. Pharmacopœia, 1890; 1 c.c. representing 1 gram of the drug; or, practically, minim for grain.

Action and uses—Aromatic, stimulant and carminative. Used in flatulent colic and hiccough.

PREPARATION.

Infusion Dill—Fl. ext. Dill, Lilly, ½ fl. oz.; Hot water, 15½ fl. ozs.; Mix—Dose ½ to 1 fl. oz.

FL. EXT. DITA BARK........................**Dose 5 to 10 m.**

Alstonia scholaris (Linn.) R. Brown.　　　**Nat. Ord.**—*Apocynaceæ.*

Synonyms—Echites scholaris Linn.

Range—India, East Indian Islands, Queensland and in Western Tropical Africa.

Part used—The bark.

Standard of strength—That of the U. S. Pharmacopœia, 1890; 1 c.c. representing 1 gram of the drug; or, practically, minim for grain.

Action and uses—Said to be used successfully in malarial fevers.

FL. EXT. DOGWOOD ....Dose 30 to 60 m.

Cornus florida Linn. **Nat. Ord.—*Cornaceæ*.**

Synonym—Boxwood.

Range—Southern New England **to Ontario and Southern Minnesota,** south to Florida and Texas.

Habitat—Dry woodlands.

Part used—The bark of the root.

Standard **of strength**—That of the U. S. Pharmacopœia, 1890; 1 c.c. representing 1 gram of the drug; or, practically, minim for grain.

Action and uses—Tonic, astringent, antiperiodic. Considered by some a valuable substitute for cinchona.

PREPARATIONS.

Tincture Dogwood—Fl. ext. Dogwood, Lilly, 4 fl. ozs.; Diluted alcohol, 12 fl. ozs.; Mix—Dose 2 to 4 fl. drs.

Wine Dogwood—Fl. ext. Dogwood, Lilly, 4 fl. ozs.; Stronger white wine, 12 fl. ozs.; Mix—Dose 2 to 4 fl. drs.

FL. EXT. DUBOISIA LEAVES ....Dose 1 to 3 m.

Duboisia myoporoides R. Brown. **Nat. Ord.—*Solanaceæ*.**

Range—Australia.

Habitat—Deep forest glens.

Part used—The leaves.

Standard of strength—That of the U. S. Pharmacopœia, 1890; 1 c.c. representing 1 gram of the drug; or, practically, minim for grain.

Action and uses—Therapeutically allied to belladonna and **often** substituted in eye practice for the same. Said to dilate the pupil **more** promptly than belladonna and the effect passes off more quickly.

FL. EXT. DWARF ELDER................. ....Dose 60 to 120 m.

Aralia hispida Vent. **Nat. Ord.—*Araliaceæ*.**

Synonym—Brittlestem.

Range—Newfoundland to Dakota, south to the mountains of North Carolina.

Habitat—Rocky and sandy places.

Part used—The root.

Standard of strength--That of the U. S. Pharmacopœia, 1890; 1 c.c. representing 1 gram of the drug; or, practically, minim for grain.

Action and uses—Diuretic and alterative. Very valuable in dropsy, gravel, suppression and other urinary disorders.

PREPARATION.

Infusion Dwarf Elder—Fl. ext. Dwarf elder, Lilly, 2 fl. ozs.; Hot water, 14 fl. ozs.; Mix—Dose 1 to 2 fl. ozs.

FL. EXT. ELDER FLOWERS .... Dose 60 to 120 m.

Sambucus **Canadensis** Linn. **Nat. Ord.—*Caprifoliaceæ*.**

Synonym—Common elder.

Range—Common in the United States east of the Rocky Mountains.

Habitat—Rich soil in open places.

Part used—The flowers.

Standard of strength—That of the U. S. Pharmacopœia, 1890; 1 c.c representing 1 gram of the drug; or, practically, minim for grain.

Action and uses—Diaphoretic, diuretic **and stimulant.** Used in erysipelas, fevers and constipation.

PREPARATIONS.

Syrup Elder Flowers—Fl. ext. Elder flowers, Lilly, 4 fl. ozs.; Syrup, 12 fl. ozs.; Mix—Dose ½ to 1 fl. oz.

Infusion Elder Flowers—Fl. ext. Elder flowers, Lilly, 2 fl. ozs.; Hot water, 14 fl. ozs.; Mix—Dose 1 to 2 fl. ozs.

FL. EXT. ELECAMPANE..................................**Dose 30 to 60 m.**
Inula Helenium Linn.　　　　　　**Nat. Ord.—*Compositæ.***

Range—Europe, Central Asia; introduced into the United States; common; cultivated.

Habitat—Roadsides and damp pastures.

Part used—The root.

Standard of strength—That of the U. S. Pharmacopœia, 1890; 1 c.c. representing 1 gram of the drug; or, practically, minim for grain.

Action and uses—Tonic and gently stimulant, diuretic and diaphoretic, expectorant and emmenagogue.

PREPARATIONS.

Syrup Elecampane—Fl. ext. Elecampane, Lilly, 4 fl. ozs.; Syrup, 12 fl. ozs.; Mix—Dose 2 to 4 fl. drs.

Infusion Elecampane—Fl. ext. Elecampane, Lilly, 2 fl. ozs.; Hot water, 14 fl. ozs.; Mix—Dose ½ to 1 fl. oz.

FL. EXT. EQUISETUM HYEMALE................**Dose 30 to 60 m.**
Equisetum hyemale Linn.　　　　　**Nat. Ord.—*Equisetaceæ.***

Synonym—Scouring rush.

Range—Europe; common in the Northern United States.

Habitat—Wet banks, along streams, marshes and lakes.

Part used—The stems.

Standard of strength—That of the U. S. Pharmacopœia, 1890; 1 c.c. representing 1 gram of the drug; or, practically, minim for grain.

Action and uses—Employed in dropsy, calculus affections, hematuria, nocturnal incontinence of urine, diabetes insipidus, hemoptysis, diarrhœa and dysentery. Also as an emmenagogue. It should not be given in feverish conditions as it is liable to render the urine bloody.

PREPARATION.

Infusion Equisetum Hyemale—Fl. ext. Equisetum hyemale, Lilly, 1 fl. oz.; Hot water, 15 fl. ozs.; Mix—Dose 1 to 2 fl. ozs.

FL. EXT. ERGOT....................................**Dose 30 to 240 m.**
Claviceps purpurea (Fries) Tulasne.　**Nat. Ord.—*Pyrenomycetes.***

Synonyms—Cordiceps purpurea Fries, Sclerotium Clavus D. C.

Range—Common in rye fields; supply chiefly from Germany, Russia and Spain.

Habitat—In the head of rye, replacing the grain.

Part used—The sclerotium.

Standard of strength—10 c.c. mixed with 90 c.c. of 95 per cent. alcohol yields a precipitate which, when separated and dried, weighs 0.4 gram.

Note—In making this important preparation the utmost care and judgment are used in every particular. The best quality of drug of the most recent crop is procured, and subjected to a cold process that perfectly exhausts the drug. The fixed oil so abundant and objectionable is not present in this preparation, which will be found entirely free from fishy or ammoniacal odor so obnoxious to patients, and which, when present, indicates decomposition of the active constituents.

Action and uses—Uterine motor stimulant and hemostatic. Aids parturition, controls internal hemorrhage, relieves local congestion and produces absorption of morbid growth.

PREPARATIONS.

Tincture Ergot—Fl. ext. Ergot, Lilly, 4 fl. ozs.; Diluted alcohol, 12 fl. ozs.; Mix—Dose 2 to 4 fl. drs.

Wine Ergot, U. S.—Fl. ext. Ergot, Lilly, 2½ fl. ozs.; Alcohol, 2 fl. ozs.; White wine, 11½ fl. ozs.; Mix—Dose for a woman in labor, 2 to 3 fl. drs., for other purposes, 1 to 4 fl. drs. repeated as required.

Infusion Ergot—Fl. ext. Ergot, Lilly, 1 fl. oz.; Hot water, 15 fl. ozs.; Mix—Dose 1 to 4 fl. ozs.

FL. EXT. ERGOT, **ETHEREAL** ....**Dose 30 to 240 m.**
Claviceps purpurea (Fries) Tulasne. **Nat. Ord.—** *Pyrenomycetes.*
Synonyms— Cordiceps purpurea Fries, Sclerotium Clavus D. C.
Range— Common in rye fields; supply chiefly from Germany, Russia and Spain.
Habitat— In the head of rye, replacing the grain.
Part used— The sclerotium.
Standard of strength— 10 c.c. mixed with 90 c.c. of 95 per cent. alcohol yields a precipitate which, when separated and dried, weighs 0.4 gram.
Note. In making this important preparation the utmost **care** and judgment are used in every particular. The best quality of drug of the most recent crop is procured, and subjected to a cold process that perfectly exhausts the drug. The fixed oil so abundant and objectionable is not present in this preparation, which will be found entirely free from fishy or ammoniacal odor so obnoxious to patients, and which, when present, indicates decomposition of the active constituents.
Action and uses— Uterine motor stimulant and hemostatic. Aids parturition, controls internal hemorrhage, relieves local congestion and produces absorption of morbid growth.

FL. EXT. EUCALYPTUS ....**Dose 10 to 60 m.**
Eucalyptus globulus Lab. **Nat. Ord.—** *Myrtaceæ.*
Synonym— Australian fever tree.
Range— Australia and Tasmania; cultivated in subtropical countries.
Habitat— Rich moist valleys and wooded slopes.
Part used— The leaves.
Standard of strength— That of the U. S. Pharmacopœia, 1890; 1 c.c. representing 1 gram of the drug; or, practically, minim for grain.
Action and uses— An excellent antiseptic, highly recommended as a dressing for wounds and ulcers. Reputed tonic, febrifuge and antiperiodic. Used also in bronchitis and asthma.

PREPARATIONS.

Tincture Eucalyptus— Fl. ext. Eucalyptus, Lilly, 4 fl. ozs.; Alcohol, 9 fl. ozs.; Water, 3 fl. ozs.; Mix—Dose 30 to 120 m.
Lotion Eucalyptus— Fl. ext. Eucalyptus, Lilly, 8 fl. ozs.; Water, 8 fl. ozs.; Glycerin, 4 fl. ozs.; Mix—To be applied to wounds and ulcers.

FL. EXT. EUPHORBIA PILULIFERA..... ....**Dose 30 to 60 m.**
Euphorbia pilulifera Linn. **Nat. Ord.—** *Euphorbiaceæ.*
Range— Florida to Mexico.
Part used— The herb.
Standard of strength— That of the U. S. Pharmacopœia, 1890; 1 c.c. representing 1 gram of the drug; **or**, practically, minim for grain.
Action and uses— Said to give prompt relief to sufferers from asthma.

FL. EXT. EUROPEAN ELDER ... .**Dose 60 to 120 m.**
Sambucus nigra Linn. **Nat. Ord.—** *Caprifoliaceæ.*
Range— Europe, Northern Africa and Southern Siberia.
Habitat— Hedges and woods; cultivated in gardens.
Part used— The flowers.
Standard of strength— That of the U. S. Pharmacopœia, 1890; 1 c.c. representing 1 gram of the drug; or, practically, minim for grain.
Action and uses— Hydragogue and cuactocathartic. Reputed valuable in epilepsy.

PREPARATION.

Infusion European Elder— Fl. ext. European elder, Lilly, 2 fl. ozs.; Hot water, 14 fl. ozs.; Mix—Dose ½ to 1 fl. oz.

WHEN ORDERING OR PRESCRIBING.

FL. EXT. EVENING PRIMROSE.... ....Dose 30 to 60 m.
Œnothera biennis Linn. **Nat. Ord.—***Onagraceæ.*

Synonyms—Onagra biennis (Linn., Scop.,—Tree primrose.
Range—Throughout the United States; naturalized in Europe.
Habitat—In fields, waste places, etc.
Part used—The herb.
Standard of strength—That of the U. S. Pharmacopœia, 1890; 1 c.c. representing 1 gram of the drug; or, practically, minim for grain.
Action and uses—Recommended as a nervine and in catarrhal affections of the respiratory and gastric mucous membranes.

FL. EXT. EYEBRIGHT................. ....Dose 10 to 20 m.
Euphrasia officinalis Linn. **Nat. Ord.—***Scrophulariaceæ.*
Synonym—E. latifolia Pursh.
Range—Europe; probably introduced into the United States; the coast of Maine and Lower Canada to the Rocky Mountains.
Part used—The leaves.
Standard of strength—That of the U. S. Pharmacopœia, 1890; 1 c.c. representing 1 gram of the drug; or, practically, minim for grain.
Action and uses—Tonic and astringent. Used with much benefit in catarrhal ophthalmia.

PREPARATION.

Infusion Eyebright—Fl. ext. Eyebright, Lilly, 2 fl. ozs.; Hot water, 14 fl. ozs.; Mix—Use as a lotion and internally in doses of ½ to 1 fl. oz.

FL. EXT. FALSE BITTERSWEET....... ....Dose 30 to 60 m.
Celastrus scandens Linn. **Nat. Ord.—***Celastraceæ.*
Synonyms—Staffvine, Climbing bittersweet.
Range—New England, Quebec, Manitoba, south to North Carolina and Kansas.
Habitat—Along streams and in thickets; climbing.
Part used—The bark.
Standard of strength—That of the U. S. Pharmacopœia, 1890; 1 c.c. representing 1 gram of the drug; or, practically, minim for grain.
Action and uses—Alterative, diuretic and diaphoretic. Used in syphilis, scrofula, leucorrhea and obstruction of the menses.

PREPARATIONS.

Tincture False Bittersweet—Fl. ext. False bittersweet, Lilly, 4 fl. ozs.; Alcohol, 5 fl. ozs.; Water, 7 fl. ozs.; Mix the alcohol and water and add the fluid extract—Dose 1 to 4 fl. drs.

Infusion False Bittersweet—Fl. ext. False bittersweet, Lilly, 1 fl. oz.; Hot water, 15 fl. ozs.; Mix—Dose 1 to 2 fl. ozs.

FL. EXT. FALSE GROMWELL.... ....Dose 15 to 30 m.
Onosmodium Virginianum (Linn.) D. C.
Nat. Ord.—*Boraginaceæ.*
Synonyms—Lithospermum Virginianum Linn.,—Corn gromwell, Job's tears.
Range—New England to Florida, Missouri and Louisiana.
Habitat—Banks and hillsides.
Standard of strength—That of the U. S. Pharmacopœia, 1890; 1 c.c. representing 1 gram of the drug; or, practically, minim for grain.
Action and uses—Diuretic and tonic.

FL. EXT. FALSE UNICORN ROOT ....**Dose 20 to 40 m.**
Chamælirium luteum (Linn.) Gray.   **Nat. Ord.—***Liliaceæ.*

Synonyms—C. Carolinianum Willd., Veratrum luteum Linn., Helonias dioica Pursh.,—Devilsbit, Starwort.

Range—New England to Georgia, west to Nebraska and Arkansas.

Habitat—Low grounds.

Part used—The rhizome.

Standard of strength—That of the U. S. Pharmacopœia, 1890; 1 c.c. representing 1 gram of the drug; or, practically, minim for grain.

Action and uses—Tonic, diuretic and vermifuge; in large doses emetic. In doses of from 10 to 15 minims of the fluid extract, repeated three or four times a day, it has been found beneficial in dyspepsia, loss of appetite and for the removal of worms. Beneficial in nocturnal emissions, the result of excesses. In diseases of the reproductive organs of females, and especially of the uterus, it is one of our most valuable agents, acting as a uterine tonic, and gradually removing abnormal conditions, while at the same time imparts tone and vigor.

PREPARATION.

Syrup False Unicorn Root—Fl. ext. False unicorn root, Lilly, 4 fl. ozs.; Syrup, 12 fl. ozs.; Mix—Dose 1 to 3 fl. drs.

FL. EXT. FENNEL SEED ....**Dose 10 to 30 m.**
Fœniculum capillaceum Gilibert.   **Nat. Ord.—***Umbelliferæ.*

Synonyms—F. vulgare Gærtn., F. Fœniculum (Linn.) Karst.

Range—Levant and Southern Europe; cultivated.

Habitat—Sandy and chalky ground.

Part used—The fruit.

Standard of strength—That of the U. S. Pharmacopœia, 1890; 1 c.c. representing 1 gram of the drug; or, practically, minim for grain.

Action and uses—Stimulant, carminative and stomachic. Used also as an adjuvant.

PREPARATION.

Infusion Fennel Seed—Fl. ext. Fennel seed, Lilly, 1 fl. oz.; Hot water, 14 fl. ozs.; Mix—Dose ½ to 1 fl. oz.

FL. EXT. FEVERBUSH BARK ... .**Dose 30 to 60 m.**
Benzoin odoriferum Nees.   **Nat. Ord.—***Laurineæ.*

Synonyms—B. Benzoin (Linn.) Coulter, Laurus Benzoin Linn., Lindera Benzoin Blume.,—Spicebush, Spicewood.

Range—Canada, southward to Florida; common.

Habitat—Moist soil, along the banks of streams.

Part used—The bark and young twigs.

Standard of strength—That of the U. S. Pharmacopœia, 1890; 1 c.c. representing 1 gram of the drug; or, practically, minim for grain.

Action and uses—Stimulant and diaphoretic.

FL. EXT. FEVERBUSH BERRIES ... .Dose 30 to 60 m.
Benzoin odoriferum Nees.   Nat. Ord.—*Laurineæ.*

Synonyms—B. Benzoin (Linn.) Coulter, Laurus Benzoin Linn., Lindera Benzoin Blume.,—Spicebush, Spicewood.

Range—Canada, southward to Florida.

Habitat—Moist soil, along the banks of streams.

Part used—The fruit—a drupe.

Standard of strength—That of the U. S. Pharmacopœia, 1890; 1 c.c. representing 1 gram of the drug; or, practically, minim for grain.

Action and uses—Aromatic, tonic and stimulant. The infusion has been successfully used in the treatment of ague and typhoid forms of fever and as an anthelmintic.

PREPARATIONS.

Syrup Feverbush Berries—Fl. ext. Feverbush berries, Lilly, 4 fl. ozs.; Syrup, 12 fl. ozs.; Mix—Dose 2 to 4 fl. drs.

Infusion Feverbush Berries—Fl. ext. Feverbush berries, Lilly, 2 fl. ozs.; Hot water, 14 fl. ozs.; Mix—Dose ½ to 1 fl. oz.

FL. EXT. FEVERFEW..................................Dose 60 to 120 m.
Chrysanthemum Parthenium (Linn.) Pers.

Nat. Ord.—*Compositæ*.

Synonyms—Matricaria Parthenium Linn., Leucanthemum Parthenium Godron.
Range—Europe; naturalized in the United States; cultivated.
Habitat—Escaped from gardens, along roadsides, etc.
Part used—The herb.
Standard of strength—That of the U. S. Pharmacopœia, 1890; 1 c.c. representing 1 gram of the drug; or, practically, minim for grain.
Action and uses—Tonic, carminative, emmenagogue, vermifuge and **stimulant.** The warm infusion is used to revent cold, flatulency, irregular menstruation, hysteria, suppression of urine, etc.

PREPARATION.

Infusion Feverfew—Fl. ext. Feverfew, Lilly, 2 fl. ozs.; Hot water, 14 fl. ozs.; Mix—Dose 1 to 2 fl. ozs.

FL. EXT. FEVERROOT ....Dose 15 to 30 m.
Triosteum perfoliatum Linn. Nat. Ord.—*Caprifoliaceæ*.

Synonyms—Horse gentian, Tinkerweed.
Range—Canada and New England to Minnesota, Iowa and Alabama.
Habitat—Rich woodlands.
Part used—The rhizome and rootlets.
Standard of strength—That of the U. S. Pharmacopœia, 1890; 1 c.c. representing 1 gram of the drug; or, practically, minim for grain.
Action and **uses**—Laxative and tonic, in large doses emetic.

PREPARATION.

Tincture Feverroot—Fl. ext. Feverroot, Lilly, 2 fl. ozs.; Alcohol, 5 fl. ozs.; Water, 9 fl. ozs.; Mix—Dose 1 to 4 fl. drs.

FL. EXT. FIVEFLOWERED GENTIAN ....Dose 10 to 30 m.
Gentiana quinquefolia Linn. Nat. Ord.—*Gentianaceæ*.

Synonyms—G. quinqueflora Lam.,—Gallweed.
Range—Maine to Ontario, Illinois and south along the mountains to Florida.
Habitat—Moist hills and boggy knolls.
Part used—The herb.
Standard of strength—That of the U. S. Pharmacopœia, 1890; 1 c.c. representing 1 gram of the drug; or, practically, minim for grain.
Action and uses—Tonic and antiperiodic. Recommended as a substitute for quinine in the treatment of fever and ague. It is not contraindicated, and may be used to advantage at any time during the fever. The fluid extract should be diluted before taking, and the dose repeated at intervals of from **one** to three hours, as the **urgency** of the **case** demands.

PREPARATION.

Syrup Fiveflowered Gentian—Fl. ext. Fiveflowered gentian, Lilly, 4 fl. ozs.; Syrup, 12 fl. ozs.; Mix—Dose ½ to 2 fl. drs.

FL. EXT. FLEABANE...................................Dose 30 to 60 m.
Erigeron Canadensis Linn. Nat. Ord.—*Compositæ*.

Synonym—Canada fleabane.
Range—North America; widely distributed over the world.
Habitat—Waste places, especially near cultivated ground.
Part used—The herb.
Standard of strength—That of the U. S. Pharmacopœia, 1890; 1 c.c. representing 1 gram of the drug; or, practically, minim for grain.
Action and uses—Astringent, tonic, diuretic and stimulant. Successfully used in the treatment of dropsies and of **various diseases of the** urinary organs.

PREPARATION.

Infusion Fleabane—Fl. ext. Fleabane, Lilly, 1 fl. oz.; Hot water, 15 fl. ozs.; Mix—Dose 1 to 2 fl. ozs.

FL. EXT. FLORIDA ALLSPICE.................................Dose 30 to 60 m.
Calycanthus floridus Linn.　　　　**Nat. Ord.—**_Calycanthaceæ._
Synonyms—Butneria florida (Linn.) Kearney,—Calycanthus, Carolina allspice, Sweetscented shrub.
Range—Virginia and southward, cultivated in gardens.
Habitat—On hillsides in rich soil.
Part used—The bark.
Standard of strength—That of the U. S. Pharmacopœia, 1890; 1 c.c. representing 1 gram of the drug; or, practically, minim for grain.
Action and uses—Aromatic and stimulant.

FL. EXT. FRINGETREE BARK..........................Dose 30 to 60 m.
Chionanthus Virginica Linn.　　　　**Nat. Ord.—**_Oleaceæ._
Synonym—Old man's beard.
Range—New Jersey and South Pennsylvania to Florida, Texas and Missouri, cultivated as an ornamental tree.
Habitat—River banks.
Part used—The bark of the root.
Standard of strength—That of the U. S. Pharmacopœia, 1890; 1 c.c. representing 1 gram of the drug; or, practically, minim for grain.
Action and uses—Aperient, alterative, tonic and febrifuge.

PREPARATIONS.

Tincture Fringetree Bark—Fl. ext. Fringetree bark, Lilly, 4 fl. ozs.; Diluted alcohol, 12 fl. ozs.; Mix—Dose 2 to 4 fl. drs.

Infusion Fringetree Bark—Fl. ext. Fringetree bark, Lilly, 1 fl. oz.; Hot water, 15 fl. ozs.; Mix—Dose 1 to 2 fl. ozs.

FL. EXT. FROSTWORT....................................Dose 60 to 120 m.
Helianthemum Canadense (Linn.) Michx.　**Nat. Ord.—**_Cistaceæ._
Synonyms—Cistus canadensis Linn.,—Rock rose.
Range—Maine to Minnesota and southward.
Habitat—Sandy or gravelly dry soil.
Part used—The herb.
Standard of strength—That of the U. S. Pharmacopœia, 1890; 1 c.c. representing 1 gram of the drug; or, practically, minim for grain.
Action and uses—Alterative and tonic. A valuable remedy in scrofula, syphilis, cancerous affections and as a gargle in scarlet fever.

PREPARATION.

Infusion Frostwort—Fl. ext. Frostwort, Lilly, 2 fl. ozs.; Hot water, 14 fl. ozs.; Mix—Dose 1 to 2 fl. ozs.

FL. EXT. GALANGAL....................................Dose 10 to 30 m.
Alpina officinarum Hance.　　　　**Nat. Ord.—**_Scitamineæ._
Synonyms—Catarrh root, Bombay root.
Range—China; near the coast.
Part used—The rhizome.
Standard of strength—That of the U. S. Pharmacopœia, 1890; 1 c.c. representing 1 gram of the drug; or, practically, minim for grain.
Action and uses—Aromatic, stimulant and stomachic.

FL. EXT. GALLS .... **Dose** 10 to 30 m.

An excrescence on the young branches of the gall oak, QUERCUS LUSI-TANICA Lam. (nat. ord.—CUPULIFERÆ) made by the sting of the gall fly, CYNIPS GALLÆ TINCTORIA Oliver (class—INSECTA; nat. ord.—HYMEN-OPTERA.)

Synonyms—Q. lusitanica Webb, var. infectoria D. C., Q. infectoria Oliver,—Dyer's oak, Nutgalls.

Range—Western Asia.

Standard of strength—That of the U. S. Pharmacopœia, 1890; 1 c.c. representing 1 gram of the drug; or, practically, minim for grain.

Action and uses—Powerful astringent.

PREPARATIONS.

Tincture Galls, U. S.—Fl. ext. Galls, Lilly, 3½ fl. ozs.; Alcohol, 3½ fl. ozs.; Glycerin, 1¼ fl. ozs.; Water, 3 fl. ozs.; Mix—Dose ½ to 2 fl. drs.

Ointment Galls—Fl. ext. Galls, Lilly, 1 fl. oz.; Lard, 7 troy ozs.; Mix and heat until the alcohol is driven off and stir till cold.

Infusion Galls—Fl. ext. Galls, Lilly, 1 fl. oz.; Hot water, 15 fl. ozs.; Mix—Dose ¼ to 1 fl. oz.

FL. EXT. GARDEN CELANDINE.............. .... **Dose** 30 to 60 m.

Chelidonium majus Linn.   **Nat. Ord.**—*Papaveraceæ.*

Synonym—Tetterwort.

Range—Europe; naturalized in North America.

Habitat—Waste and uncultivated grounds.

Part used—The herb.

Standard of strength—That of the U. S. Pharmacopœia, 1890; 1 c.c. representing 1 gram of the drug; or, practically, minim for grain.

Action and uses—Purgative, diuretic and diaphoretic. Used in scrofula, cutaneous diseases and affections of the spleen. Reputed especially valuable in jaundice.

PREPARATIONS.

Tincture Garden Celandine—Fl. ext. Garden celandine, Lilly, 4 fl. ozs.; Diluted alcohol, 12 fl. ozs.; Mix—Dose 2 to 4 fl. drs.

Infusion Garden Celandine—Fl. ext. Garden celandine, Lilly, 1 fl. oz.; Hot water, 15 fl. ozs.; Mix—Dose 1 to 2 fl. ozs.

FL. EXT. GARLIC..................... .... **Dose** 15 to 30 m.

Allium sativum Linn.   **Nat. Ord.**—*Liliaceæ.*

Synonym—Clove garlic.

Range—Sicily, Italy, Southern France; cultivated.

Habitat—Semi-wild on the edges of desert places.

Part used—The bulb.

Standard of strength—That of the U. S. Pharmacopœia, 1890; 1 c.c. representing 1 gram of the drug; or, practically, minim for grain.

Action and uses—Stimulant, diuretic and diaphoretic. Used also as a vermifuge.

FL. EXT. GELSEMIUM, U. S........... .... **Dose** 5 to 10 m.

Gelsemium sempervirens (Linn.) Aiton. **Nat. Ord.**—*Loganaceæ.*

Synonyms—G. nitidum Michx., Bignonia sempervirens Linn.,—Yellow jessamine, Wild jessamine, Woodbine.

Range—Eastern Virginia to Florida and Texas.

Habitat—Low grounds, swamps.

Part used—The root.

Standard of Strength—0.5 per cent. of total alkaloids, estimated gravimetrically.

Action and uses—POISONOUS. A powerful motordepressant, antispasmodic and diaphoretic. It is indicated in all conditions of exalted nerve function and contraindicated whenever there is a weak heart. Its especial field is in remittent and typhomalarial fevers and cerebrospinal meningitis. Valuable in insomnia, delirium tremens, spasmodic cough, neuralgia of the fifth nerve, afterpain, ovarian neuralgia, etc. In most of these affections the dose must be pushed so as to induce some physiological symptoms but its action should not be carried beyond the production of drooped eyelids, diplopia and muscular debility (Potter).

Antidotes—Morphine the most complete antagonist. Digitalis, ammonia, alcohol and xanthoxylum fraxineum are valuable. Emetics, heat, faradization to the respiratory muscles and artificial respiration are of prime importance. Tannic acid and caustic alkalies are chemically incompatible.

PREPARATION.

Tincture Gelsemium, U. S.—Fl. ext. Gelsemium, Lilly, 2½ fl. ozs.; Alcohol, 13½ fl. ozs.; Mix—Dose 10 to 20 m.

FL. EXT. GENTIAN, U. S. .... **Dose 10 to 30 m.**
Gentiana lutea Linn. **Nat. Ord.**—*Gentianaceæ.*
Range—Mountainous Europe.
Habitat—Open grassy places on mountain slopes.
Part used—The root.
Standard of strength—That of the U. S. Pharmacopœia, 1890; 1 c.c. representing 1 gram of the drug; or, practically, minim for grain.
Action and uses—An agreeable bitter tonic. Largely used in dyspepsia and debility with loss of appetite.

PREPARATIONS.

Tincture Gentian—Fl. ext. Gentian, Lilly, 2 fl. ozs.; Diluted Alcohol, 14 fl. ozs.; Mix—Dose 3 to 6 fl. drs.

FL. EXT. GENTIAN COMP. .... **Dose 10 to 20 m.**
Standard of strength—One pint represents Gentian, 12½ troy ounces; Bitter orange peel, 4½ troy ounces; Cardamon, 1½ troy ounces.
Action and uses—This is an elegant tonic bitter much used in dyspepsia and as an addition to tonic mixtures in debilitated conditions of the digestive organs and in convalescence to improve the appetite.

PREPARATIONS.

Tincture Gentian Comp., U. S.—Fl. ext. Gentian comp., Lilly, 2 fl. ozs.; Diluted alcohol, 14 fl. ozs.; Mix—Dose 1 to 2 fl. drs.

Syrup Gentian Comp.—Fl. ext. Gentian comp., Lilly, 4 fl. ozs.; Syrup, 12 fl. ozs.; Mix—Dose 1 to 2 fl. drs.

Wine Gentian Comp.—Fl. ext. Gentian comp., Lilly, 1 fl. oz.; Sherry wine, 15 fl. ozs.; Mix—Dose ½ to 1 fl. oz.

FL. EXT. GERMAN CHAMOMILE. .... **Dose 30 to 60 m.**
Matricaria Chamomilla Linn. **Nat. Ord.**—*Compositæ.*
Synonyms—Chrysanthemum Chamomilla Meyer, Chamomilla officinalis Koch.
Range—Europe and Western Asia; cultivated in the United States.
Habitat—In waste and cultivated ground as a weed.
Part used—The inflorescence.
Standard of strength—That of the U. S. Pharmacopœia, 1890; 1 c.c. representing 1 gram of the drug; or, practically, minim for grain.
Action and uses—A mild tonic; in large doses emetic. Employed in Germany as an antispasmodic and anthelmintic.

PREPARATION.

Infusion German Chamomile—Fl. ext. German chamomile, Lilly, 1 fl. oz.; Hot water, 15 fl. ozs.; Mix—Dose 1 to 2 fl. ozs.

FL. EXT. GINGER............Dose 2 to 10 m., in sweetened water.

Zingiberis officinale Roscoe.   **Nat. Ord.**—*Scitamineæ.*

Range—India; cultivated in tropical countries.

Habitat—Not known in a truly wild state.

Part used—The rhizome.

Standard of strength—That of the U. S. Pharmacopœia, 1890; 1 c.c. representing 1 gram of the drug; or, practically, minim for grain.

Action and uses—Stimulant and carminative.

PREPARATIONS.

Tincture Ginger, U. S.—Fl. ext. Ginger, Lilly, 3¼ fl. ozs.; Alcohol, 12¾ fl. ozs.; Mix—Dose 10 to 40 m.

Syrup Ginger, U. S.—Fl. ext. Ginger, Lilly, 1 fl. oz.; Calcium phosphate, ½ troy oz.; Water, 11½ fl. ozs.; Sugar, 26 troy ozs.; Mix the fluid extract and the calcium phosphate. When the alcohol has evaporated add the water, filter and dissolve the sugar in the filtrate. Finally add sufficient water to make two pints—Dose 1 to 4 fl. drs.

FL. EXT. GINGER, SOLUBLE......................Dose 2 to 10 m.

Zingiberis officinale Roscoe.   **Nat. Ord.**—*Scitamineæ.*

Range—India; cultivated in tropical countries.

Habitat—Not known in a truly wild state.

Part used—The rhizome.

Standard of strength—One pint represents 8 troy ounces Jamaica ginger.

Action and uses—Stimulant and carminative. This preparation will make clear mixtures with syrup or wine and will be found convenient for making syrup ginger, U. S., ginger ale, syrup for mineral water, etc.

PREPARATION.

Syrup Ginger, U. S.—Fl. ext. Ginger, soluble, Lilly, 1 fl. oz.; Syrup, 15 fl. ozs.; Mix—Dose 1 to 4 fl. ozs.

FL. EXT. GOLDEN ROD.........................Dose 30 to 60 m.

Solidago odora Aiton.   **Nat. Ord.**—*Compositæ.*

Synonym—Sweetscented golden rod.

Range—Canada to Florida and Texas, chiefly near the coast, but as far interior as Kentucky.

Habitat—Dry or sandy soil.

Part used—The leaves and inflorescence.

Standard of strength—That of the U. S. Pharmacopœia, 1890; 1 c.c. representing 1 gram of the drug; or, practically, minim for grain.

Action and uses—Aromatic, stimulant, carminative and diaphoretic. Used in flatulent colic, nausea, convalescence from severe diarrhea, dysentery or cholera morbus.

PREPARATIONS.

Tincture Golden Rod—Fl. ext. Golden rod, Lilly, 4 fl. ozs.; Alcohol, 5 fl. ozs.; Water, 7 fl. ozs.; Mix—Dose 2 to 4 fl. drs.

Infusion Golden Rod—Fl. ext. Golden rod, Lilly, 1 fl. oz.; Hot water, 15 fl. ozs.; Mix—Dose 1 to 2 fl. ozs.

FL. EXT. GOLDEN SEAL, U. S.....................Dose 30 to 60 m.

Hydrastis Canadensis Linn.   **Nat. Ord.**—*Ranunculaceæ.*

Synonyms—Hydrastis, U. S.,—Yellow root, Orange root, Yellow puccoon.

Range—New York to Minnesota and southward.

Habitat—Rich woodlands.

Part used—The rhizome and roots.

Standard of strength—2 per cent. of pure hydrastine.

NOTE—For lotions and injections the fluid extract golden seal, non-alcoholic, Lilly, is a very much better preparation.

Action and uses—Simple bitter and tonic to the stomach, antiperiodic, a mild laxative and an antiseptic. Used locally and internally in all forms of catarrh, especially that of the stomach, duodenum, gall ducts, bladder, uterus and vagina. Internally in glandular swelling, constipation from sluggish liver and deficiency of other intestinal secretions. Valuable as an injection in gonorrhœa, gleet and chronic nasal catarrh and also in syphilitic affections of the nose throat and nares. Highly recommended for unhealthy ulcers and sores, apatise, rectal fissure, hemorrhoids, conjunctivitis, etc.

PREPARATIONS.

Tincture Golden Seal, U. S.—Fl. ext. Golden seal, Lilly, 3¾ fl. ozs. Alcohol, 6¼ fl. ozs.; Water, 6¼ fl. ozs.; Mix—Dose 1 to 2 fl. drs.

Wine Golden Seal—Fl. ext. Golden seal, Lilly, 2 fl. ozs.; Sherry wine, 13 fl. ozs.; Alcohol, 1 fl. oz.; Mix—Dose 2 to 4 fl. drs.

Golden Seal Bitters—Fl. ext. Golden seal, Lilly, 1 fl. oz.; Fl. ext. Orange peel, bitter, Lilly, 2 fl. ozs.; Fl. ext. Prickly ash bark, Lilly, ½ fl. oz.; Diluted alcohol, 12 fl. ozs.; Sugar, 4 troy ozs.; Dissolve the sugar in the diluted alcohol and add the fluid extracts.

FL. EXT. GOLDEN SEAL, Nonalcoholic. Dose 30 to 60 m.
(Glyceritum Hydrastis U. S.)

Hydrastis Canadensis Linn. **Nat. Ord.**—*Ranunculaceæ.*

Synonyms—Hydrastis, U. S.,—Yellow root, Orange root, Yellow puccoon.

Range—New York to Minnesota and southward.

Habitat—Rich woodlands.

Part used—The rhizome and roots.

Standard of strength—That of the U. S. Pharmacopœia, 1890; 1 c.c. representing 1 gram of the drug; or, practically, minim for grain. In this preparation the resin and other inert matter is eliminated while the hydrastine and berberine are retained in natural combination.

NOTE—This is the official Glyceritum of Hydrastis.

Action and uses—Simple bitter and tonic to the stomach, antiperiodic, a mild laxative and an antiseptic. Used locally and internally in all forms of catarrh, especially that of the stomach, duodenum, gall ducts, bladder, uterus and vagina. Internally in glandular swelling, constipation from sluggish liver and deficiency of other intestinal secretions. Valuable as an injection in gonorrhœa, gleet and chronic nasal catarrh and also in syphilitic affections of the nose throat and nares. Highly recommended for unhealthy ulcers and sores, epithe, rectal fissure, hemorrhoids, conjunctivitis, etc.

PREPARATION.

Injection or Lotion Golden Seal—Fl. ext. Golden seal, nonalcoholic, Lilly, 1 fl. oz.; Water, 7 fl. ozs.; Or the proportions may be varied to suit the case.

FL. EXT. GOLDTHREAD, see appendix, page 331.

FL. EXT. GRAINS OF PARADISE .... Dose 10 to 20 m.
Amomum Granum-paradisi Afzelius.
Nat. Ord.—*Scitamineæ.*

Synonyms—A. Melegueta Roscoe,—Guinea grains, Malaguetta pepper.

Range—Coast regions of Western Tropical Africa.

Part used—The seed.

Standard of strength—That of the U. S. Pharmacopœia, 1890; 1 c.c. representing 1 gram of the drug; or, practically, minim for grain.

Action and uses—Stimulant and aromatic.

PREPARATION.

Tincture Grains of Paradise—Fl. ext. Grains of Paradise, Lilly, 2 fl. ozs.; Alcohol, 14 fl. ozs.; Mix—Dose 1 to 2 fl. drs.

WHEN ORDERING OR PRESCRIBING.

FL. EXT. GRAVEL PLANT.........................Dose 30 to 60 m.
Epigea repens Linn. **Nat. Ord.**—*Ericaceæ.*
Synonyms—Trailing arbutus, Ground laurel.
Range—North America; Newfoundland to Minnesota, south to Florida.
Habitat—In sandy woods or in rocky soil, especially in the shade of pines.
Part used—The leaves.
Standard of strength—That of the U. S. Pharmacopœia, 1890; 1 c.c. representing 1 gram of the drug; or, practically, minim for grain.
Action and uses—Diuretic and astringent. Beneficial in lithic acid gravel and all diseases of the urinary organs. It substitutes uva ursi.

PREPARATIONS.

Infusion Gravel Plant—Fl. ext. Gravel plant, Lilly, 1 fl. oz.; Hot water, 15 fl. ozs.; Mix—Dose 1 to 2 fl. ozs.

Infusion Gravel Plant Comp.—Fl. ext. Gravel plant, Lilly, 1 fl. oz.; Fl. ext. Juniper berries, Lilly, 2 fl. ozs.; Nitrate potassium, 1 dr.; Hot water, 13 fl. ozs.; Mix—Dose 1 to 2 fl. ozs.

FL. EXT. GREEN OSIER BARK.....................Dose 30 to 60 m.
Cornus circinata L. Heritier. Nat. Ord.—*Cornaceæ.*
Synonyms—C. rugosa Lam.,—Roundleaved dogwood.
Range—Nova Scotia to Dakota, south to Virginia and Missouri.
Habitat—Rich or sandy soil, or on rocks.
Part used—The bark.
Standard of strength—That of the U. S. Pharmacopœia, 1890; 1 c.c. representing 1 gram of the drug; or, practically, minim for grain.
Action and uses—Astringent, tonic and febrifuge.

FL. EXT. GRINDELIA, U. S..........................Dose 30 to 60 m.
Grindelia robusta Nutt. *and C. squarrosa* Dunal.
Nat. Ord.—*Compositæ.*
Synonym—Gum plant.
Range—Western United States, west of the Rocky Mountains.
Habitat—In salt marshes and on alkaline soil.
Part used—The leaves and inflorescence.
Standard of strength—That of the U. S. Pharmacopœia, 1890; 1 c.c. representing 1 gram of the drug; or, practically, minim for grain.
Action and uses—Antispasmodic and motor-depressant. Especially efficacious in spasmodic asthma, bronchitis and whooping cough. Useful in dyspnœa, hay fever and chronic cystitis. Used as a sedative lotion in poisoning by rhus tox. and for skin diseases in which itching or burning sensations occur.

PREPARATIONS.

Tincture Grindelia—Fl. ext. Grindelia, Lilly, 4 fl. ozs., Alcohol, 9 fl. ozs.; Water, 3 fl. ozs.; Mix—Dose 2 to 4 fl.drs.

Infusion Grindelia—Fl. ext. Grindelia, Lilly, 2 fl. ozs.; Hot water, 14 fl. ozs.; Mix—Dose ½ to 1 fl. oz.

FL. EXT. GRINDELIA, soluble, see Appendix, page 332.

FL. EXT. GRINDELIA COMP..........................Dose 30 to 60 m.
Standard of strength—One pint represents Grindelia, 10 troy ounces; Senna, Rhubarb, of each, 3 troy ounces.
Action and uses—Applicable in cases where grindelia alone constipates the patient. Antispasmodic and motor-depressant. Especially efficacious in spasmodic asthma, bronchitis and whooping cough. Useful in dyspnœa, hay fever and chronic cystitis.

PREPARATIONS.

Tincture Grindelia Comp.—Fl. ext. Grindelia comp., Lilly, 4 fl. ozs.; Alcohol, 9 fl. ozs.; Water, 3 fl. ozs.; Mix—Dose 2 to 4 fl. drs.
Infusion Grindelia Comp.—Fl. ext. Grindelia comp., Lilly, 2 fl. ozs.; Hot water, 14 fl. ozs.; Mix—Dose ½ to 1 fl. oz.

FL. EXT. GROUND **IVY**, see Appendix, page 332.

FL. EXT. GUACO **LEAVES**.................................... Dose 15 to 30 m.
Mikania Guaco Humboldt and Bonpland. Nat. Ord.—*Compositæ*.
Synonym—Huaco.
Range—Tropical America.
Part used—The leaves.
Standard of strength—That of the U. S. Pharmacopœia, 1890; 1 c.c.
representing 1 gram of the drug; or, practically, minim for grain.
Action and uses—Reputed valuable in the treatment of cholera and
diarrhœa, also in chronic rheumatism.

FL. **EXT. GUAIAC RESIN**...................................Dose 15 to 60 m.
Guaiacum officinale Linn. Nat. Ord.—*Zygophylleæ*.
Synonyms—Lignum vita, Pockwood.
Range—Bahamas and West Indies; Tropical America.
Part used—The resin of the wood.
Standard of strength—One pint represents 8 troy ounces of purified guaiac resin.
Action and uses—Diaphoretic, expectorant and alterative. A very
efficient remedy in tonsilitis, 15 to 30 minim doses of the tincture or
ammoniated tincture in milk to abate the inflammation or abort the
disease. The ammoniated tincture in water makes an excellent
gargle. Valuable also in neuralgic dysmenorrhea, amenorrhea, chronic
rheumatism, gout, lumbago and sciatica.

PREPARATIONS.

Tincture Guaiac, U. S.—Fl. ext. Guaiac, Lilly, 6½ fl. ozs.; Alcohol,
9½ fl. ozs.; Mix—Dose 1 to 2 fl. drs.

Tincture Guaiac Ammoniated, U. S.—Fl. ext. Guaiac, Lilly, 6½
fl. ozs.; Aromatic spirit of ammonia, 9½ fl. ozs.; Mix—Dose 1 to 2 fl. drs.

Infusion Guaiac—Fl. ext. Guaiac, Lilly, 1 fl. oz.; Hot water, 15 fl.
ozs.; Mix—Dose 1 to 2 fl. ozs.

FL. EXT. GUAIAC WOOD. ....Dose 30 to 120 m.
Guaiacum officinale Linn. *and G. sanctum* Linn.
Nat. Ord.—*Zygophylleæ*.
Synonyms—Lignum vita, Pockwood.
Range—Bahamas and West Indies, Tropical America.
Part used—The heart wood.
Standard of strength—That of the U. S. Pharmacopœia, 1890; 1 c.c.
representing 1 gram of the drug; or, practically, minim for grain.
Action and uses—Diaphoretic, expectorant and alterative. Valuable
in neuralgic dysmenorrhea, amenorrhea, chronic rheumatism, gout,
lumbago and sciatica.

PREPARATION.

Infusion Guaiac Wood—Fl. ext. Guaiac wood, Lilly, 1 fl. oz.; Hot
water, 15 fl. ozs., Mix—Dose 1 to 4 fl. ozs.

FL. EXT. GUARANA, **U. S**.....................Dose 60 to 120 m.
Paullinia Cupana Kunth. Nat. Ord.—*Sapindaceæ*.
Synonym—P. sorbilis Martius.
Range—Northern and Western Brazil.
Habitat—Moist forests and along wooded river banks.
Part used—Dried paste made chiefly from the crushed seeds.
Standard of Strength—4.5 per cent. of caffeine.
Action and uses—Astringent, stimulant and stomachic. Valuable in
nervous sick headache and the cephalalgia sometimes following menstru-
ation and that following dissipation. Apparently contra-indicated in
neuralgia, chronic headache and in all cases where it is undesirable to
excite the heart, increase arterial tension or increase the temperature.

PREPARATION.

Syrup Guarana—Fl. ext. Guarana, Lilly, 4 fl. ozs.; Syrup, 12 fl. ozs.;
Mix—Dose ½ to 1 fl. oz.

WHEN ORDERING OR PRESCRIBING.

FL. EXT. HAIRCAP MOSS.........................Dose 60 to 120 m.

Polytrichum juniperinum Hedwig.

Class—*Musci;* **Nat. Ord.—***Bryaceæ.*

Synonyms—Robinsrye, Bearsbed.

Range—United States.

Habitat—Moist ground, rocks etc., in shady places.

Part used—The whole plant.

Standard of strength—That of the U. S. Pharmacopœia, 1890; 1 c.c. representing 1 gram of the drug; or, practically, minim for grain.

Action and uses—A powerful diuretic. In doses of 2 fluid ounces of the infusion every half hour it has been known to remove from a dropsical patient from twenty to forty pounds of water in twentyfour hours. It may be combined with hydragogue cathartics if desired. Useful also in phosphatic gravel and urinary obstructions.

PREPARATION.

Infusion Haircap Moss—Fl. ext. Haircap moss, Lilly, 2 fl. ozs.; Hot water, 14 fl. ozs.; Mix—Dose 1 to 2 fl. ozs.

FL. EXT. HARDHACK ....Dose 30 to 60 m.

Spiræa tomentosa Linn. **Nat. Ord.—***Rosaceæ.*

Range—Nova Scotia to the mountains of Georgia, west to Minnesota and Kansas.

Habitat—Low grounds.

Part used—The herb.

Standard of strength—That of the U. S. Pharmacopœia, 1890; 1 c.c. representing 1 gram of the drug; or, practically, minim for grain.

Action and uses—Astringent and tonic. Valuable in summer complaint of children and diarrhœa. Efficient as a tonic in debility and convalescence from bowel and stomach troubles.

PREPARATION.

Infusion Hardhack—Fl. ext. Hardhack, Lilly, 2 fl. ozs.; Hot water, 14 fl. ozs.; Mix—Dose ½ to 1 fl. oz.

FL. EXT. HEMLOCK BARK ....Dose 15 to 60 m.

Tsuga Canadensis (Linn.) Carr. **Nat. Ord.—***Compositæ.*

Synonyms—Pinus Canadensis Linn., Abies Canadensis Michx.

Range—Nova Scotia to Delaware and along the mountains to **Alabama,** west to Michigan and Minnesota.

Habitat—Hilly or rocky woodlands.

Part used—The bark.

Standard of strength—That of the U. S. Pharmacopœia, 1890; 1 c.c. representing 1 gram of the drug; or, practically, minim for grain.

Action and uses—Astringent. Recommended in the treatment **of** chronic diarrhœa and the later stages of dysentery and cholera infantum. It may usually substitute tannin, matico and rhatany.

PREPARATION.

Infusion Hemlock Bark—Fl. ext. Hemlock bark, Lilly, 2 fl. ozs.; Hot water, 14 fl. ozs.; Mix—Dose 2 to 4 fl. drs.

FL. EXT. HENBANE, U. S.....................Dose 5 to 10 m.

Hyoscyamus niger Linn. **Nat. Ord.—***Solanaceæ.*

Synonym—Hyoscyamus, U. S.

Range—Europe, Asia and Africa; naturalized in the Northeastern United States; cultivated.

Habitat—Sandy soil, along roadsides and in waste places.

Part used—The leaves and inflorescence.
Standard of strength—0.1 per cent. of alkaloid, estimated by titration with acid.
Action and uses—NARCOTIC POISON. Anodyne and antispasmodic. Its action is similar to belladonna. It is chiefly used as an anodyne and hypnotic when opium is contra-indicated and for children. It is the remedy in acute mania with high motor excitement, obstinate insomnia, hallucinations and chronic mania.
Antidotes—In poisoning by this drug tannic acid and emetics should be used, then morphine, physostigmine or pilocarpine for the nervous disturbance. Caustic alkalies decompose atropine and are therefore incompatible with preparations of belladonna.

PREPARATION.

Tincture Henbane, U. S.—Fl. ext. Henbane, Lilly, 2½ fl. ozs.; Alcohol, 10½ fl. ozs.; Water, 3½ fl. ozs.; Mix—Dose 30 to 60 m.

FL. EXT. HOPS.................................Dose 10 to 30 m.
Humulus Lupulus Linn.   **Nat. Ord.**—*Urticaceæ.*
Range—North America, Europe, Asia; cultivated.
Habitat—Along banks of streams, in rich soil.
Part used—The strobiles.
Standard of strength—That of the U. S. Pharmacopœia, 1890; 1 c.c. representing 1 gram of the drug; or, practically, minim for grain.
Action and uses—Tonic, anodyne and feebly narcotic.

PREPARATIONS.

Tincture Hops, U. S.—Fl. ext. Hops, Lilly, 3¼ fl. ozs.; Alcohol, 12¾ fl. ozs.; Mix—Dose 1 to 3 fl. drs.

Infusion Hops—Fl. ext. Hops, Lilly, ½ fl. oz.; Hot water, 15½ fl. ozs.; Mix—Dose 1 to 2 fl. ozs.

FL. EXT. HOREHOUND..........................Dose 30 to 60 m.
Marrubium vulgare Linn.   **Nat. Ord.**—*Labiatæ.*
Range—Europe, Central Asia; naturalized and cultivated in the United States.
Habitat—Waste places near cultivated ground.
Part used—The leaves and inflorescence.
Standard of strength—That of the U. S. Pharmacopœia, 1890; 1 c.c. representing 1 gram of the drug; or, practically, minim for grain.
Action and uses—Stimulant, tonic, expectorant and diuretic. Used in the form of syrup in coughs, colds, chronic catarrh, asthma and all pulmonary affections.

PREPARATION.

Syrup Horehound—Fl. ext. Horehound, Lilly, 4 fl. ozs.; Syrup, 12 fl. ozs.; Mix—Dose 2 to 4 fl. drs.

FL. EXT. HOREHOUND **COMP.**....................Dose 30 to 60 m.
Standard of strength—One pint represents Horehound, Jersey tea, Elecampane, Spikenard, Comfrey and Cherry bark, of each, 2½ troy ounces; Blood root, 1¼ troy ounce.
Action and uses—Pectoral. Used for obstinate coughs and pulmonary complaints generally.

PREPARATION.

Syrup Horehound Comp.—Fl. ext. Horehound comp., Lilly, 4 fl. ozs.; Syrup, 12 fl. ozs.; Mix—Dose 2 to 4 fl. drs.

FL. EXT. HORSE CHESTNUTS ....Dose 1 to 5 m.
Æsculus Hippocastanum Linn.   **Nat. Ord.—***Sapindaceæ.*
Range—Asia; naturalized in Europe and in the United States; culti-
vated as an ornamental and shade tree.
Part used—The nut.
Standard of strength—That of the U. S. Pharmacopœia, 1890; 1 c.c.
representing 1 gram of the drug; or, practically, minim for grain.
Action and uses—Narcotic.

PREPARATION.

Tincture Horse Chestnuts—Fl. ext. Horse chestnuts, Lilly, 2
fl. ozs.; Alcohol, 10½ fl. ozs.; Water, 3½ fl. ozs.; Mix—Dose 10 to 40 m.

FL. EXT. HORSE CHESTNUT BARK... ....Dose 60 to 120 m.
Æsculus Hippocastanum Linn.   **Nat. Ord.—***Sapindaceæ.*
Range—Asia; naturalized in Europe and in the United States; cultivated
as an ornamental and shade tree.
Part used—The bark.
Standard of strength—That of the U. S. Pharmacopœia, 1890; 1 c.c.
representing 1 gram of the drug; or, practically, minim for grain.
Action and uses—Tonic, astringent, febrifuge, narcotic and anti-
septic. In intermittent fevers good results have followed its use.

PREPARATION.

Infusion Horsechestnut Bark—Fl. ext. Horsechestnut bark,
Lilly, 2 fl. ozs.; Hot water, 14 fl. ozs.; Mix—Dose 1 to 2 fl. ozs.

FL. EXT. HORSE NETTLE BERRIES.............Dose 30 to 240 m
Solanum Carolinense Linn.   **Nat. Ord.—***Solanaceæ.*
Range—Connecticut, west to Iowa, south to Florida and Texas.
Habitat—Sandy soil and waste grounds.
Part used—The fresh berries.
Standard of strength—That of the U. S. Pharmacopœia, 1890; 1 c.c.
representing 1 gram of the drug; or, practically, minim for grain.
Action and uses—Anodyne, antispasmodic and diuretic. It has
proven especially valuable in controlling convulsions of epilepsy. It
seems necessary in epilepsy to push the dose rapidly up to the point of
drowsiness if not stupor in the patient in order to obtain the desired impression and there appears to be no danger in this as harmful effects have
not been observed even when the largest doses have been repeated at
short intervals.
Note—Send for booklet, "Medical and Botanical Information of Horse
Nettle and its Use in the Treatment of Epilepsy," Eli Lilly & Company,
Indianapolis Ind., U. S. A.

FL. EXT. HORSE NETTLE ROOT............ .....Dose 30 to 240 m.
Solanum Carolinense Linn.   **Nat Ord.—***Solanaceæ.*
Range—Connecticut, west to Iowa, south to Florida and Texas.
Habitat—Sandy soil and waste grounds.
Part used—The root.
Standard of strength—That of the U. S. Pharmacopœia, 1890; 1 c.c.
representing 1 gram of the drug; or, practically, minim for grain.
Action and uses—Anodyne, antispasmodic and diuretic. It has
proven especially valuable in controlling convulsions of epilepsy. It
seems necessary in epilepsy to push the doses rapidly up to the point of
drowsiness if not stupor in the patient in order to obtain the desired
impression and there appears to be no danger in this as harmful effects
have not been observed even when the largest doses have been repeated
at short intervals.
Note—Send for booklet, "Medical and Botanical Information of Horse
Nettle and its Use in the Treatment of Epilepsy," Eli Lilly & Company,
Indianapolis, Ind., U. S. A.

FL. EXT. HORSEMINT .... Dose 30 to 60 m.
Monarda punctata Linn.　　　　　**Nat. Ord.—*Labiatæ*.**
Synonym—Origanum.
Range—New York to Minnesota and Colorado, south to Florida and Texas.
Habitat—Sandy grounds, banks of streams, etc.
Part used—The herb.
Standard **of strength**—That of the U. S. Pharmacopœia, 1890; 1 c.c. representing 1 gram of the drug; or, practically, minim for grain.
Action **and uses**—Stimulant, carminative and sudorific. Used in nausea, flatulence, vomiting and as a diuretic.

PREPARATION.

Infusion Horsemint—Fl. ext. Horsemint, Lilly, 1 fl. oz.; Hot water, 15 fl. ozs.; Mix—Dose 1 to 2 fl. ozs.

FL. EXT. HYDRANGEA .... Dose 60 to 120 m.
Hydrangea arborescens Linn.　　　　　**Nat. Ord.—*Saxifragaceæ*.**
Synonyms—Wild hydrangea, Sevenbarks.
Range—Pennsylvania, south to Florida, west to Iowa and Missouri.
Habitat—Rocky banks.
Part used—The root.
Standard of strength—That of the U. S. Pharmacopœia, 1890; 1 c.c. representing 1 gram of the drug; or, practically, minim for grain.
Action and uses—Valuable in removing urinary calculi while in the form known as gravel, removing these deposits by its own specific action on the bladder while they are small enough to pass through the urethra.

PREPARATION.

Syrup Hydrangea—Fl. ext. Hydrangea, Lilly, 4 fl. ozs.; Syrup, 12 fl. ozs.; Mix—Dose ½ to 1 fl. oz.

FL. EXT. HYSSOP .... Dose 30 to 60 m.
Hyssopus officinalis Linn.　　　　　**Nat. Ord.—*Labiatæ*.**
Range—Southern Europe; naturalized in the United States; cultivated in gardens.
Part used—The herb.
Standard of strength—That of the U. S. Pharmacopœia, 1890; 1 c.c. representing 1 gram of the drug, or, practically, minim for grain.
Action and uses—Stimulant, aromatic, carminative and tonic. Useful in asthma, coughs and other affections of the chest.

PREPARATIONS.

Syrup Hyssop—Fl. ext. Hyssop, Lilly, 4 fl. ozs.; Syrup, 12 fl. ozs.; Mix—Dose 2 to 4 fl. drs.

Infusion Hyssop—Fl. ext. Hyssop, Lilly, 1 fl. oz.; Hot water, 15 fl. ozs.; Mix—Dose 1 to 2 fl. ozs.

FL. EXT. IGNATIA BEAN .... Dose 1 to 5 m.
Strychnos Ignatia Lindley.　　　　　**Nat. Ord.—*Loganiaceæ*.**
Synonyms—Ignatiana Philippinica Loureiro., I. amara Linn.—Bean of St. Ignatius.
Range—Philippine Islands; introduced in Cochin China.
Part used—The seed.
Standard of Strength—1.5 per cent. of alkaloid, estimated gravimetrically.
Action and uses—VIOLENT POISON. It stimulates digestion. An excellent nerve tonic; of value as a tonic in general functional atony and relaxation; of value in paralysis depending upon a depressed state

of the spinal or other motor centers. When there is inflammation or irritation of these latter, it should not be employed, as it may do great injury by increasing the irritation. It has been recommended in lead paralysis. Its value in amaurosis from abuse of alcohol and tobacco is undisputed. Headache and giddiness associated with nerve troubles which manifest themselves in the eye, are frequently relieved, though the nerve be atrophied and the eye be blind. As a respiratory stimulant in dyspnea dependent upon pulmonic affections, such as chronic bronchitis, emphysema and phthisis, it is considered of great value. It is useful in dyspepsia or constipation, or diarrhea connected with atony of visceral muscular coat, in local paralysis as prolapse of the rectum, atonic retention of urine or incontinence, loss of voluntary motion, infantile paralysis.

Antidotes—Tannic acid or a soluble salt of iodine, then emetics or the stomach pump, followed by absolute quiet. Antagonists are chloral, tobacco, chloroform or ether inhalations. The bladder must be frequently evacuated to prevent reabsorption. Artificial respiration.

FL. EXT. INDIAN TURNIP........ ....**Dose 15 to 30 m.**
Arisæma triphyllum (Linn.) Torr.   **Nat. Ord.—***Araceæ.*

Synonyms—Arum triphyllum Linn.,—Wake robin, Dragon root, Jack in the pulpit.

Range—Nova Scotia to Florida, west to Minnesota and Eastern Kansas.

Habitat—Rich woodlands, shaded river banks.

Part used—The tuber.

Standard of strength—That of the U. S. Pharmacopœia, 1890; 1 c.c. representing 1 gram of the drug; or, practically, minim for grain.

Action and uses—Expectorant and diaphoretic. Used to advantage in asthma, chronic catarrh, chronic rheumatism and various other affections connected with the cachectic state of the system.

PREPARATION.

Syrup Indian Turnip—Fl. ext. Indian turnip, Lilly, 4 fl. ozs.; Syrup, 12 fl. ozs.; Mix—Dose 1 to 2 fl. drs.

FL. EXT. IPECAC, U. S.... ....**Dose.** { Expectorant, 1 to 5 m.
                                              { Emetic, 15 to 30 m.
Cephælis Ipecacuanha (Brotero) A. Richard.

                                              Nat. Ord.—*Rubiaceæ.*

Synonym—Callicocca Ipecacuanha Brotero.

Range—Brazil to Bolivia and New Granada; cultivated in India.

Habitat—Moist, shady woods.

Part used—The root.

Standard of strength—2 per cent. of alkaloid, estimated by titration with acid.

Action and uses—Emetic, expectorant and diaphoretic.

PREPARATIONS.

Syrup Ipecac, U. S.—Fl. ext. Ipecac, Lilly. 1½ fl. oz.; Syrup, 13½ fl. ozs.; Glycerin, 1½ fl. ozs.; Acetic acid, 75 m.; Mix—Dose, expectorant, 5 to 20 m.; emetic, ½ to 1 fl. dr. repeated.

Wine Ipecac, U. S.—Fl. ext. Ipecac, Lilly, 1⅝ fl. ozs.; Alcohol, 1½ fl. ozs.; White wine, 12¾ fl. ozs.; Mix—Dose, expectorant, 5 to 10 m. repeated every half hour or hour. Not eligible as an emetic as the contained alcohol counteracts the emetic action of the drug.

FL. EXT. IPECAC AND OPIUM.....................**Dose 5 to 10 m.**

Synonyms—Tr. Ipecac and Opium, U. S.,—Fluid Dover's.

Standard of strength—One pint represents Ipecac and Opium, of each, 1⅝ troy ounces; or each minim is equivalent to one grain Dover's powder. The morphine strength is six grains in each fluid ounce.

Action and uses—Valuable in all cases where Dover's powder is indicated and often more convenient to administer.

FL. EXT. IPECAC AND **SENEGA**.................... **Dose 5 to 15 m.**
Standard of strength—One pint represents Ipecac, 5½ troy ounces;
Senega, 10½ troy ounces.
Action and uses—Combines the expectorant effect of senega with the
relaxing effect of ipecac.

PREPARATION.

Syrup Ipecac and Senega—Fl. ext. Ipecac and senega, Lilly, 4 fl.
ozs.; Syrup, 12 fl. ozs.; Mix—Dose ½ to 1 fl. dr.

FL. EXT. JABORANDI, **U. S.**................ ...... Dose 15 to 30 m.
Pilocarpus Selloanus Engler (Rio Janeiro Jaborandi) and *P. Jaborandi*
Holmes (Pernambuco Jaborandi).   **Nat. Ord.**—*Rutaceæ.*
Synonym—Pilocarpus, U. S.
Range—Brazil.
Habitat—Forest clearings on **hill slopes.**
Part used—The leaflets.
Standard of Strength—0.5 per **cent. of alkaloid, estimated grav-**
imetrically.
Action and uses—POISONOUS IN OVERDOSES. A powerful diaphoretic
and sialagogue. Efficient in dropsies, especially in the renal form, in
uremia, pleuritis, meningitis and other inflammations of the serous
membranes. A valuable remedy in Bright's disease but from its depressant action must be employed with great caution. Contra-indicated
where the heart, from any cause, is weak. In agalactia it stimulates the
secretion of the milk and often gives relief in parotitis.
Antidotes—Atropine is the antagonist, morphine **controls the nausea.**
Caustic alkalies and salts of the metals generally are **chemically incom-**
patible.

PREPARATIONS.

Tincture Jaborandi—Fl. ext. Jaborandi, Lilly, 2 fl. ozs.; Diluted
alcohol, 14 fl. ozs.; Mix—Dose 2 to 4 fl. drs.

Infusion Jaborandi—Fl. ext. Jaborandi, Lilly, 2 fl. ozs.; Hot water,
14 fl. ozs.; Mix—Dose 2 to 4 fl. drs.

FL. EXT. JALAP.......................... Dose 15 to 30 m.
Ipomœa Jalapa Nutt.   **Nat. Ord.**—*Convolvulaceæ.*
Synonyms—I. Purga **Hayne, Convolvulus** Purga Wenderoth, Exo-
gonium Purga Benth.
Range—Eastern Mexico.
Habitat—Shady woods in vegetable mold.
Part used—The tuberous root.
Standard of Strength—12 per cent. of resin.
Action and uses—Hydragogue cathartic. Valuable as an ordinary
cathartic and when free catharsis is desirable **in cerebral lesions, kidney**
diseases and cardiac affections.

PREPARATION.

Tincture Jalap—Fl. ext. Jalap, Lilly, 3 fl. ozs.; Alcohol, 13 fl. ozs.;
Mix—Dose 1 to 3 fl. drs.

WHEN ORDERING OR PRESCRIBING.

FL. EXT. JAMAICA DOGWOOD.................. ....Dose 30 to 60 m.

Piscidia Erythrina Jacq. **Nat. Ord.**—*Leguminosæ.*

Range—West Indies.

Part used—The root bark.

Standard of strength—That of the U. S. Pharmacopœia, 1890; 1 c.c. representing 1 gram of the drug; or, practically, minim for grain.

Action and uses—Anodyne and narcotic. Recommended as a substitute for opium. It is claimed to have many of the valuable properties of that drug without disagreeable after effects or the formation of a habit.

PREPARATION.

Tincture Jamaica Dogwood—Fl. ext. Jamaica dogwood, Lilly, 4 fl. ozs.; Diluted alcohol, 12 fl. ozs.; Mix—Dose 2 to 4 fl. drs.

FL. EXT. JAMBUL SEED ....Dose 10 to 30 m.

Eugenia Jambolana Linn. **Nat. Ord.**—*Myrtaceæ.*

Range—East Indies and Queensland.

Part used—The seed.

Standard of strength—That of the U. S. Pharmacopœia, 1890; 1 c.c. representing 1 gram of the drug; or, practically, minim for grain.

Action and uses—Reputed valuable in diabetes, possessing the property of arresting the formation of sugar. Late reports confirm its value.

FL. EXT. JERSEY TEA................... ....Dose 60 to 120 m.

Ceanothus Americanus Linn. **Nat. Ord.**—*Rhamnaceæ.*

Synonyms—Red root, Wild snowball.

Range—New England, south to Florida; west to Minnesota and Texas.

Habitat—Open woodlands and along river banks.

Part used—The leaves.

Standard of strength—That of the U. S. Pharmacopœia, 1890; 1 c.c. representing 1 gram of the drug; or, practically, minim for grain.

Action and uses—Astringent, expectorant, sedative and antispasmodic. Used in gonorrhœa, dysentery, asthma, chronic bronchitis, whooping cough and pulmonary affections.

PREPARATION.

Infusion Jersey Tea—Fl. ext. Jersey tea, Lilly, 2 fl. ozs.; Hot water, 14 fl. ozs.; Mix—Dose 1 to 2 fl. ozs.

FL. EXT. JEWEL WEED ....Dose 30 to 60 m.

Impatiens aurea Muhl. **Nat. Ord.**—*Balsaminaceæ.*

Synonyms—I. pallida Nutt,—Snapweed, Wild celandine, Balsam weed, Pale touch-me-not.

Range—New England, south to Georgia; west to Dakota and Arkansas.

Habitat—Rich damp soils, along water courses.

Part used—The herb.

Standard of strength—That of the U. S. Pharmacopœia, 1890; 1 c.c. representing 1 gram of the drug; or, practically, minim for grain.

Action and uses—Aperient, diuretic. Recommended in jaundice, hepatitis and dropsy.

PREPARATION.

Infusion Jewel Weed—Fl. ext. Jewel weed, Lilly, 2 fl. ozs.; Hot water, 14 fl. ozs.; Mix—Dose ½ to 1 fl. oz.

FL. EXT. JOHNSWORT .... **Dose 30 to 60 m.**
Hypericum perforatum Linn.   **Nat. Ord.—***Hypericacew*.
Synonym—St. John's wort.
Range—Europe, Northern Africa, portions of Asia; naturalized in North America.
Habitat—In fields and along roadsides.
Part used—The inflorescence.
Standard of strength—That of the U. S. Pharmacopœia, 1890; 1 c.c. representing 1 gram of the drug; or, practically, minim for grain.
Action and uses—Astringent, sedative, diuretic and vermifuge. Used in suppression of urine, chronic urinary affections, diarrhea, dysentery, worms, jaundice, menorrhagia, hysteria, depressing nervous affections, hemoptysis and other hemorrhages. Externally as an ointment in hard tumors, caked breasts and bruises.

PREPARATIONS.

Ointment Johnswort—Fl. ext. Johnswort, Lilly, 1 fl. oz.; Lard, 2 troy ozs. Melt the lard, add the fluid extract. When the alcohol has evaporated stir till cold.

Infusion Johnswort—Fl. ext. Johnswort, Lilly, 2 fl. ozs.; Hot water, 14 fl. ozs.; Mix—Dose ½ to 1 fl. oz.

FL. EXT. JUDAS TREE .... **Dose 60 to 120 m.**
Cercis Canadensis Linn.   **Nat. Ord.—***Leguminosæ*.
Synonym—Red bud.
Range—New York to Florida, west to Southern Minnesota, Kansas and Louisiana.
Habitat—Rich woodlands.
Part used—The bark.
Standard of strength—That of the U. S. Pharmacopœia, 1890; 1 c.c. representing 1 gram of the drug; or, practically, minim for grain.
Action and uses—Astringent. Recommended in treatment of chronic diarrhea and dysentery. The injection is valuable in gleet, leucorrhea and all chronic catarrhal conditions; especially where an atonic condition of the mucous membrane exists.

PREPARATIONS.

Tincture Judas Tree—Fl. ext. Judas tree, Lilly, 2 fl. ozs.; Diluted alcohol, 14 fl. ozs.; Mix—Dose 2 to 4 fl. drs.

Injection Judas Tree—Fl. ext. Judas tree, Lilly, 1 fl. oz.; Glycerin, ½ fl. oz.; Water, 14½ fl. ozs.

FL. EXT. JUNIPER BERRIES .... **Dose 60 to 120 m.**
Juniperus communis Linn.   **Nat. Ord.—***Coniferæ*.
Range—Europe, Asia, Northern Africa; in North America, Canada, Northern United States, along the Rocky Mountains to Mexico.
Habitat—Dry sterile hills.
Part used—The fruit.
Standard of strength—That of the U. S. Pharmacopœia, 1890; 1 c.c. representing 1 gram of the drug; or, practically, minim for grain.
Action and uses—Gently stimulant and diuretic. Chiefly used with more powerful diuretics in dropsical complaints but is unquestionably valuable in scorbutic and cutaneous diseases, catarrh of the bladder and atonic conditions of the alimentary canal and uterus.

PREPARATIONS.

Compound Spirits of Juniper—Fl. ext. Juniper Berries, Lilly, 2 fl. ozs.; Fl. ext. Lovage, Lilly, 1 fl. oz.; Holland gin, 11 fl. ozs.; Syrup or honey, 2 fl. ozs.; Mix—Dose ½ to 1 fl. oz.

Infusion Juniper Berries—Fl. ext. Juniper Berries, Lilly, 2 fl. ozs.; Hot water, 14 fl. ozs.; Mix—Dose 1 to 2 fl. ozs.

FL. EXT. KAMALA............... ....**Dose 60 to 180 m.**
Mallotus Philippinensis (Linn.) Mueller.
                                    Nat. Ord.—*Euphorbiaceæ.*
Synonyms—Croton Philippinensis Lam.
Range—Abyssinia, Southern Arabia, Southern Asia, Australia and East Indies.
Habitat—Mountain sides to 5000 feet above the sea level.
Part used—The glands and hairs from the capsules.
Standard of strength—That of the U. S. Pharmacopœia, 1890, 1 c.c. representing 1 gram of the drug; or, practically, minim for grain.
Action and uses—Purgative and vermifuge. Long successfully used in India and later in Europe and America in the treatment of tapeworm. The worm is usually expelled dead at the third or fourth stool. Should the first dose fail to operate on the bowels it may be repeated in four hours.

FL. EXT. KAVA KAVA............ ....**Dose 15 to 60 m.**
Piper methysticum Forster.   **Nat. Ord.—***Piperaceæ.*
Synonyms—Macropiper methysticum Miquel,—Ava kava.
Range—South Sea Islands.
Part used—The root.
Standard of strength—That of the U. S. Pharmacopœia, 1890, 1 c.c. representing 1 gram of the drug; or, practically, minim for grain.
Action and uses—In small doses said to be tonic and stimulant; in large doses it intoxicates producing drowsiness accompanied by incoherent dreams. It has been employed as a pleasant remedy in bronchitis, rheumatism, gout, gonorrhœa and gleet, and has been recommended as a powerful sudorific. It has been found useful in chronic catarrhal affections of the various organs, and in chronic inflammation of the neck of the bladder. It is considered one of the most efficacious diuretics.

PREPARATION.

Tincture Kava Kava—Fl. ext. Kava kava, Lilly, 2 fl. ozs.; Alcohol, 10 fl. ozs.; Water, 4 fl. ozs.; Mix the alcohol and water and add the fluid extract—Dose 2 to 4 fl. drs.

FL. EXT. KINO....... ....**Dose 10 to 30 m.**
Pterocarpus Marsupium Roxburgh.   **Nat. Ord.—***Leguminosæ.*
Range—East Indies and India.
Habitat—In forests.
Part used—The inspissated juice.
Standard of strength—One pint represents eight troy ounces of kino.
Action and uses—A powerful astringent. Is much used for the suppression of morbid discharges and diarrhœa not attended with febrile excitement or inflammation. It is also used in chronic dysentery when astringents are admissable, in leucorrhœa, diabetes and in passive hemorrhages, especially of the uterus.

PREPARATION.

Tincture Kino, U. S.—Fl. ext. Kino, Lilly, 3½ fl. ozs.; Alcohol, 6½ fl. ozs.; Water, 6½ fl. ozs.; Mix—Dose 1 to 2 fl. drs.

FL. EXT. KOLA NUT... ....**Dose 30 to 60 m.**
Kola acuminata R. Brown.   **Nat. Ord.—***Sterculiaceæ.*
Synonyms—Sterculia acuminata Beau.,—Cola.
Range—Tropical Western Africa.
Part used—The seed.
Standard of Strength—1 per cent. of pure caffeine.
Action and uses—Kola nuts are valued very highly by the natives of Africa for their stimulating action. Sufficient has been ascertained concerning their medicinal properties to entitle them to use in the same manner as guarana, tea, coffee, and cocoa for sustaining fatigue and aiding digestion. It is said that kola nuts are used successfully in neutralizing the intoxicating effects of alcohol.

STANDARD FLUID EXTRACTS. 73

FL. EXT. KOUSSO, U. S. ....Dose 1-2 to 1 fl. oz.
Hagenia Abyssinica (Bruce) Gmelin. **Nat. Ord.**—*Rosaceæ*.
Synonyms—Brayera anthelmintica Kunth, Banksia Abyssinica Bruce,—Brayera.
Range—Abyssinia.
Habitat—Tablelands 3000-8000 feet above sea level.
Part used—The female inflorescence.
Standard of strength—That of the U. S. Pharmacopœia, 1890; 1 c.c. representing 1 gram of the drug; or, practically, minim for grain.
Action and uses—An efficient remedy in tape worm, acting as a poison to the worm. A dose of the infusion should be taken in the morning on an empty stomach, a light meal having been made the previous evening. Should it not act on the bowels in three or four hours, a brisk cathartic should be administered.

PREPARATION.

Infusion Kousso—Fl. ext. Kousso, Lilly, 2 fl. ozs.; Hot water, 14 fl. ozs.; Mix—Dose 4 fl. ozs.

FL. EXT. LABRADOR TEA .... Dose 30 to 60 m.
Ledum Grœnlandicum Œder. **Nat. Ord.**—*Ericaceæ*.
Synonyms—L. latifolium Ait.,—James tea.
Range—New England to Pennsylvania, Michigan, Minnesota and northward.
Habitat—Cold bogs and mountain woods.
Part used—The leaves.
Standard of strength—That of the U. S. Pharmacopœia, 1890; 1 c.c. representing 1 gram of the drug; or, practically, minim for grain.
Action and uses—Pectoral and tonic.

FL. EXT. LACTUCARIUM .. .. Dose 10 to 30 m.
Lactuca virosa Linn. **Nat. Ord.**—*Compositæ*.
Range—Southern and Central Europe; naturalized in parts of North America.
Habitat—Fields and waste places.
Part used—The concrete milk-juice.
Standard of strength—That of the U. S. Pharmacopœia, 1890; 1 c.c. representing 1 gram of the drug; or, practically, minim for grain.
Action and uses—Hypnotic and anodyne.

PREPARATION.

Syrup Lactucarium, U. S.—Fl. ext. Lactucarium, Lilly, 6½ fl. drs.; Syrup, sufficient to make 16 fl. ozs.; Mix—Dose 2 to 4 fl. drs.

FL. EXT. LADIES' SLIPPER, U. S......... .. .. Dose 10 to 15 m.
Cypripedium pubescens Swartz, *and C. parviflorum* Salisbury. **Nat. Ord.**—*Orchidaceæ*.
Synonyms—American valerian.
Range—Newfoundland to Georgia, west to Minnesota and Eastern Kansas.
Habitat—Bogs and low woods.
Part used—The rhizome.
Standard of strength—That of the U. S. Pharmacopœia, 1890; 1 c.c. representing 1 gram of the drug; or, practically, minim for grain.
Action and uses—Tonic, nervine and antispasmodic. Useful in chorea, hysteria, nervous headache and in all cases of nervous irritability and excitability.

PREPARATIONS.

Tincture Ladies' Slipper—Fl. ext. Ladies' slipper, Lilly, 2 fl. ozs.; Diluted alcohol, 14 fl. ozs.; Mix—Dose 1 to 2 fl. drs.

Syrup Ladies' Slipper—Fl. ext. Ladies' slipper, Lilly, 4 fl. ozs.; Syrup, 12 fl. ozs.; Mix—Dose ½ to 1 fl. dr.

WHEN ORDERING OR PRESCRIBING.

FL. EXT. LARGE FLOWERING SPURGE............**Dose 5 to 20 m.**

Euphorbia corollata Linn.   **Nat. Ord.**—*Euphorbiaceæ.*

Synonyms—Blooming spurge, Emetic root.

Range—New York to Florida, west to Minnesota and Louisiana.

Habitat—Rich or sandy soil.

Part used—The root.

Standard of strength—That of the U. S. Pharmacopœia, 1890; 1 c.c. representing 1 gram of the drug; or, practically, minim for grain.

Action and uses—Emetic and cathartic, in small doses diaphoretic and expectorant. Four minims of fluid extract every three hours act as a diaphoretic. In doses of three minims it acts as an expectorant. The emetic dose is from 15 to 20 minims. Valuable in dropsical diseases, especially hydrothorax and ascites.

FL. EXT. LARKSPUR SEED   ... .**Dose 2 to 5 m.**

Delphinium Consolida Linn.   **Nat. Ord.**—*Ranunculaceæ.*

Synonyms—Knight's spur, Lark's claw.

Range—Europe; naturalized in the United States.

Habitat—Old grain fields, along roadsides.

Part used—The seed.

Standard of strength—That of the U. S. Pharmacopœia, 1890; 1 c.c. representing 1 gram of the drug; or, practically, minim for grain.

Action and uses—Diuretic, emetic and **emmenagogue**. Valuable in spasmodic asthma and dropsy.

PREPARATIONS.

Tincture Larkspur Seed—Fl. ext. Larkspur seed, Lilly, 2 fl. ozs.; Alcohol, 14 fl. ozs.; Mix—Dose 20 to 40 m.

Infusion Larkspur Seed—Larkspur seed, Lilly, 1 fl. oz.; Hot water, 15 fl. ozs.; Mix—Dose ½ to 1 fl. dr.

FL. EXT. LAVENDER FLOWERS............... ....**Dose 30 to 60 m.**

Lavandula officinalis Chaix.   **Nat. Ord.**—*Labiatæ.*

Synonyms—L. vera D. C.,—Garden lavender, Spike lavender.

Range—Southern Europe; extensively cultivated.

Habitat—Dry hilly soil.

Part used—The flower.

Standard of strength—That of the U. S. Pharmacopœia, 1890; 1 c.c. representing 1 gram of the drug; or, practically, minim for grain.

Action and uses—Aromatic, stimulant, tonic.

PREPARATIONS.

Tincture Lavender Flowers—Fl. ext. Lavender flowers, Lilly, 2 fl. ozs.; Alcohol, 10½ fl. ozs.; Water, 3½ fl. ozs.; Mix—Dose 2 to 4 fl. drs.

Infusion Lavender Flowers—Fl. ext. Lavender flowers, Lilly, 1 fl. oz.; Hot water, 15 fl. ozs.; Mix—Dose 1 to 2 fl. ozs.

FL. EXT. LAVENDER COMP.

For preparing Tincture Lavender Comp., U. S.

Standard of strength—One pint represents Cinnamon, 2½ troy ozs.; Nutmeg, Red saunders, of each, 1½ troy ozs.; Cloves, ¾ troy oz.; Oil lavender flowers, 1 fl. oz.; Oil rosemary, 2 fl. drs.

PREPARATION.

Tincture Lavender Comp., U. S.—Fl. ext. Lavender comp., Lilly, 2 fl. ozs.; Alcohol, 10½ fl. ozs.; Water, 3½ fl. ozs.; Mix—Dose 30 to 60 m.

FL. EXT. LEMON **BALM**................................Dose 30 to 60 m.
Melissa officinalis Linn **Nat. Ord.**—*Labiatæ*.
Synonyms—Balm, Sweet Balm.
Range—Asia Minor, Southern Europe, naturalized and cultivated in the
United States.
Habitat—Waste places near cultivated grounds, sparingly escaped from
gardens.
Part used—The leaves and inflorescence.
Standard of strength—That of the U. S. Pharmacopœia, 1890; 1 c.c.
representing 1 gram of the drug; or, practically, minim for grain.
Action and uses—Aromatic, diaphoretic, emmenagogue. In infusion
it promotes the action of diaphoretic medicines.

PREPARATION.

Infusion Lemon Balm—Fl. ext. Lemon balm, Lilly, 2 fl. ozs.; Hot
water, 14 fl. ozs.; Mix—Dose ½ to 1 fl. oz.

FL. EXT. LEMON PEEL.......................................**Dose 30 to 60 m.**
Citrus Limonum Risso. Nat. Ord.—*Rutaceæ*.
Range—Northern India; cultivated in subtropical countries.
Habitat—In wild state, on mountain slopes to an elevation of 4000 feet.
Part used—The rind.
Standard of strength—That of the U. S. Pharmacopœia, 1890; 1 c.c.
representing 1 gram of the drug; or, practically, minim for grain.
Action and uses—Aromatic and **tonic**.

PREPARATION.

Syrup Lemon Peel—Fl. ext. Lemon peel, Lilly, 2 fl. ozs.; Syrup, 14
fl. ozs.; Mix—Dose ½ to 1 fl. dr.

FL. EXT. LETTUCE...................................... **Dose 30 to 60 m.**
Lactuca sativa Linn. **Nat. Ord.**—*Compositæ*.
Range—Original native country unknown; commonly cultivated in gar-
dens of both Europe and the United States.
Part used—The leaves.
Standard of strength—That of the U. S. Pharmacopœia, 1890; 1 c c.
representing 1 gram of the drug; or, practically, minim for grain.
Action and uses—Anodyne, narcotic, sedative.

PREPARATION.

Syrup Lettuce—Fl. ext. Lettuce, Lilly, 2 fl. ozs.; Syrup, 14 fl. ozs.;
Mix—Dose ½ to 1 fl. oz.

FL. EXT. LEVANT WORMSEED.......................Dose 10 to 30 m.
Artemisia pauciflora Weber. Nat. Ord.—*Compositæ*.
Synonyms—A. maritima Linn., var. Stechmanniana Besser.—Santonica,
U. S.
Range—Lower Volga and Don regions, steppes and desert plains of
Southern Russia, Russian Turkestan; cultivated.
Habitat—Near salt marshes, in alkaline soil.
Part used—The unexpanded flower heads.
Standard of strength—That of the U. S. Pharmacopœia, 1890; 1 c.c.
representing 1 gram of the drug; or, practically, minim for grain.
Action and uses—Used almost exclusively as a vermicide for lumbri-
coids and ascarides. In smaller doses it is stomachic and stimulant.

PREPARATIONS.

Tincture Levant Wormseed—Fl. ext. Levant wormseed, Lilly, 2
fl. ozs.; Alcohol, 14 fl. ozs.; Mix—Dose 1 to 4 fl. drs.

Infusion Levant Wormseed—Fl. ext. Levant wormseed, Lilly, 1
fl. oz.; Hot water, 15 fl. ozs.; Mix—Dose ½ to 1 fl. oz.

FL. EXT. LICORICE, U. S. ....Dose 60 to 120 m.
Glycyrrhiza glabra Linn. *and G. glabra var. glandulifera* (Waldstein et Kittaibel) Regel et Herder. **Nat. Ord.—***Leguminosæ.*

Synonyms—G. glandulifera Waldstein et Kittaibel.

Range—Southern Europe, Asia Minor and Northern Asia; cultivated in Europe.

Habitat—Moist sandy soil.

Part used—The root.

Standard of strength—That of the U. S. Pharmacopœia, 1890; 1 c.c. representing 1 gram of the drug; or, practically, minim for grain.

Action and uses—An excellent demulcent. The infusion is used in catarrhal affections and diarrhea. It is particularly useful as an adjuvant to cough syrups, but in this respect it is inferior to YERBAZIN, Lilly.

PREPARATIONS.

Syrup Licorice—Fl. ext. Licorice, Lilly, 4 fl. ozs.; Syrup, 12 fl. ozs.; Mix—Used as a vehicle.

Infusion Licorice—Fl. ext. Licorice, Lilly, 1 fl. oz.; Hot water, 15 fl. ozs.; Mix—Dose 2 to 4 fl. ozs.

FL. EXT. LICORICE, For Quinine.
From Glycyrrhiza glabra Linn. *and G. glabra var. glandulifera* (Waldstein and Kittaibel) Regel et Herder.

NOTE—This preparation contains the sweet principle of **Licorice** and is miscible in all proportions with water, syrup or glycerin.

Standard of strength—That of the U. S. Pharmacopœia, 1890; 1 c.c. representing 1 gram of the drug; or, practically, minim for grain.

Action and uses—This preparation is used almost exclusively for the purpose of masking the bitterness of quinine. For this purpose, however, it is inferior to YERBAZIN, Lilly.

PREPARATION.

Syrup Licorice, For Quinine—Fl. ext. Licorice, for quinine, Lilly, 2 fl. ozs.; Syrup, 14 fl. ozs.; Mix—Used as a vehicle.

Directions—Suspend the quinine in the syrup, taking care to break the crystals as little as possible. By thoroughly mixing, the quinine will remain suspended for a long time without developing the bitter taste. In no case should the quinine be dissolved with acids or alcohol, as the bitter taste is at once developed thereby. Cinchonidia or other bitter or nauseous medicines may also be disguised with this syrup.

FL. EXT. LICORICE, for syrup, see appendix, p age 332.

FL. EXT. LIFE EVERLASTING ....Dose 30 to 60 m.
Gnaphalium obtusifolium Linn. **Nat. Ord.—***Compositæ.*

Synonym—G. polycephalum Michx.

Range—Canada to Wisconsin, south to Texas; common.

Habitat—Old fields, open woods, dry ground.

Part used—The herb.

Standard of strength—That of the U. S. Pharmacopœia, 1890; 1 c.c. representing 1 gram of the drug; or, practically, minim for grain.

Action and uses—Astringent and diaphoretic. It has been used to advantage in ulceration of the throat. A warm infusion may be used in fevers to produce diaphoresis, and is of service in quinsy, pulmonary complaints, leucorrhea, etc.

PREPARATION.

Infusion Life Everlasting—Fl. ext. Life everlasting, Lilly, 1 fl. oz.; Hot water, 15 fl. ozs.; Mix—Dose 1 to 2 fl. ozs.

FL. EXT. LIFE ROOT ....Dose 30 to 60 m.

Senecio aureus Linn.

Synonyms—Golden senecio, False valerian, Ragwort.

Range—Newfoundland to British **Columbia**, south to Florida and Texas, along the sierra Nevada, California.

Habitat—Swamps and wet banks, usually in shaded ground.

Part used—The herb.

Standard of strength—That of the U. S. Pharmacopœia, 1890; 1 c.c. representing 1 gram of the drug; or, practically, minim for grain.

Action and uses—Diuretic, pectoral, diaphoretic and **tonic**. It exerts a peculiar influence upon the female reproductive organs and is efficacious in promoting the menstrual flow. Valuable in amenorrhœa and dysmenorrhœa; it has also proven a valuable diuretic in gravel and other urinary affections.

PREPARATIONS.

Syrup Life Root—Fl. ext. Life root, Lilly, 4 fl. ozs.; Syrup, 12 fl. ozs.; Mix—Dose 2 to 4 fl. drs.

Infusion Life Root—Fl. ext. Life root, Lilly, 2 fl. ozs.; Hot water, 14 fl. ozs.; Mix—Dose ½ to 1 fl. oz.

FL. EXT. LILY OF THE VALLEY, U. S...............Dose 5 to 15 m.

Convallaria majalis Linn.   **Nat. Ord.**-*Liliaceæ*.

Synonym—Convallaria, U. S.

Range—Europe, Northern Asia; in the United States on high mountains of Virginia to South Carolina; cultivated in gardens.

Part used—The rhizome.

Standard of strength—That of the U. S. Pharmacopœia, 1890; 1 c.c. representing 1 gram of the drug; or, practically, minim for grain.

Action and uses—Cathartic, anthelmintic and, in large doses, emetic. In organic heart disease its effects are equal to those of digitalis without the cumulative effects of that drug; the urine is increased, serous deposits are rapidly absorbed, and nervousness is diminished.

PREPARATION.

Tincture Lily of the Valley—Fl. ext. Lily of the valley, Lilly, 2 fl. ozs.; Diluted alcohol, 14 fl. ozs.; Mix—Dose ½ to 2 fl. drs.

FL. EXT. LIONSFOOT..............................Dose 30 to 60 m.

Prenanthes alba Linn.   **Nat. Ord.**—*Compositæ*.

Synonyms—Naialus alba Hook, —Canker root.

Range—Canada, New England to Saskatchewan, Illinois and Georgia.

Habitat—Open oak woods and sandy or gravelly soil.

Part used—The herb.

Standard of strength—That of the U. S. Pharmacopœia, 1890; 1 c.c. representing 1 gram of the drug; or, practically, minim for grain.

Action and uses—Used as an antidote to the bites of poisonous insects and serpents. Has been successfully used in the bite of rattle snake; also used in dysentery.

PREPARATION.

Infusion Lionsfoot—Fl. ext. Lionsfoot, Lilly, 2 fl. ozs.; Hot water, 14 fl. ozs.; Mix—Dose ½ to 1 fl. oz.

FL. EXT. LIPPIA MEXICANA, (Concentrated Tincture.)
Dose 30 to 60 m.

Lippia dulcis Trev.   **Nat. Ord.**—*Verbenaceæ*.

Range—Mexico.

Part used—The leaves.

Standard of strength—One pint represents 4 troy ounces of the drug.

Action and uses—Demulcent and expectorant. Said to be alterative to the bronchial mucous membrane. Used in chronic bronchitis and acute catarrhal affections of the respiratory tract.

FL. EXT. LIVERWORT................... ....Dose 30 to 120 m.
Hepatica tribola Chaix.   **Nat. Ord.—*Ranunculaceæ*.**

Synonyms- H. Hepatica (Linn.) Karst., Anemone Hepatica Linn.

Range—From the Atlantic to Missouri, Minnesota and northward.

Habitat—In woodlands.

Part used—The herb.

Standard of strength—That of the U. S. Pharmacopœia, 1890; 1 c.c. representing 1 gram of the drug; or, practically, minim for grain.

Action and uses—A mild, mucilaginous astringent. Useful in fevers, hepatic complaints etc.

PREPARATIONS.

Syrup Liverwort—Fl. ext. Liverwort, Lilly, 4 fl. ozs.; Syrup, 12 fl. ozs.; Mix—Dose 2 to 4 fl. drs.

Infusion Liverwort—Fl. ext. Liverwort, Lilly, 4 fl. ozs.; Hot water, 12 fl. ozs.; Mix—Dose 2 to 4 fl. drs.

FL. EXT. LOBELIA COMP. .... Dose 5 to 20 m.

Standard of strength—One pint represents Lobelia herb, 8 troy ounces; Skunk cabbage and Bloodroot, of each, 4 troy ounces.

Action and uses—Emetic, expectorant and antispasmodic.

PREPARATION.

Tincture Lobelia Comp,—Fl. ext. Lobelia comp., Lilly, 2 fl. ozs.; Alcohol, 8½ fl. ozs.; Water, 5½ fl. ozs.; Mix the alcohol and water and add the fluid extract—Dose ½ to 2 fl. drs.

FL. EXT. LOBELIA HERB, U. S. .. . ... Dose 1 to 5 m.
Lobelia inflata Linn.   **Nat. Ord.—*Lobeliaceæ*.**

Synonyms—Indian tobacco, Pukeweed, Emetic herb.

Range—Hudson's Bay to Saskatchewan, south to Georgia and Arkansas.

Habitat—Open dry grounds.

Part used—The herb.

Standard of strength—That of the U. S. Pharmacopœia, 1890; 1 c.c. representing 1 gram of the drug; or, practically, minim for grain.

Action and uses—POISONOUS IN OVER DOSES. Emetic but should never be used as such the effect being too lasting and distressing. Its principal use is in paroxysmal spasmodic asthma and dry tickling cough, as an antispasmodic but should be cautiously used. As an enema in strangulated hernia it is safer than tobacco and quite as efficient.

Antidotes—Tannic acid to form the insoluble tannate. Strychnine to antagonize its action on the nervous system. Alcohol, digitalis, belladonna and ergot antagonize its effect on the circulation. Caustic alkalies are incompatible.

PREPARATIONS.

Tincture Lobelia, U. S.—Fl. ext. Lobelia herb, Lilly, 2½ fl. ozs.; Alcohol, 6¾ fl. ozs.; Water, 6¾ fl. ozs.; Mix—Dose, as an expectorant, 5 to 30 m.; as a nauseant and antispasmodic, 30 to 60 m.

Vinegar Lobelia Herb—Fl. ext. Lobelia herb, Lilly, 1½ fl. ozs.; Diluted acetic acid, 14½ fl. ozs.; Mix—Dose, as an expectorant, 10 to 60 m.; as a nauseant and antispasmodic, 1 to 2 fl. drs.

FL. EXT. LOBELIA SEED.................. Dose 1-2 to 2 m.
Lobelia inflata Linn.   **Nat. Ord.—*Lobeliaceæ*.**

Synonyms—Indian tobacco, Pukeweed, Emetic herb.

Range—Hudson's Bay to Saskatchewan, south to Georgia and Arkansas.

Habitat—Open dry grounds.

Part used—The seed.

Standard of strength—That of the U. S. Pharmacopœia, 1890; 1 c.c. representing 1 gram of the drug; or, practically, minim for grain.

Action and uses—POISONOUS IN OVER DOSES. Emetic but should

---

never be used as such the effect being too lasting and distressing. Its principal use is in paroxysmal spasmodic asthma and dry tickling cough, as an antispasmodic, but should be cautiously used. As an enema in strangulated hernia it is safer than tobacco and quite as efficient.

Antidotes—Tannic acid to form the insoluble tannate. Strychnine to antagonize its action on the nervous system. Alcohol, digitalis, belladonna and ergot antagonize its effect on the circulation. Caustic alkalies are incompatible.

PREPARATION.

Tincture Lobelia Seed—Fl. ext. Lobelia seed, Lilly, 2 fl. ozs.; Alcohol, 10½ fl. ozs.; Water, 3½ fl. ozs.; Mix—Dose, as an expectorant, 5 to 30 m.; as a nauseant and antispasmodic, 30 to 60 m.

FL. EXT. LOGWOOD .... Dose **30 to 60 m.**

Hæmatoxylon Campechianum Linn. Nat. Ord.—*Leguminosæ.*

Synonym—Peachwood.

Range—Central America, Mexico; naturalized in West Indies.

Part used—The heart wood.

Standard of strength—That of the U. S. Pharmacopœia, 1890; 1 c.c. representing 1 gram of the drug; or, practically, minim for grain.

Action and uses—Mild astringent, without irritating properties, and well adapted to the treatment of the relaxed condition of the bowels which sometimes succeeds cholera infantum. It is occasionally used with advantage in chronic diarrhea and dysentery.

PREPARATION.

Infusion Logwood—Fl. ext. Logwood, Lilly, 1 fl. oz.; Hot water, 15 fl. ozs.; Mix—Dose 1 to 2 fl. ozs.

FL. EXT. LOVAGE .... Dose **30 to 60 m.**

Levisticum officinale Koch. Nat. Ord.—*Umbelliferæ.*

Synonym—Ligusticum Levisticum Linn.

Range—Mountainous districts of Southern Europe; cultivated in Germany.

Part used—The root.

Standard of strength—That of the U. S. Pharmacopœia, 1890; 1 c.c. representing 1 gram of the drug; or, practically, minim for grain.

Action and uses—Stimulant, carminative, diaphoretic and emmenagogue.

PREPARATION.

Infusion Lovage—Fl. ext. Lovage, Lilly, 2 fl. ozs.; Hot water, 14 fl. ozs.; Mix—Dose ½ to 1 fl. oz.

FL. EXT. LUNGMOSS...... Dose **15 to 30 m.**

Sticta pulmonaria Acharius. Fungi, Class—*Ascomycetes.* Nat. Ord.—*Lichenes.*

Synonym—Tree lungwort.

Part used—The thallus.

Standard of strength—That of the U. S. Pharmacopœia, 1890; 1 c.c. representing 1 gram of the drug; or, practically, minim for grain.

Action and **uses**—Tonic and demulcent. Used in pulmonary complaints.

PREPARATION.

Infusion Lungmoss—Fl. ext. Lungmoss, Lilly, 1 fl. oz.; Hot water, 15 fl. ozs.; Mix—Dose ½ to 1 fl. oz.

FL. EXT. LUPULIN...................................Dose 10 to 15 m.
Humulus Lupulus Linn. **Nat. Ord.—***Urticaceæ.*
Range—North America, Europe, Asia; cultivated.
Habitat—Along banks of streams, borders of woods in rich soil.
Part used—The granular powder separated from the strobiles.
Standard of strength—That of the U. S. Pharmacopœia, 1890; 1 c.c. representing 1 gram of the drug; or, practically, minim for grain.
Action and uses—Tonic and moderately narcotic. Used with advantage in delirium tremens, and wakefulness in connection with nervous irritation; it does not disorder the stomach **nor** cause constipation, as with opium; also useful in after pains, to suppress venereal desires, and to allay the pain attendant on gonorrheal disease.

PREPARATION.
Tincture Lupulin—Fl. ext. Lupulin, Lilly, 2 fl. ozs.; Alcohol, 14 fl. ozs.; Mix—Dose 1 to 2 fl. drs.

FL. EXT. LUPULIN COMP.......................Dose 15 to 30 m.
Standard of strength—One pint represents Lupulin, Lettuce and Scullcap, of each, 5½ troy ounces.
Action and uses—Mildly narcotic, nervine and antispasmodic.

FL. EXT. MACE....................................Dose 5 to 15 m.
Myristica fragrans Houttuyn. **Nat. Ord.—***Myristicaceæ.*
Synonyms—M. aromatica Lam., M. moschata Thunb., M. officinalis Linn. f.
Range—Molucca Islands; cultivated in tropical countries.
Habitat—On light soil in moist shady places.
Part used—The arillode of the seed.
Standard of strength—That of the U. S. Pharmacopœla, 1890; 1 c.c. representing 1 gram of the drug; or, practically, minim for grain.
Action and uses—Aromatic, stimulant and in large doses narcotic. Used mostly as a condiment.

PREPARATION.
Tincture Mace—Fl. ext. Mace, Lilly, 2 fl. ozs.; Alcohol, 14 fl. ozs.; Mix—Dose ½ to 1 fl. dr.

G. EXT. MAGNOLIA BARK........................Dose 30 to 60 m.
Magnolia **Virginiana** Linn. **Nat. Ord.—***Magnoliaceæ.*
Synonyms—M. Virginiana var. glauca Linn., M. glauca Linn.
Range—Near Cape Ann and New York to Pennsylvania, southward, near the coast.
Habitat—In swamps.
Part used—The bark.
Standard of strength—That of the U. S. Pharmacopœia, 1890; 1 c.c. representing 1 gram of the drug; or, practically, minim for grain.
Action and uses—An aromatic bitter tonic and diaphoretic useful in chronic rheumatism, remittent and intermittent fever. In the latter, freely used it will arrest the paroxysm.

FL. EXT. MAIDENHAIR..........................Dose 30 to 60 m.
Adiantum pedatum Linn. **Nat. Ord.—***Filices.*
Synonym—Rockfern.
Range—North Carolina to California and northward.
Habitat—Cool damp woods.
Part used—The fronds.
Standard of strength—That of the U. S. Pharmacopœia, 1890; 1 c.c. representing 1 gram of the drug; or, practically, minim for grain.
Action and uses—Refrigerant, expectorant, tonic and demulcent. Used in pulmonary catarrh. Reputed valuable in pleurisy and jaundice.

PREPARATION.
Tincture Maidenhair—Fl. ext. Maidenhair, Lilly, 2 fl. ozs.; Alcohol, 14 fl. ozs.; Mix—Dose ½ to 1 fl. oz.

STANDARD FLUID EXTRACTS.

81

FL. EXT. MALE FERN .... Dose 60 to 240 m.
Dryopteris Filix mas Schott. *and D. Marginalis* Gray.
Nat. Ord. — *Filices.*
Synonyms—Aspidium Filix-mas Swartz and A. marginale Swartz.
Range—Europe; in United States, Northern Michigan to Dakota and Colorado.
Habitat—Cool rocky woods.
Part used—The rhizome.
Standard of strength—That of the U. S. Pharmacopœia, 1890; 1 c.c. representing 1 gram of the drug; or, practically, minim for grain.
Action and uses—Used for the expulsion of tape-worm. The patient should live upon milk and a little bread for one day, and the following morning take a full dose of the fluid extract, repeating it in two or three hours. At noon the patient may resume the use of food, and in the evening a brisk cathartic should be given.

FL. MANACA .... Dose 5 to 15 m.
Brunfelsia Hopeana (Hook.) Benth.   Nat. Ord.—*Solanaceæ*
Synonym—Franciscea uniflora Don.
Range—Brazil is the source of the supply.
Part used—The root.
Standard of strength—That of the U. S. Pharmacopœia, 1890; 1 c.c. representing 1 gram of the drug; or, practically, minim for grain.
Action and uses—Diuretic, diaphoretic, alterative, antisyphilitic and emmenagogue. Reputed valuable in subacute and chronic rheumatism.

FL. EXT. MANDRAKE, U. S. .... Dose 5 to 15 m.
Podophyllum peltatum Linn.   Nat. Ord.—*Berberidaceæ.*
Synonyms—May apple, Wild lemon, Raccoon berry.
Range—North America; common.
Habitat—Rich woodlands.
Part used—The rhizome.
Standard of Strength—4 per cent. of resin.
Action and uses—Cathartic, emetic, alterative, hydragogue and sialagogue. In bilious or typhoid febrile diseases, it is very valuable as a cathartic or emetocathartic, often breaking up the disease at once. It is especially valuable in chronic hepatitis, arousing the liver to healthy action. In alterative doses it has been used successfully in scrofula, rheumatism and syphilitic diseases. In constipation it acts upon the bowels without disposing them to subsequent costiveness.

PREPARATION.

Tincture Mandrake—Fl. ext. Mandrake, Lilly, 2 fl. ozs.; Alcohol, 11½ fl. ozs.; Water, 2½ fl. ozs.; Mix the alcohol and water and add the fluid extract—Dose 2 to 4 drs.

FL. EXT. MANDRAKE COMP. .... Dose 10 to 20 m.
Standard of strength—One pint represents Mandrake, 6 troy ounces Jalap, 6 troy ounces; Senna, 4 troy ounces; Potassium carbonate, 120 grains, and aromatics.
Action and uses—Laxative and cathartic.

PREPARATION.

Tincture Mandrake Comp.—Fl. ext. Mandrake comp., Lilly, 2 fl. ozs.; Alcohol, 8 fl. ozs.; Water, 6 fl. ozs.; Mix the alcohol and water and add the fluid extract—Dose 2 to 4 drs.

FL. EXT. MANGO FRUIT .... Dose 30 to 60 m.
Garcinia Mangostana Linn.   Nat. Ord.—*Guttiferæ.*
Synonym—Wild mangosteen.
Range—Chiefly found in India and the East Indies; cultivated.
Part used—The fruit.
Standard of strength—That of the U. S. Pharmacopœia, 1890; 1 c.c. representing 1 gram of the drug; or, practically, minim for grain.
Action and uses—Astringent. Used in sore throat, nasal catarrh, diarrhea, dysentery, leucorrhea, etc.

FL. EXT. MANZANITA **LEAVES** .... **Dose 30 to 60 m.**
Arctostaphylos glauca Lindley.   **Nat. Ord.**—*Ericaceæ.*
Synonym—Bearberry.
Range—Mountains of California.
Habitat—Dry rocky places.
Part used—The leaves.
Standard of strength—That of the U. S. Pharmacopœia, 1890; 1 c.c. representing 1 gram of the drug; or, practically, minim for grain.
Action and uses—Astringent, tonic and diuretic. Indicated in diabetes, incontinence of urine, catarrh of the bladder, gleet, leucorrhœa and menorrhagia.

PREPARATION.

Tincture Manzanita—Fl. ext. Manzanita leaves, Lilly, 4 fl. ozs.; Diluted alcohol, 12 fl. ozs.; Mix—Dose 2 to 4 fl. drs.

FL. EXT. MARSHMALLOW HERB .... Dose 60 to 120 m.
Althæa officinalis Linn.   **Nat. Ord.**—*Malvaceæ.*
Range—Europe, **Western and Northern Asia; cultivated in** Europe and the United States.
Habitat—Salt marshes.
Part used—The herb.
Standard of strength—That of the U. S. Pharmacopœia, 1890; 1 c.c. representing 1 gram of the drug; or, practically, minim for grain.
Action and uses—Demulcent and diuretic. The infusion is valuable in treatment of diseases of the mucous tissues, as hoarseness, catarrh, pneumonia, gonorrhœa, vesical catarrh, etc., and in nearly all affections of the kidneys and bladder.

PREPARATION.

Infusion Marshmallow Herb—Fl. ext. Marshmallow herb, Lilly, 1 fl. oz.; Hot water, 15 fl. ozs.; Mix—Dose 2 to 4 fl. ozs.

FL. EXT. MARSHMALLOW ROOT .... **Dose 60 to 120 m.**
Althæa officinalis Linn.   **Nat. Ord.**—*Malvaceæ.*
Range—Europe, **Western and Northern Asia; cultivated in Europe and** the United States.
Habitat—Salt marshes.
Part used—The root.
Standard of strength—That of the U. S. Pharmacopœia, 1890; **1 c.c.** representing 1 gram of the drug; or, practically, minim for grain.
Action and uses—Demulcent and diuretic. The **infusion is valuable** in treatment of diseases of the mucous tissues, as **hoarseness, catarrh,** pneumonia, gonorrhœa, vesical catarrh, etc., and in **nearly all affections** of the kidneys and bladder.

PREPARATION.

Infusion Marshmallow Root—Fl. ext. Marshmallow root, Lilly, 1 fl. oz.; Hot water, 15 fl. ozs.; Mix—Dose 2 to 4 fl. ozs.

FL. EXT. **MASTERWORT** .... Dose 30 to 60 m.
Heracleum lanatum Michx.   Nat. Ord.—*Umbelliferæ.*
Synonym—Cow parsnip.
Range—Newfoundland to the Pacific, southward to North Carolina, Kentucky and Kansas.
Habitat—Wet ground.
Part used—The root.
Standard of strength—That of the U. S. Pharmacopœia, 1890; 1 c.c. representing 1 gram of the drug; or, practically, minim for grain.
Action and uses—Stimulant, carminative and antispasmodic. Used in flatulency and dyspepsia. Also recommended in asthma, amenorrhœa, dysmenorrhœa, etc.

PREPARATION.

Infusion Masterwort—Fl. ext. Masterwort, Lilly, 1 fl. oz.; Hot water, 15 fl. ozs.; Mix—Dose 1 to 2 fl. ozs.

FL. EXT. MATICO . . . . **Dose 30 to 60 m.**
Piper angustifolium Ruiz et Pavon. **Nat. Ord.**—*Piperaceæ.*
Synonyms—P. elongatum Vahl., Artanthe elongata Miquel.
Range—Peru and other parts of tropical South America; cultivated.
Habitat—Moist woodlands.
Part used—The leaves.
Standard of strength—That of the U. S. Pharmacopœia, 1890; 1 c.c. representing 1 gram of the drug; or, practically, minim for grain.
Action and uses—Diuretic, stimulant and tonic. Matico is used externally to check hemorrhage. In the form of fluid extract, it has been highly recommended in hemorrhage and diseases of the mucous membranes, including gonorrhea and leucorrhea.

PREPARATIONS.

Tincture Matico, U. S.—Fl. ext. Matico, Lilly, 1½ fl. ozs.; Alcohol, 10 fl. ozs.; Water, 5½ fl. ozs.; Mix—Dose 2 to 4 fl. drs.

Matico Bitters—Fl. exts. Matico, Gentian, Orange peel and Allspice, Lilly, of each, ½ fl. oz.; Syrup, 4 fl. ozs.; Diluted alcohol, 10 fl. ozs.; Mix—Dose ½ fl. oz.

Infusion Matico—Fl. ext. Matico, Lilly, 1 fl. oz.; Hot water, 15 fl. ozs.; Mix—Dose 1 to 2 fl. ozs.

FL. EXT. MERCURY WEED. . . . . **Dose 15 to 20 m.**
Mercurialis annua Linn. **Nat. Ord.**—*Euphorbiaceæ.*
Range—Europe.
Part used—The herb.
Standard of strength—That of the U. S. Pharmacopœia, 1890; 1 c.c. representing 1 gram of the drug; or, practically, minim for grain.
Action and uses—Purgative and emmenagogue. It has some repute as a diuretic and is used in the treatment of syphilis.

FL. EXT. MEZEREUM, **U. S.** . . . . **Not used internally.**
Daphne Mezereum Linn. **Nat. Ord.**—*Thymelæaceæ.*
Synonyms—Mezereum officinarum Meyer,—Mezereon, Olive spurge.
Range—Europe and Siberia; escaped from cultivation in Northeastern United States and Canada.
Habitat—Hilly woodlands.
Part used—The bark.
Standard of strength—That of the U. S. Pharmacopœia, 1890; 1 c.c. representing 1 gram of the drug; or, practically, minim for grain.
Action and uses—Sialagogue and an acrid irritant poison. Laxative and diuretic in small doses but rarely employed alone. Its principal use is as a local irritant.

PREPARATIONS.

Liniment Mustard Comp., U. S.—Fl. ext. Mezereum, Lilly, 3¼ fl. ozs.; Camphor, 1 avd. oz.; Castor oil, 2¼ fl. ozs.; Volatile oil mustard, 230 m.; Alcohol, sufficient to make one pint; Dissolve the camphor and oils in the alcohol and add the fluid extract.

Ointment Mezereum—Fl. ext. Mezereum, Lilly, 4 fl. ozs.; Yellow wax, 2 avd. ozs.; Lard, 13½ avd. ozs.; Melt the lard and wax together on a water bath, add the fluid extract, heat until the alcohol is driven off, remove from the fire and stir till cold.

FL. EXT. MISTLETOE......................................Dose 30 to 60 m.
Phoradendron flavescens (Pursh) Nutt.
                                 Nat. Ord.—*Loranthaceæ.*
Synonyms—Viscum flavescens Pursh,—American mistletoe.
Range—New Jersey to Southern Indiana, Missouri and southward.
Habitat—Parasitic on various deciduous trees.
Part used—Leaves and young twigs.
Standard of strength—That of the U. S. Pharmacopœia, 1890; 1 c.c.
representing 1 gram of the drug; or, practically, minim for grain.
Action and uses—It is said to be narcotic, antispasmodic and tonic;
has been found beneficial in epilepsy, insanity, paralysis and other
nervous diseases.   It has been recommended as an oxytocic, claiming
the advantage over ergot of being more prompt and certain.

PREPARATIONS.

Tincture Mistletoe—Fl. ext. Mistletoe, Lilly, 4 fl. ozs.; Alcohol.
9 fl. ozs.; Water, 3 fl. ozs.; Mix—Dose 2 to 4 fl. drs.

Infusion Mistletoe—Fl. ext. Mistletoe, Lilly, 1 fl. oz.; Hot water, 15
fl. ozs.; Mix—Dose 1 to 2 fl. ozs.

FL. EXT. MOTHERWORT......................................Dose 30 to 60 m.
Leonurus Cardiaca Linn.   **Nat. Ord.—***Labiatæ.*
Range—Europe; naturalized in the United States.
Habitat—Waste ground, along roadsides and near dwellings.
Part used—The herb.
Standard of strength—That of the U. S. Pharmacopœia, 1890; 1 c.c.
representing 1 gram of the drug; or, practically, minim for grain.
Action and uses—Emmenagogue, nervine, antispasmodic and laxa-
tive.   Usually given in warm infusion in amenorrhea from colds, and in
suppressed lochia; also in hysteria.   Recommended in nervous com-
plaints peculiar to females.

PREPARATIONS.

Tincture Motherwort—Fl. ext. Motherwort, Lilly, 2 fl. ozs.; Alcohol, 5 fl. ozs.; Water, 9 fl. ozs.; Mix the alcohol and water and add the
fluid extract—Dose 1 to 4 fl. drs.

Infusion Motherwort—Fl. ext. Motherwort, Lilly, 1 fl. oz.; Hot
water, 15 fl. ozs.; Mix—Dose 1 to 2 fl. ozs.

FL. EXT. MOUNTAIN ASH......................................Dose 10 to 30 m.
Sorbus Americana Marsh.   **Nat. Ord.—***Rosaceæ.*
Synonyms—S. microcarpa Pursh, Pyrus Americana D. C.,—American
mountain ash.
Range—Newfoundland to North Carolina, west to Northern Michigan
and Minnesota.
Habitat—Swamps and mountain woods; cultivated.
Part used—The bark.
Standard of strength—That of the U. S. Pharmacopœia, 1890; 1 c.c.
representing 1 gram of the drug; or, practically, minim for grain.
Action and uses—Tonic and astringent.   Used in infusion as a gargle
in acute affections of the tonsils and pharynx.

PREPARATION.

Infusion Mountain Ash—Fl. ext. Mountain ash, Lilly, 1 fl. oz.;
Hot water, 15 fl. ozs.; Mix—Dose ½ to 1 fl. oz.

FL. EXT. MOUNTAIN LAUREL......................................Dose 10 to 40 m.
Kalmia latifolia Linn.   **Nat. Ord.—***Ericaceæ.*
Synonyms—Broad leaved laurel, Calico bush.
Range—Canada, Maine, along mountains to Florida, west to Ohio, Ken-
tucky and Tennessee.

Habitat—Rocky hills and damp soil.

Part used—The leaves.

Standard of strength—That of the U. S. Pharmacopœia, 1890; 1 c.c. representing 1 gram of the drug; or, practically, minim for grain.

Action and uses—In overdoses narcotic poison. Antisyphilitic, sedative and astringent. Valuable in primary and secondary syphilis, febrile and inflammatory diseases. Also in active hemorrhages, diarrhea and flux. This remedy should always be used with prudence, and the dose diminished or suspended if unfavorable symptoms occur.

PREPARATION.

Infusion Mountain Laurel—Fl. ext. Mountain laurel, Lilly, 1 fl. oz.; Hot water, 15 fl. ozs.; Mix—Dose 2 to 4 fl. drs.

FL. EXT. MOUNTAIN SAGE....................Dose 60 to 120 m.
Artemisia frigida Willd. **Nat. Ord.**—*Compositæ.*

Synonyms—Sierra salvia, Sage brush.

Range—Northern Asia; North America, from Saskatchewan to Minnesota and Western Texas, west to Idaho, Nevada and New Mexico.

Habitat—Dry hills and rocks.

Part used—The leaves and inflorescence.

Standard of strength—That of the U. S. Pharmacopœia, 1890; 1 c.c. representing 1 gram of the drug; or, practically, minim for grain.

Action and uses—Largely used by the people of the mountainous regions of Western United States in mountain fever and all malarial diseases.

PREPARATION.

Infusion Mountain Sage—Fl. ext. Mountain sage, Lilly, 2 fl. ozs.; Hot water, 14 fl. ozs.; Mix—Dose 1 to 2 fl. ozs.

FL. EXT. MUGWORT....................Dose 60 to 120 m.
Artemisia vulgaris Linn. **Nat. Ord.**—*Compositæ.*

Range—Europe; naturalized in the United States and Canada.

Habitat—Waste places near dwellings, along roadsides.

Part used—The herb.

Standard of strength—That of the U. S. Pharmacopœia, 1890; 1 c.c. representing 1 gram of the drug; or, practically, minim for grain.

Action and uses—Anthelmintic, tonic, antispasmodic. Said to be beneficial in epilepsy, hysteria and amenorrhea.

PREPARATION.

Infusion Mugwort—Fl. ext. Mugwort, Lilly, 1 fl. oz.; Hot water, 15 fl. ozs.; Mix—Dose 2 to 4 fl. ozs.

FL. EXT. MULLEIN LEAVES....................Dose 60 to 120 m.
Verbascum Thapsus Linn. **Nat. Ord.**—*Scrophulariaceæ.*

Range—Europe; naturalized in the United States, a common weed.

Habitat—In waste ground, along roadsides, etc.

Part used—The leaves.

Standard of strength—That of the U. S. Pharmacopœia, 1890; 1 c.c. representing 1 gram of the drug; or, practically, minim for grain.

Action and uses—Demulcent, diuretic, anodyne and antispasmodic. The infusion is useful in coughs, catarrh, hemoptysis, diarrhea and dysentery.

PREPARATION.

Infusion Mullein Leaves—Fl. ext. Mullein leaves, Lilly, 2 fl. ozs.; Hot water, 14 fl. ozs.; Mix—Dose 1 to 2 fl. ozs.

WHEN ORDERING OR PRESCRIBING.

FL. EXT. MUSK ROOT .... Dose 2 to 10 m.

Ferula Sumbul (Kauffman) Hooker.   **Nat. Ord.—*Umbelliferæ.***

Synonyms—Euryangium Sumbul Kauffman,—Sumbul, U. S.,—Jatamansi.

Range—Central and Northeastern Asia.

Habitat—In mountainous districts.

Part used—The root.

Standard of strength—That of the U. S. Pharmacopœia, 1890; 1 c.c. representing 1 gram of the drug; or, practically, minim for grain.

Action and uses—Nervous stimulant and tonic. It has been recommended in low typhus fevers, in gastric spasm, hysteria, delirium tremens, diarrhœa, dysentery, leucorrhœa, gleet, chlorosis, asthma and chronic bronchitis.

PREPARATION.

Tincture Musk Root, U. S.—Fl. ext. Musk root, Lilly, 1½ fl. ozs.; Alcohol, 14½ fl. ozs.; Mix—Dose 20 to 60 m.

FL. EXT. MUSTARD SEED .... Dose, diluted, 10 to 20 m.

Sinapis nigra (Linn.) Koch.   **Nat. Ord.—*Cruciferæ.***

Synonyms—Brassica nigra Koch.,—Black mustard.

Range—Asia and Southern Europe; naturalized in the United States.

Habitat—Rich soil near cultivated ground, along roadsides and fences.

Part used—The seed.

Standard of strength—That of the U. S. Pharmacopœia, 1890; 1 c.c. representing 1 gram of the drug; or, practically, minim for grain.

Action and uses—Internally it may be employed as an emetic in indigestion or narcotic poisoning. Externally as an addition to liniments in muscular rheumatism, neuralgia, etc.

FL. EXT. MYRRH .... Dose 10 to 20 m.

Commiphora Myrrha (Nees) Engler.   **Nat. Ord.—*Burseraceæ.***

Synonyms—Balsamodendron Myrrha Nees,—Myrrha, U. S.

Range—Eastern Africa and Arabia.

Habitat—Sandy soil; in Southwestern Arabia found in acacia and euphorbia growths.

Part used—The gum resin.

Standard of strength—That of the U. S. Pharmacopœia, 1890; 1 c.c. representing 1 gram of the drug; or, practically, minim for grain.

Action and uses—Seldom used internally; used externally as an application to stimulate indolent and foul ulcers and promote the exfoliation of bones. Diluted with water it is applied to spongy gums, aphthous sore mouth, etc. Internally expectorant and emmenagogue.

PREPARATION.

Tincture Myrrh, U. S.—Fl. ext. Myrrh, Lilly, 3¾ fl. ozs.; Alcohol 12¼ fl. ozs.; Mix—Dose 15 to 30 m.

FL. EXT. MYRRH AND CAPSICUM .... Dose, diluted, 5 to 10 m.

Standard of strength—One pint represents Myrrh, 12 troy ounces; Capsicum, 3 troy ounces.

Action and uses—Used almost exclusively for preparing Number Six, or Rheumatism drops.

PREPARATION.

Number Six—Fl. ext. Myrrh and capsicum, Lilly, 2 fl. ozs.; Alcohol, 14 fl. ozs.; Mix—Dose 20 to 60 m.

FL. EXT. NETTLE ROOT.................... ....Dose 15 to 30 m.
Urtica dioica Linn. **Nat. Ord.**—*Urticaceæ.*

Synonym—Stinging nettle.

Range—Europe; naturalized in North America, Canada, New England to South Carolina, west to Minnesota and Missouri.

Habitat—Waste places, along roadsides.

Part used—The root.

Standard of strength—That of the U. S. Pharmacopœia, 1890; 1 c.c. representing 1 gram of the drug; or, practically, minim for grain.

Action and uses—Valuable in diarrhea, dysentery, hemorrhoids, hemorrhages, gravel and scorbutic affections. The compound syrup is an excellent remedy in bowel complaints of either children or adults.

PREPARATIONS.

Syrup Nettle Root—Fl. ext. Nettle root, Lilly, 4 fl. ozs.; Syrup, 12 fl. ozs.; Mix—Dose 1 to 2 fl. drs.

Syrup Nettle Root Comp.—Fl. exts. Nettle root and Cherry bark, Lilly, of each, 2 fl. ozs.; Fl. ext. Blackberry root, Lilly, 1 fl. oz.; Syrup, 11 fl. ozs.; Mix—Dose 1 to 2 fl. drs.

FL. EXT. NUTMEG................ ....Dose 5 to 20 m.
Myristica fragrans Houttuyn. **Nat. Ord.**—*Myristicaceæ.*

Synonyms—M. aromatica Lam., M. moschata Thunb., M. officinalis Linn. f.,—Myristica, U. S.

Range—Molucca Islands; cultivated in tropical countries.

Habitat—On light soil in moist shady places.

Part used—The seed.

Standard of strength—That of the U. S. Pharmacopœia, 1890; 1 c.c. representing 1 gram of the drug; or, practically, minim for grain.

Action and uses—Narcotic and intoxicant. Mostly used as a condiment.

FL. EXT. NUX VOMICA, U. S. ....Dose 1 to 3 m.
Strychnos Nux Vomica Linn. **Nat. Ord.**—*Loganaceæ.*

Range—India and East Indian Islands.

Part used—The seed.

Standard of strength—100 c.c. contains 1.5 grains of total alkaloids.

Action and uses—POISONOUS IN OVER DOSES. It stimulates digestion. An excellent nerve tonic; of value as a tonic in general functional atony and relaxation; of value in paralysis depending upon a depressed state of the spinal or other motor centers. When there is inflammation or irritation of these latter, it should not be employed, as it may do great injury by increasing the irritation. It has been recommended in lead paralysis. Its value in amaurosis from abuse of alcohol and tobacco is undisputed. Headache and giddiness, associated with nerve troubles which manifest themselves in the eye, are frequently relieved, though the nerve be atrophied and the eye be blind. As a respiratory stimulant in dyspnea dependent upon pulmonic affections, such as chronic bronchitis, emphysema and phthisis, it is considered of great value. It is useful in dyspepsia or constipation, or diarrhea connected with atony of visceral muscular coat, in local paralysis as prolapse of the rectum, atonic retention of urine or incontinence, loss of voluntary motion, infantile paralysis.

Antidotes—Tannic acid or a soluble salt of iodine, then emetics or the stomach pump followed by absolute quiet. Antagonists are chloral, tobacco, chloroform or other inhalations. The bladder must be frequently evacuated to prevent reabsorption. Artificial respiration.

PREPARATION.

Tincture Nux Vomica, U. S.—Fl. ext. Nux vomica, Lilly, 3¼ fl. ozs.; Alcohol, 75%, 9½ fl. ozs.; Water, 3¼ fl. ozs. Mix—Dose 5 to 20 m.

WHEN ORDERING OR PRESCRIBING.

FL. EXT. OPIUM, AQUEOUS (Tr. Opii Deodorata, U. S.)

Dose 10 to 15 m.

Standard of strength—6 grains of morphine in each fluid ounce.

Action and uses—Narcotic Poison. Like opium but producing less cerebral distress than laudanum and not so liable to constipate.

Antidotes—Atropine is the antagonist but must be used with caution; otherwise, belladonna narcosis will be substituted for that of opium. Three doses, of 1-120 grain each, given hypodermically every fifteen minutes, are usually sufficient. Caffeine is often resorted to in the form of strong black coffee frequently administered. Potassium permanganate is said to be a perfect chemical antidote, but it must be promptly administered. The measures chiefly indicated are to evacuate the stomach, maintain circulation and respiration, faradization of the chest muscles, cold affusion and evacuation of the bladder.

FL. EXT. OPIUM, CAMPHORATED ....For making Paregoric.

Standard of strength—1.96 grains of morphine in each fluid ounce; thus being eight times the strength of Tr. Opium Camphorated, U. S. Each fluid ounce of the latter preparation contains 0.245 grains of morphine.

PREPARATION.

Tincture Opium Camphorated, U. S., (Paregoric)—Fl. ext. Opium, camphorated, Lilly, 2 fl. ozs.; Diluted alcohol, 14 fl. ozs.; Mix—Dose, for infants, 5 to 20 m.; for adults, 60 to 120 m.

FL. EXT. OPIUM, CONCENTRATED.

CAUTION—This preparation is used solely for conveniently producing the weaker preparations of opium.

Standard of strength—24 grains of morphine in each fluid ounce.

Antidotes—Atropine is the antagonist but must be used with caution; otherwise, belladonna narcosis will be substituted for that of opium. Three doses, of 1-120 grain each, given hypodermically every fifteen minutes, are usually sufficient. Caffeine is often resorted to in the form of strong black coffee frequently administered. Potassium permanganate is said to be a perfect chemical antidote, but it must be promptly administered. The measures chiefly indicated are to evacuate the stomach, maintain circulation and respiration, faradization of the chest muscles, cold affusion and evacuation of the bladder.

PREPARATIONS.

Tincture Opium, U. S.—Fl. ext. Opium, concentrated, Lilly, 4 fl. ozs.; Diluted alcohol, 12 fl. ozs.; Mix—Dose 5 to 15 m.

Vinegar Opium, U. S.—Fl. ext. Opium, concentrated, Lilly, 4 fl. ozs.; Fl. ext. Nutmeg, Lilly, ½ fl. ozs.; Sugar, 8½ avd. ozs.; Diluted acetic acid, sufficient to make one pint. Mix and agitate till the sugar is dissolved—Dose 5 to 15 m.

Wine Opium, U. S.—Fl. ext. Opium, concentrated, Lilly, 4 fl. ozs.; Fl. exts. Cinnamon and Cloves, Lilly, of each, 75 m.; Alcohol, 1½ fl. ozs.; White wine, 10 fl. ozs.; Mix and filter—Dose 5 to 15 m.

FL. EXT. ORANGE PEEL, BITTER ....Dose 15 to 30 m.

Citrus vulgaris Risso.   Nat. Ord.—*Rutaceæ.*

Synonym—Aurantii Amari, U. S.

Range—Northern India; cultivated in subtropical countries.

Part used—The rind of the fruit.

Standard of strength—That of the U. S. Pharmacopœia, 1890, 1 c.c. representing 1 gram of the drug; or, practically, minim for grain.

Action and uses—A mild bitter tonic and aromatic.

PREPARATIONS.

Tincture Orange Peel, Bitter, U. S.—Fl. ext. Orange peel, bitter, Lilly, 3¼ fl. ozs.; Diluted alcohol, 12¾ fl. ozs.; Mix—Dose 2 to 4 fl. drs.

Syrup Orange Peel, Bitter—Fl. ext. Orange peel, bitter, Lilly, 2 fl. ozs.; Syrup, 14 fl. ozs.; Mix—Dose 1 to 2 fl. drs. The official syrup is prepared from the peel of the sweet orange.

FL. EXT. ORANGE PEEL, SWEET, for syrup......Dose 30 to 60 m.

Citrus Aurantium Linn.   Nat. Ord.—*Rutaceæ.*

Synonym—Aurantii Dulcis, U. S.

Range—Northern India; cultivated in subtropical countries. (Orange of commerce.)

Part used—The rind of the fruit.

Standard of strength—That of the U. S. Pharmacopœia, 1890; 1 c.c. representing 1 gram of the drug; or, practically, minim for grain.

Action and uses—Aromatic. Used as an adjuvant.

PREPARATIONS.

Syrup Orange, U. S.—Fl. ext. Orange peel, sweet, Lilly, 2½ fl. ozs.; Syrup, 29½ fl. ozs.

Tincture Orange Peel, U. S.—Fl. ext. Orange peel, sweet, Lilly, 3½ fl. ozs.; Alcohol, 12½ fl. ozs.

Elixir Orange—Simple Elixir—Fl. ext. Orange peel, sweet, Lilly, 1 fl. ozs.; Alcohol, 16 fl. ozs.; Syrup, 20 fl. ozs.; Water, 16 fl. ozs.; Mix the alcohol, syrup and water and add the fluid extract.

FL. EXT. ORANGE PEEL COMP.

Standard of strength—One pint represents Sweet orange peel, 12 troy ounces; Coriander, 2 troy ounces; Cardamom, ⅔ troy ounce; Cinnamon, 1 troy ounce; Anise, ⅔ troy ounce.

Action and uses—An elegant aromatic adjuvant.

PREPARATION.

Elixir Orange Peel Comp.—Fl. ext. Orange peel comp., Lilly, 2 fl. ozs.; Alcohol, 4 fl. ozs.; Water, 7 fl. ozs.; Syrup 5 fl. ozs.

FL. EXT. ORRIS ROOT..................Dose 5 to 15 m.

Iris Florentina Linn.   Nat. Ord.—*Irideæ.*

Synonym—White flag.

Range—Italy and other parts of Southern Europe; cultivated.

Part used—The rhizome.

Standard of strength—That of the U. S. Pharmacopœia, 1890; 1 c.c. representing 1 gram of the drug; or, practically, minim for grain.

Action and uses—Formerly esteemed as a diuretic. Its principal use, however, is in perfumery, cosmetics, sachets, etc., for its odor.

FL. EXT. PANSY........................ ...Dose 30 to 60 m.

Viola tricolor Linn.   Nat. Ord.—*Violaceæ.*

Range—Northern Asia, Europe; naturalized in the United States, New York to Iowa, Kansas and southward.

Habitat—Dry or sandy woodlands.

Part used—The herb.

Standard of strength—That of the U. S. Pharmacopœia, 1890; 1 c.c. representing 1 gram of the drug; or, practically, minim for grain.

Action and uses—Pectoral, emollient, laxative and vulnerary. Recommended in some forms of eczema, also in bronchitis.

FL. EXT. PAWPAW SEED..................Dose 15 to 30 m.

Asimina triloba (Linn.) Dunal.   Nat. Ord.—*Anonaceæ.*

Synonym—Anona triloba Linn.

Range—New York and Pennsylvania to Illinois, Southeastern Nebraska and southward.

Habitat—Rich woodlands, along banks of streams.

Part used—The seed.

Standard of strength—That of the U. S. Pharmacopœia, 1890; 1 c.c. representing 1 gram of the drug; or, practically, minim for grain.

Action and uses—Emetic.

FL. EXT. PAREIRA BRAVA, U. S..................Dose 60 to 120 m.
Chondodendron tomentosum Ruiz et Pavon.
        Nat. Ord.—*Menispermaceæ.*
Synonyms—Pareira U. S.,—Velvet leaf, Ice vine.
Range—Peru and Brazil.
Habitat—Hilly woodlands.
Part used—The root.
Standard of strength—That of the U. S. Pharmacopœia, 1890; 1 c.c. representing 1 gram of the drug; or, practically, minim for grain.
Action and uses—Used with advantage in chronic cystitis, in irritable bladder and in chronic gonorrhea, and appears to exert a stimulant action upon the mucous membrane of the whole genito-urinary apparatus. It is said, also, to be tonic and slightly aperient, so that it is specially valuable in urinary diseases, where there is feebleness of digestion and a tendency to costiveness.

PREPARATION.

Infusion Pareira Brava—Fl. ext. Pareira brava, Lilly, 1 fl. oz.; Hot water 15 fl. ozs.; Mix—Dose 1 to 2 fl. ozs.

FL. EXT. PARSLEY ROOT ....Dose 30 to 60 m.
Carum Petroselinum Bentham.   **Nat. Ord.**—*Umbelliferæ.*
Synonyms—Petroselinum sativum Hoffm., Apium Petroselinum Linn.
Range—Southern Europe; cultivated extensively.
Part used—The root.
Standard of strength—That of the U. S. Pharmacopœia, 1890; 1 c.c. representing 1 gram of the drug; or, practically, minim for grain.
Action and uses—Aperient and diuretic and is occasionally used in dropsical and nephritic affections. Very useful in dropsy, especially that following scarlatina and other exanthematous diseases.

PREPARATION.

Infusion Parsley Root—Fl. ext. Parsley root, Lilly, 2 fl. ozs.; Hot water, 14 fl. ozs.; Mix—Dose ½ to 1 fl. oz.

FL. EXT. PARSLEY SEED ....Dose 30 to 60 m.
Carum Petroselinum Benth.   **Nat. Ord.**—*Umbelliferæ.*
Synonyms—Petroselinum sativum Hoffm., Apium Petroselinum Linn.
Range—Southern Europe; cultivated extensively.
Part used—The fruit.
Standard of strength—That of the U. S. Pharmacopœia, 1890; 1 c.c. representing 1 gram of the drug; or, practically, minim for grain.
Action and uses—Aperient and diuretic, and is occasionally used in dropsical and nephritic affections. Very useful in dropsy, especially that following scarlatina and other exanthematous diseases.

PREPARATION.

Infusion Parsley Seed—Fl. ext. Parsley seed, Lilly, 2 fl. ozs.; Hot water, 14 fl. ozs.; Mix—Dose ½ to 1 fl. oz.

FL. EXT. PASSION FLOWER.................Dose 15 to 30 m.
Passiflora incarnata Linn.   **Nat. Ord.**—*Passifloraceæ.*
Synonym—Maypops.
Range—Virginia to Florida, west to Missouri and Arkansas.
Habitat—Dry soil.
Part used—The leaves, inflorescence and younger portions of the vine.
Standard of strength—That of the U. S. Pharmacopœia, 1890; 1 c.c. representing 1 gram of the drug; or, practically, minim for grain.
Action and uses—Neurotic, antispasmodic, soporific, anodyne and sedative. It is claimed to exert a special influence over the ganglia of the thorax, pelvis and abdominal regions and to quiet the excitement of the medulla oblongata. Recommended in insomnia, neuralgia, tetanus, chorea and nervous headache.

FL. EXT. PEACH LEAVES.................................Dose 30 to 60 m.

Prunus Persicaria (Linn.) Seibold and Tuccarini.
Nat. Ord.—*Rosaceæ*.

Synonyms—Amygdalus Persica Linn., Persica vulgaris D. C.

Range—Southwestern Asia; cultivated throughout a large part of temperate and warm temperate zones.

Part used—The leaves.

Standard of strength—That of the U. S. Pharmacopœia, 1890; 1 c.c. representing 1 **gram** of the drug; or, practically, minim for grain.

Action and uses—Sedative and laxative.

PREPARATION.

Syrup Peach Leaves—Fl. ext. Peach leaves, Lilly, 4 fl. ozs.; Syrup, 12 fl. ozs.; Mix—Dose 2 to 4 fl. drs.

FL. EXT. PELLITORY.

Anacyclus Pyrethrum (Linn.) D. C.   **Nat. Ord.**—*Compositæ*.

Synonyms—Anthemis Pyrethrum Linn.,—Pyrethrum, U. S.,—Pellitory of Spain, Spanish chamomile.

Range—Northern Africa, especially Algeria.

Habitat—Highlands between the coast and the desert.

Part used—The root.

Standard of strength—That of the U. S. Pharmacopœia, 1890; 1 c.c. representing 1 **gram** of the drug; or, practically, minim for grain.

Action and uses—Not used internally. A powerful local irritant, acting as a rubefacient when externally applied. The decoction has been used as a gargle in relaxation of the uvula. The root chewed has been found valuable for neuralgic and rheumatic affections of the head and face and palsy of the tongue.

PREPARATIONS.

Tincture Pellitory, U. S.—Fl. ext. Pellitory, Lilly, 3¼ fl. ozs.; Alcohol, 12¾ fl. ozs.; Use externally

Infusion Pellitory—Fl. ext. Pellitory, Lilly, 1 fl. oz.; Hot water, 15 fl. ozs.; Mix—Use as a gargle **in palsy of the** tongue or throat and in relaxation of the uvula.

FL. EXT. PENNYROYAL............................Dose 60 to 30 m.

Hedeoma pulegioides (Linn.) Persoon.   **Nat. Ord.**—*Labiatæ*.

Synonyms—Cunila pulegioides Linn.,—Tickweed, Squawmint.

Range—Common from New **England to** Dakota and southward.

Habitat—Sandy or dry **soil, in woodlands and along roadsides.**

Part used—The leaves **and inflorescence.**

Standard of strength—That of the U. S. Pharmacopœia, 1890; 1 c.c. representing 1 gram of the drug; or, practically, minim for grain.

Action and uses—Stimulant, carminative, diaphoretic and emmenagogue. The warm infusion used freely will promote perspiration, restore suppressed lochia and excite the menstrual discharge when recently checked; a large draught to be taken at bedtime, the feet being previously bathed in warm water.

PREPARATION.

Infusion Pennyroyal—Fl. ext. Pennyroyal, Lilly, 2 fl. ozs.; Hot water, 14 fl. ozs.; Mix—Dose 1 to 3 fl. ozs.

FL. EXT. PEONY..Dose 15 to 30 m.

Pæonia officinalis Linn.   **Nat. Ord.**—*Ranunculaceæ*.

Synonym—Double peony.

Range—Southern Europe; introduced in the United States; cultivated extensively as an ornamental plant.

Part used—The root stock.

Standard of strength—That of the U. S. Pharmacopœia, 1890; 1 c.c. representing 1 gram of the drug; or, practically, minim for grain.

Action and uses—Tonic and antispasmodic. Employed with success in chorea, spasms and various nervous affections.

PREPARATION.

Infusion Peony—Fl. ext. Peony, Lilly, 1 fl. oz.; Hot water, 15 fl. ozs.; Mix—Dose ½ to 1 fl. oz.

FL. EXT. PEPPERMINT.................... Dose 60 to 120 m.

Mentha piperita Linn. Nat. Ord.—*Labiatæ.*

Range—Asia, Europe and North America; common, escaped from cultivation.

Habitat—Along brooks and in wet places.

Part used—The leaves and inflorescence.

Standard of strength—That of the U. S. Pharmacopœia, 1890; 1 c.c. representing 1 gram of the drug; or, practically, minim for grain.

Action and uses—A powerful diffusive stimulant. Antispasmodic, carminative and stomachic. Used in the treatment of gastrodynia, flatulent colic, hysteria and spasms or cramps of the stomach.

PREPARATIONS.

Spirit Peppermint, U. S.—Fl. ext. Peppermint, Lilly, 1½ fl. drs.; Oil peppermint, 12½ fl. drs.; Alcohol, 14½ fl. ozs.; Mix and filter—Dose 5 to 15 drops on sugar.

Infusion Peppermint—Fl. ext. Peppermint, Lilly, 1 fl. oz.; Hot water, 15 fl. ozs.; Mix—Dose 2 to 4 fl. ozs.

FL. EXT. PICHI .... Dose 10 to 40 m.

Fabiana imbricata Ruiz et Pavon. Nat. Ord.—*Solanaceæ.*

Range—Chili and Argentine Republic.

Habitat—Sandy fields and on dry hills.

Part used—The leaves, inflorescence and young twigs.

Standard of strength—That of the U. S. Pharmacopœia, 1890; 1 c.c. representing 1 gram of the drug; or, practically, minim for grain.

Action and uses—Valued in urinary disorders. Has also been used in dyspepsia and with much success in vesical catarrh.

PREPARATION.

Infusion Pichi—Fl. ext. Pichi, Lilly, 1 fl. oz.; Hot water, 15 fl. ozs.; Mix—Dose ½ to 1 fl. oz.

FL. EXT. PIMENTO .... Dose 10 to 40 m.

Pimenta officinalis Lindley. Nat. Ord.—*Myrtaceæ.*

Synonyms—Eugenia Pimenta D. C.,—Pimenta U. S.,—Allspice.

Range—Tropical America; cultivated in Jamaica on limestone hills near the coast.

Part used—The nearly ripe fruit.

Standard of strength—That of the U. S. Pharmacopœia, 1890; 1 c.c. representing 1 gram of the drug; or, practically, minim for grain.

Action and uses—Aromatic stimulant, and is used as a condiment to stimulate the digestive organs when they are suffering from exhaustion. Used to relieve flatulence and to correct the tendency of purgatives to gripe.

FL. EXT. PINK ROOT, **U. S.**...................Dose 60 to 120 m.

Spigelia Marylandica Linn.   **Nat. Ord.** - *Loganaceæ.*

Synonyms—Lonicera Marylandica Linn.,—Spigelia U. S.

Range—New Jersey to Wisconsin and Texas.

Habitat—Rich soil in the borders of woods.

Part used—The rhizome and roots.

Standard of strength—That of the U. S. Pharmacopœia, 1890; 1 c.c. representing 1 gram of the drug; or, practically, minim for grain.

Action and uses—Anthelmintic. An efficient remedy in case of the round worms or lumbricoids, and in moderate doses entirely safe, but in over doses it has narcotic properties. A brisk cathartic should follow its use.

PREPARATION.

Infusion Pink Root—Fl. ext. Pink root, Lilly, 1 fl. oz.; Hot water, 15 fl. ozs.; Mix—Dose 1 to 4 fl. ozs.

FL. EXT. PINK ROOT AND SENNA ....Dose **60 to 240 m.**

Standard of strength—One pint represents Pink root, 10 troy ounces; Senna, 6 troy ounces; Potassium carbonate, ½ troy ounce; Oil anise, Oil caraway, of each, 20 m.

Action and uses—Anthelmintic and cathartic. The doses for children are from 30 to 60 m., repeated every four hours until it purges.

FL. EXT. PIPSISSEWA, **U. S.**.........................**Dose 30 to 60 m.**

Chimaphila umbellata (Linn.) Nutt.   **Nat. Ord.**—*Ericaceæ.*

Synonyms—Pyrola umbellata Linn., Chimaphila U. S.,—Prince's pine.

Range—United States and northern continents.

Habitat—In dry woods, especially in pine forests.

Part used—The leaves.

Standard of strength—That of the U. S. Pharmacopœia, 1890; 1 c.c. representing 1 gram of the drug; or, practically, minim for grain.

Action and uses—Tonic, diuretic, astringent and alterative. Prof. Geo. B. Wood has commended it highly in external scrofula, asserting that he had large experience with it, and that in power over the disease it stands next to cod liver oil and the preparations of iodine and iron. Dr. John King states that the decoction alone has cured ascites, and been advantageous in strangury, chronic gonorrhœa and catarrh of the bladder. In urinary disorders it may be used as a substitute for uva ursi.

PREPARATIONS.

Syrup Pipsissewa—Fl. ext. Pipsissewa, Lilly, 4 fl. ozs.; Syrup, 12 fl. ozs.; Mix—Dose 2 to 4 fl. drs.

Infusion Pipsissewa—Fl ext. Pipsissewa, Lilly, 1 fl. oz.; Hot water, 15 fl. ozs.; Mix—Dose 1 to 2 fl. ozs.

FL. EXT. PLAINTAIN LEAVES.... ....Dose 120 to 240 m.

Plantago major Linn.   **Nat. Ord.**—*Plantaginaceæ.*

Range—Europe; introduced in most parts of the United States from Europe but native from Lake Superior, Northern Minnesota and northward.

Habitat—In waste places, around dwellings and along roadsides.

Part used—The leaves.

Standard of strength—That of the U. S. Pharmacopœia, 1890; 1 c.c. representing 1 gram of the drug; or, practically, minim for grain.

Action and uses—Alterative, diuretic and antiseptic. Highly recommended in syphilitic, mercurial and scrofulous diseases; also beneficial in menorrhagia, leucorrhœa, diarrhœa, dysentery and hemorrhoids.

PREPARATION.

Infusion Plantain Leaves—Fl. ext. Plantain leaves, Lilly, 2 fl. ozs.; Hot water, 14 fl. ozs.; Mix—Dose 2 to 4 fl. ozs.

FL. EXT. PLEURISY ROOT, U. S........ ....**Dose 20 to 60 m.**
Asclepias tuberosa Linn.   **Nat. Ord.—**Asclepiadeæ.
Synonyms— Asclepias U. S.,—Butterflyweed, Wind root.
Range—Canada, United States; common, especially southward.
Habitat—Dry fields, borders of thickets.
Part used—The root.
Standard of strength—That of the U. S. Pharmacopœia, 1890; 1 c.c.
representing 1 gram of the drug; or, practically, minim for grain.
Action and uses—Diaphoretic and expectorant. Used in infusion
for promoting perspiration and expectoration in diseases of the respira-
tory organs, especially pleurisy, inflammation of the lungs and catarrhal
affections. It is also reputed carminative, tonic, diuretic and antispasmodic.

PREPARATIONS.

Tincture Pleurisy Root—Fl. ext. Pleurisy root, Lilly, 2 fl. ozs.;
Diluted alcohol, 14 fl. ozs.; Mix—Dose 2 to 4 fl. drs.

Syrup Pleurisy Root Comp.—Fl. ext. Pleurisy root, Lilly, 2
ozs.; Fl. exts. Ipecac and Opium aqueous, Lilly, of each, ½ fl. oz.; Syrup,
8 fl. ozs.; Mix—Dose 1 to 2 fl. drs.

Infusion Pleurisy Root—Fl. ext. Pleurisy root, Lilly, 1 fl. oz.;
Hot water, 15 fl. ozs.; Mix—Dose 1 to 2 fl. ozs.

FL. EXT. POISON OAK.   Dose 2 to 10 m.
Rhus radicans Linn.   Nat. Ord.—Anacardiaceæ.
Synonyms—R. toxicodendron radicans Marsh.,—Rhus toxicodendron
U. S.
Range—Widely distributed over the United States.
Habitat—Near cultivated fields, abundant on sandy banks of streams,
in the borders of woods and thickets.
Part used—The fresh leaves.
Standard of strength—That of the U. S. Pharmacopœia, 1890; 1 c.c.
representing 1 gram of the drug; or, practically, minim for grain.
Action and uses—In large doses irritant narcotic. In small doses
nervous stimulant, diuretic, diaphoretic and laxative. Recommended
in chronic paralysis, chronic rheumatism and cutaneous diseases.

PREPARATION.

Tincture Poison Oak—Fl. ext. Poison oak, Lilly, 2 fl. ozs.; Alcohol,
10½ fl. ozs.; Water, 5½ fl. ozs.; Mix—Dose 20 to 60 m.

FL. EXT. POKE BERRIES.......... .... Dose 30 to 60 m.
Phytolacca decandra Linn.   Nat. Ord.—Phytolaccaceæ.
Synonyms— Garget, Pigeon berry, Coakum.
Range—North America; naturalized in Southern Europe and West
Indies.
Habitat—In rich soil in waste places.
Part used—The fruit.
Standard of strength—That of the U. S. Pharmacopœia, 1890; 1 c.c.
representing 1 gram of the drug; or, practically, minim for grain.
Action and uses—Recommended in chronic rheumatism. It has
been used with variable results in obesity. In some cases the flesh has
been reduced remarkably without apparent ill effects on the general
health.

PREPARATIONS.

Tincture Poke Berries—Fl. ext. Poke berries, Lilly, 4 fl. ozs.; Diluted alcohol, 12 fl. ozs.; Mix—Dose 2 to 4 fl. drs.

Syrup Poke Berries—Fl. ext. Poke berries, Lilly, 4 fl. ozs.; Syrup,
12 fl. ozs.; Mix—Dose 2 to 4 fl. drs.

FL. EXT. POKE ROOT, **U. S**................Dose { Alterative, 1 m. / Emetic, 30 m.

Phytolacca decandra Linn.   **Nat. Ord.**—*Phytolaccaceæ.*

Synonym—Phytolacca radix U. S.,—Garget, Pigeon berry, Coakum.

Range—North America; naturalized in Southern Europe and West Indies.

Habitat—In rich soil in waste places.

Part used—The fruit.

Standard of strength—That of the U. S. Pharmacopœia, 1890; 1 c.c. representing 1 gram of the drug; or, practically, minim for grain.

Action and uses—Emetic, cathartic and alterative. Highly useful in syphilitic, scrofulous, rheumatic and cutaneous diseases; hence, it is an important ingredient in SUCCUS ALTERANS, Lilly.

PREPARATIONS.

Tincture Poke Root—Fl. ext. Poke root, Lilly, 2 fl. ozs.; Alcohol, 9 fl. ozs.; Water, 5 fl. ozs.; Mix—Dose 1 to 2 fl. drs.

Syrup Poke Root—Fl. ext. Poke root, Lilly, 4 fl. ozs.; Syrup; 12 fl. ozs.; Mix—Dose ½ to 1 fl. dr.

FL. EXT. POMEGRANATE ROOT BARK..........**Dose 60 to 120 m.**

Punica Granatum Linn.   **Nat. Ord.**—*Lythrarieæ.*

Synonym—Granatum U. S.

Range—Mediterranean region, Eastern, Western and Southern Asia; cultivated in subtropical countries.

Part used—The root bark.

Standard of strength—That of the U. S. Pharmacopœia, 1890; 1 c.c. representing 1 gram of the drug; or, practically, minim for grain.

Action and uses—Employed for the removal of the tape worm, in which it is said to destroy the worm in three hours. The infusion should be followed by a brisk cathartic. The infusion is also used as an astringent gargle in sore throat, and as an injection in gonorrhœa, leucorrhœa, etc.

PREPARATION.

Infusion Pomegranate Root Bark—Fl. ext. Pomegranate root bark, Lilly, 1 fl. oz.; Hot water, 15 fl. ozs; Mix—Dose 2 to 4 fl. ozs.

FL. EXT. POPPY HEADS.   ....Dose 30 to 120 m.

Papaver somniferum Linn.   **Nat. Ord.**—*Papaveraceæ.*

Synonym—Opium poppy.

Range—Western Asia; cultivated in India, China, Japan, Persia, Egypt and Asiatic Turkey.

Habitat—Not known in the original wild state.

Part used—The capsules or fruit.

Standard of strength—That of the U. S. Pharmacopœia, 1890; 1 c.c. representing 1 gram of the drug; or, practically, minim for grain.

Action and uses—Anodyne and mildly narcotic. Used to calm irritation and to promote rest.

PREPARATION.

Syrup Poppy Heads—Fl. ext. Poppy heads, Lilly, 4 fl. ozs.; Syrup, 12 fl. ozs.; Mix—Dose 1 to 2 fl. drs.

FL. EXT. PRICKLY ASH BARK...... ...Dose, in syrup, **10** to 30 m.

    Nat. Ord.—*Rutaceæ.*

Xanthoxylum Americanum Miller *and* **X.** *Clava-Herculis* Linn.

Synonyms—Xanthoxylum=Zanthoxylum, X. Caroliniana Lam.=X. Clava-Herculis Linn.,—Xanthoxylum U. S.,—Toothache tree, Yellow wood.

Range—Of X. Americanum—Northern, Middle and Western States; of X. Clava-Herculis—Virginia, Western Texas and probably into Mexico.

Habitat—Of X. Americanum—rocky hillsides, frequently in rich soil, along the banks of streams; of X. Clava-Herculis—dry sandy soil, especially near the coast.

Part used—The bark.

Standard of strength—That of the U. S. Pharmacopœia, 1890; 1 c.c. representing 1 gram of the drug; or, practically, minim for grain.

Action and uses—Stimulant, tonic, alterative and sialagogue. Valuable as a sialagogue in paralysis of the tongue and mouth. Highly beneficial in chronic rheumatism, colic, syphilis, hepatic derangements and wherever stimulating alterative treatment is required. It is an important ingredient in STUCUS ALTERANS, Lilly. The acridity of this drug requires it to be largely diluted for internal administration.

PREPARATIONS.

Tincture Prickly Ash Bark—Fl. ext. Prickly ash bark, Lilly, 2 fl. ozs.; Alcohol, 5½ fl. ozs.; Water, 8½ fl. ozs.; Mix the alcohol and water and add the fluid extract—Dose ½ to 2 fl. drs.

Syrup Prickly Ash Bark—Fl. ext. Prickly ash bark, Lilly, 4 fl. ozs.; Syrup, 14 fl. ozs.; Mix—Dose ½ to 2 fl. drs.

Infusion Prickly Ash Bark—Fl. ext. Prickly ash bark, Lilly, 1 fl. oz.; Hot water, 15 fl. ozs.; Mix—Dose 1 to 4 fl. drs

FL. EXT. PRICKLY ASH BERRIES...... Dose, in syrup, 10 to 30 m.

Xanthoxylum Americanum Miller and *X. Clava-Herculis* Linn.
Nat. Ord.— *Rutaceæ.*

Synonyms—Xanthoxylum = Zanthoxylum, X. Carolinianum Lam. = X. Clava-Herculis Linn.,—Toothache tree, Yellow wood.

Range—Of X. Americanum—Northern, Middle and Western States; of X. Clava-Herculis—Virginia, Western Texas and probably into Mexico.

Habitat—Of X. Americanum—rocky hillsides, frequently in rich soil, along the banks of streams; of X. Clava-Herculis—dry sandy soil, especially near the coast.

Part used—The fruit.

Standard of strength—That of the U. S. Pharmacopœia, 1890; 1 c.c. representing 1 gram of the drug; or, practically, minim for grain.

Action and uses—Stimulant, carminative and antispasmodic, acting especially on mucous tissues. Useful in all nervous diseases, spasms of the bowels, flatulency and in diarrhœa; also in tympanitic distension of the bowels during peritoneal inflammation. Used internally as an injection, to which 10 to 20 drops of laudanum may be added. It has been used successfully in Asiatic cholera. Combined with fluid extract poke berries it is invaluable in chronic rheumatism.

PREPARATION.

Tincture Prickly Ash Berries—Fl. ext. Prickly ash berries, Lilly, 2 fl. ozs.; Alcohol, 10½ fl. ozs.; Water, 3½ fl. ozs.—Dose ½ to 2 fl. drs

FL. EXT. PULSATILLA.... ....Dose 2 to 3 m.

Anemone Pulsatilla Linn. and *A. pratensis* Linn.
Nat. Ord.— *Ranunculaceæ.*

Synonyms—Pulsatilla U. S.,—Pasque flower, Meadow anemone.

Range—Europe, Siberia; in North America on the prairies of Illinois and Missouri, thence northward and westward.

Part used—The herb.

Standard of strength—That of the U. S. Pharmacopœia, 1890; 1 c.c. representing 1 gram of the drug; or, practically, minim for grain.

Action and uses—POISONOUS IN OVER DOSES. Dr. J. M. Scudder states that its most important use is to allay irritation of the nervous system in persons of feeble health, giving sleep and rest. On men and women who have become nervous from sedentary habits, as well as the nervousness of masturbaters, or from excessive use of tobacco, he has found its action certain. It is the remedy for nervous women, where there is debility and faulty nutrition of the nerve centers; useful in headache and neuralgia. In amenorrhea, the result of cold or emotional excitement, it is used with advantage.

Antidotes—Alcohol, opium and digitalis are the physiological antagonists. The caustic alkalies, tannic acid and metallic salts are incompatible.

PREPARATION.

Tincture Pulsatilla—Fl. ext. Pulsatilla, Lilly, 4 fl. ozs.; Diluted alcohol, 12 fl. ozs.; Mix—Dose 5 to 15 m.

FL. EXT. PUMPKIN SEED ....Dose 1-2 to 2 fl. ozs.
Curcubita Pepo Linn. **Nat. Ord.**—*Cucurbitaceæ*.
Range—Tropical Asia, the Mediterranean Basin and America; cultivated extensively.
Habitat—Rich sandy soil, not known in the original wild state.
Part used—The seed.
Standard of strength—That of the U. S. Pharmacopœia, 1890; 1 c.c. representing 1 gram of the drug; or, practically, minim for grain.
Action and uses—Anthelmintic. Used principally in the treatment of tape worm. The infusion should be taken on a fasting stomach, repeated in two hours and in two hours more followed by a dose of castor oil.

PREPARATION.

Infusion Pumpkin Seed—Fl. ext. Pumpkin seed, Lilly, 4 fl. ozs.; Hot water, 12 fl. ozs.; Mix—Dose 2 to 8 fl. ozs.

FL. EXT. QUASSIA, U. S. ....Dose 5 to 10 m.
Picræna excelsa (Swartz) Lindley. **Nat. Ord.**—*Simarubœ*.
Synonyms—Quassia excelsa Swartz, Simaruba excelsa D. C.
Range—Jamaica and Caribbean Islands.
Part used—The wood.
Standard of strength—That of the U. S. Pharmacopœia, 1890; 1 c.c. representing 1 gram of the drug; or, practically, minim for grain.
Action and uses—Useful whenever a simple tonic impression is desired. The infusion, given as an injection, is recommended for the removal of ascarides. A strong decoction of quassia sweetened with brown sugar or molasses, is recommended as an effectual poison for flies.

PREPARATIONS.

Tincture Quassia, U. S.—Fl. ext. Quassia, Lilly, 1½ fl. ozs.; Alcohol, 4½ fl. ozs.; Water, 9¼ fl. ozs.; Mix the alcohol and water and add the fluid extract—Dose ½ to 1 fl. drs.

Infusion Quassia—Fl. ext. Quassia, Lilly, 1 fl. oz.; Hot water, 15 fl. ozs.; Mix—Dose 1 to 2 fl. drs.

FL. EXT. QUEBRACHO, U. S. ....Dose 15 to 60 m.
Aspidosperma Quebracho Schlecht. **Nat. Ord.**—*Apocynaceæ*.
Range—Argentine Republic.
Part used—The bark.
Standard of strength—That of the U. S. Pharmacopœia, 1890; 1 c.c. representing 1 gram of the drug; or, practically, minim for grain.
Action and uses—Quebracho bark is said to be used as an antiperiodic in Chili and has frequently attracted much attention as a remedy in cardiac and asthmatic dyspnœa.

FL. EXT. QUEEN OF THE MEADOW ....Dose 30 to 60 m.
Eupatorium purpureum Linn. **Nat. Ord.**—*Compositæ*.
Synonyms—E. trifoliatum Linn.—Gravel root, Trumpet weed.
Range—New Brunswick to Saskatchewan, Florida and westward in wooded districts to New Mexico, Utah and British Columbia.
Habitat—Low or wet grounds.
Part used—Root stock and rootlets.
Standard of strength—That of the U. S. Pharmacopœia, 1890; 1 c.c. representing 1 gram of the drug; or, practically, minim for grain.
Action and uses—Diuretic, tonic, stimulant and astringent. Valuable in dropsical affections, strangury, gravel and all chronic urinary diseases; hematuria, gout and rheumatism. Appears to exert specific influence upon chronic affections of the kidneys and bladder.

PREPARATION.

Infusion Queen of the Meadow—Fl. ext. Queen of the meadow, Lilly, 1 fl. oz.; Hot water, 15 fl. ozs.; Mix—Dose 1 to 2 fl. ozs.

FL. EXT. RAGWEED.............................Dose 30 to 60 m.

Ambrosia artemisiæfolia Linn.   Nat. Ord.—*Compositæ*.

Synonym—Ambrosia.

Range—Nova Scotia, Saskatchewan, Texas, California and Washington. West Indies, Mexico to Brazil.

Habitat—Dry ground; common as a weed.

Part used—The leaves and inflorescence.

Standard of strength—That of the U. S. Pharmacopœia, 1890; 1 c.c. representing 1 gram of the drug; or, practically, minim for grain.

Action and uses—Stimulant, astringent and antiphlogistic.

FL. EXT. RASPBERRY LEAVES...............Dose 20 to 40 m.

Rubus strigosus Michx.   Nat. Ord.—*Rosaceæ*.

Synonym—R. Idæus Linn. var. strigosus Maxim.

Range—Labrador to New Jersey, south to North Carolina, west to Minnesota and Missouri.

Habitat—Thickets and hills.

Part used—The leaves.

Standard of strength—That of the U. S. Pharmacopœia, 1890; 1 c.c. representing 1 gram of the drug; or, practically, minim for grain.

Action and uses—Astringent, said to be an excellent remedy in diarrhœa, dysentery, cholera infantum, relaxed condition of intestines in children, passive hemorrhages from the stomach, bowels or uterus, and in colliquative diarrhœa.

PREPARATIONS.

Syrup Raspberry Leaves—Fl. ext. Raspberry leaves, Lilly, 4 fl. ozs.; Syrup, 12 fl. ozs.; Mix—Dose 2 to 4 fl. drs.

Infusion Raspberry Leaves—Fl. ext. Raspberry leaves, Lilly, 2 fl. ozs.; Hot water, 14 fl. ozs.; Mix—Dose ½ to 1 fl. oz.

FL. EXT. RED OAK BARK........................Dose 5 to 10 m.

Quercus rubra Linn.   Nat. Ord.—*Cupuliferæ*.

Range—From the Atlantic to Eastern Minnesota and Eastern Kansas.

Habitat—Common in both rich and poor soils.

Part used—The inner bark.

Standard of strength—That of the U. S. Pharmacopœia, 1890; 1 c.c. representing 1 gram of the drug; or, practically, minim for grain.

Action and uses—Astringent and mildly tonic. It is seldom used internally. The cold infusion is used as an injection or astringent wash for sores or ulcers.

PREPARATION.

Infusion Red Oak Bark—Fl. ext. Red oak bark, Lilly, 1 fl. oz.; Water, 15 fl. ozs.

FL. EXT. RED SAUNDERS.

Pterocarpus santalinus Linn. f.   Nat. Ord.—*Leguminosæ*.

Synonym—Santalum rubrum U. S.

Range—India and East Indies.

Habitat—Mountainous districts, hillsides, etc.

Part used—The wood.

Standard of strength—That of the U. S. Pharmacopœia, 1890; 1 c.c. representing 1 gram of the drug; or, practically, minim for grain.

Action and uses—Used as a coloring agent.

PREPARATION.

Tincture Red Saunders—Fl. ext. Red saunders, Lilly, 2 fl. ozs.; Alcohol, 14 fl. ozs.

FL. EXT. RHATANY, **U. S.**...................................**Dose 10 to 60 m.**
Krameria triandra Ruiz et **Pavon and** *K. Ixina* Linn.
Nat. Ord.—*Polygaleæ.*

Synonyms—K. tomentosa St. Hil.=K. Ixina Linn.,—Krameria U. S.

Range—Peru, Bolivia, New Granada, Brazil and northward.

Habitat—Barren sandy declivities, up to 8000 feet above the sea level.

Part used—The root.

Standard of strength—That of the U. S. Pharmacopœia, 1890; 1 c.c.
representing 1 gram of the drug; or, practically, minim for grain.

Action and uses—Gentle tonic and powerful astringent. Used in
chronic diarrhea, menorrhagia, some forms of leucorrhea and in all cases
where kino and catechu are beneficial.

PREPARATIONS.

Tincture Rhatany, U. S.—Fl. ext. Rhatany, Lilly, 3¾ **fl. ozs.; Al-**
cohol, 9½ fl. ozs.; Water, 3¼ fl. ozs.; Mix—Dose ½ to 4 fl. drs.

Syrup Rhatany, U. S.—Fl. ext. Rhatany, U. S., Lilly, 7 fl. ozs.;
Syrup, 9 fl. ozs.; Mix—Dose 20 to 50 m., for a child one to two years old.

Infusion Rhatany—Fl. ext. Rhatany, Lilly, 1 fl. oz.; Hot water, 15
fl. ozs.; Mix—Dose 1 to 2 fl. ozs.

FL. EXT. RHUBARB, U. S....... Dose $\begin{cases} \text{As a laxative, 5 to 10 m.} \\ \text{As a cathartic, 20 to 30 m.} \end{cases}$
Rheum officinale Baillon. **Nat. Ord.—***Polygonaceæ.*

Range—Western and Central China.

Habitat—Growing best in light sandy soil on elevated regions.

Part used—The root.

Standard of Strength—100 c.c. contain 30 gm. of extractive.

Action and uses—Rhubarb combines astringent properties with its
undoubted cathartic effects. When taken in considerable doses, it not
only stimulates the peristaltic movement of the small intestines,
more especially the duodenum, but it moistens and softens the feces
and increases the secretion of bile. Its astringent action renders it
useful in most forms of diarrhea, depending upon the presence of indi-
gestible matters in the alimentary canal, and where removal of the exciting cause is sufficient to effect a cure. It is a good tonic in some forms
of dyspepsia and forms a good purgative for children.

PREPARATIONS.

Tincture Rhubarb, U. S.—Fl. ext. Rhubarb, Lilly, 3¼ fl. ozs.; Fl.
ext. Cardamom, Lilly, ½ fl. ozs.; Alcohol, 24 fl. ozs.; Water, 7¼ fl. ozs.;
Mix—Dose 1 to 4 fl. drs.

Syrup Rhubarb, U. S.—Fl. ext. Rhubarb, Lilly, 3¼ fl. ozs.; Spirit
Cinnamon, U. S., 1 fl. dr.; Potassium carbonate, 146 grs.; Glycerin,
Water, of each, 12 fl. drs.; syrup, sufficient to make 2 pints; Dissolve the
potassium carbonate in the water, add to the fluid extracts and spirit of
cinnamon, then add the glycerin and syrup—Dose 1 to 2 fl. drs.

Wine Rhubarb—Fl. ext. Rhubarb, Lilly, 3½ fl. ozs.; Fl. ext. Calamus,
Lilly, ½ fl. oz.; Stronger white wine (U. S. 1880), 28½ fl. ozs.; Mix—
4 fl. drs.

FL. EXT. RHUBARB, AROMATIC................**Dose 20 to 60 m.**

Standard of strength—One pint represents Rhubarb, 6¼ troy
ounces; Cloves, Cassia, Cinnamon, of each, 1¼ troy ounces; Nutmeg, ⅝
troy ounce.

Action and uses—Used mostly to make the U. S. tincture from which
the official syrup is prepared, or the latter can be made directly from the
fluid extract.

WHEN ORDERING OR PRESCRIBING.

PREPARATIONS.

Tincture Rhubarb, Aromatic, U. S.—Fl. ext. Rhubarb, aromatic, Lilly, 8 fl. ozs.; Diluted alcohol, 8 fl. ozs.; Mix—Dose 1 to 2 fl. drs.

Syrup Rhubarb, Aromatic, U. S.—Fl. ext. Rhubarb, aromatic, Lilly, 1½ fl. ozs.; Diluted alcohol, 1¼ fl. ozs.; Syrup, 13½ fl. ozs.; Mix—Dose 1 to 4 fl. drs.

FL. EXT. RHUBARB AND POTASSIUM COMP.
For preparing neutralizing cordial.

Standard of strength—One pint represents Rhubarb, 8 troy ounces; Golden seal, Cinnamon, of each, 4 troy ounces; Oil peppermint, 30 m.; Potassium carbonate, 1 troy ounce.

Action and uses—The neutralizing cordial prepared from this extract is an agreeable laxative, antacid and tonic. Used in cases of obstinate constipation, acidity of the stomach, dyspepsia, and as a laxative in pregnancy, and where piles are present. It is valuable in diarrhea, dysentery, cholera morbus, cholera infantum.

PREPARATION.

Neutralizing Cordial—Fl. ext. Rhubarb and potassium comp., Lilly, 2 fl. ozs.; Syrup, 7 fl. ozs.; Diluted alcohol or brandy, 7 fl. ozs.; Mix—Dose, for an adult, ½ fl. oz. every half hour, hour or two hours according to the urgency; for a child in proportion to its age.

FL. EXT. RHUBARB AND SENNA. . . . . Dose 30 to 60 m.
Standard of strength—One pint represents Rhubarb, 4 troy ounces; Senna, 12 troy ounces; Potassium carbonate, ½ troy ounce; and aromatics.
Action and uses—Laxative and cathartic.

FL. EXT. RHUBARB, SWEET. . . . . Dose 30 to 60 m.
Standard of strength—One pint represents Rhubarb, 6½ troy ounces; Licorice root, Anise, of each, 2 drams; Cardamom, 30 grains.
Action and uses—Laxative and cathartic. Used principally for preparing the sweet tincture of rhubarb.

PREPARATION.

Tincture Rhubarb, Sweet, U. S.—Fl. ext. Rhubarb, sweet, Lilly, 4 fl. ozs.; Diluted alcohol, 12 fl. ozs.; Mix—Dose 2 to 5 fl. drs.

FL. EXT. RHUS AROMATICA . . . . Dose 20 to 30 m.
Rhus aromatica Ait.   **Nat. Ord.**—*Anacardiaceæ.*

Synonyms—R. Canadensis Marsh., Toxicodendron crenatum Mill.,—Stink bush, Skunk bush.

Range—Western Vermont to Minnesota and southward.

Habitat—Dry rocky banks.

Part used—The bark.

Standard of strength—That of the U. S. Pharmacopeia, 1890; 1 c.c. representing 1 gram of the drug; or, practically, minim for grain.

Action and uses—This remedy is highly recommended in the treatment of diabetes, uterine hemorrhage, hematuria, enuresis and diseases of the genito-urinary organs generally. It has been successfully used in atonic diarrhea, dysentery, etc.

PREPARATIONS.

Tincture Rhus Aromatica—Fl. ext. Rhus aromatica, Lilly, 4 fl. ozs.; Alcohol, 9 fl. ozs.; Water, 3 fl. ozs.; Mix—Dose ½ to 2 fl. drs.

Syrup Rhus Aromatica—Fl. ext. Rhus aromatica, Lilly, 4 fl. ozs.; Syrup, 12 fl. ozs.; Mix—Dose ½ to 2 fl. drs.

FL. EXT. ROSINWEED ....Dose 10 to 30 m.
Silphium laciniatum Linn. **Nat. Ord.**—*Compositæ.*
Synonyms—Compass plant, Polar plant.
Range—Michigan to Dakota, south to Alabama, Kansas and Texas.
Habitat—Prairies.
Part used—The root.
Standard of strength—That of the U. S. Pharmacopœia, 1890; 1 c.c.,
representing 1 gram of the drug; or, practically, minim for **grain.**
Action and uses—Tonic, diuretic and expectorant. Beneficial in
intermittent fever; in dry obstinate cough, asthma and pulmonary
catarrhal diseases. Said to **cure** heaves in horses.

PREPARATIONS.

Tincture Rosinweed—Fl. ext. Rosinweed, Lilly, 4 fl. ozs.; Alcohol,
12 fl. ozs., Mix—Dose 1 to 2 fl. drs.

Syrup Rosinweed—Fl. ext. Rosinweed, Lilly, 4 fl. ozs.; Syrup, 12 fl.
ozs.; Mix—Dose 1 to 2 fl. drs.

FL. EXT. **RUE**.............. ....Dose 15 to 30 m.
Ruta graveolens Linn. **Nat. Ord.**—*Rutaceæ.*
Range—Throughout Southern **Europe,** Canary Islands; cultivated.
Habitat—Waste stony ground.
Part used—The leaves.
Standard of strength—That **of the U. S.** Pharmacopœia, 1890; 1 c.c.
representing 1 gram of the drug; or, **practically,** minim for grain.
Action and uses—Emmenagogue, cephalic, anthelmintic **and** antispas-
modic. In large doses it is an acrid narcotic poison and causes abortion,
accompanied by inflammation of the stomach and bowels. It appears to
have a tendency to the uterus in moderate doses, proving emmenagogue.
It has been successfully used in flatulent colic, hysteria and epilepsy,
and is an excellent vermifuge.

PREPARATION.

Infusion Rue—Fl. ext. Rue, Lilly, 1 fl. oz.; Hot water, 15 fl. ozs.; Mix—
Dose ½ to 1 fl. oz.

FL. EXT. SAGE.............. ....Dose 30 to 60 m.
Salvia officinalis Linn. **Nat. Ord.**—*Labiatæ.*
Range—Southern **Europe;** cultivated in gardens in the United States.
Habitat—Dry soil.
Part used—The **leaves.**
Standard of strength—That of the U. S. Pharmacopœia, 1890; 1 c.c.
representing 1 gram of the drug; or, practically, minim for grain.
Action and uses—Feebly tonic and astringent, diaphoretic and expectorant. The infusion is beneficial in flatulence connected with
gastric debility, restrains the exhausting sweats of hectic fever, a valuable diaphoretic in some febrile diseases; it is recommended in sperma-
torrhœa, and to check excessive venereal desires. The infusion may be
used as a gargle for inflammation and ulceration of the throat and relaxed uvula, either alone or combined with vinegar, honey, alum **or**
sumach berries.

PREPARATION.

Infusion Sage—Fl. ext. Sage, Lilly, 1 fl. oz.; Hot water, 15 fl. ozs.;
Mix—Dose 1 to 2 fl. ozs.

FL. EXT. SAMPSON SNAKEROOT................. Dose 30 to 60 m.
Gentiana ochroleuca Fræl.   **Nat. Ord.**—*Gentianaceæ.*
Synonyms—G. villosa Linn.
Range—Pennsylvania to Florida and Louisiana.
Habitat—Dry or damp grounds.
Part used—The root.
Standard of strength—That of the U. S. Pharmacopœia, 1890; 1 c.c.
representing 1 gram of the drug; or, practically, minim for grain.
Action and uses—Bitter tonic, anthelmintic and astringent. Useful
as a tonic to enfeebled mucous tissues in chronic catarrhal affections,
mucous diarrhea, etc.

PREPARATION.

Infusion Sampson Snakeroot—Fl. ext. Sampson snakeroot,
Lilly, 1 fl. oz.; Hot water, 15 fl. ozs.; Mix—Dose 1 to 2 fl. ozs.

FL. EXT. SANDALWOOD .... Dose 30 to 120 m.
Santalum album Linn.   **Nat. Ord.**—*Santalaceæ.*
Synonym—White saunders.
Range—India and Islands of the East Indian Archipelago; cultivated in
India.
Habitat—Dry open places in hilly districts, hedge rows, not in forests.
Part used—The wood.
Standard of strength—That of the U. S. Pharmacopœia, 1890; 1 c.c.
representing 1 gram of the drug; or, practically, minim for grain.
Action and uses—Regarded by some physicians superior to copaiba
in gonorrhea and without its inconveniences.

FL. EXT. SARSAPARILLA, U. S.................. Dose 30 to 60 m.
Smilax officinalis Kunth., *S. medica* Chamisso et Schlecht., *S.
papyraceæ* Duhamel and other undetermined species of *Smilax.*
    Nat. Ord.—*Liliaceæ.*
NOTE—The species *S. medica* and *S. officinalis* are thought to furn-
ish nearly all of the sarsaparilla of the market.
Range—Tropical America, from Mexico to Brazil; cultivated.
Habitat—Forests of river valleys and of mountainous or hilly districts,
some species extending into altitudes of 8000 feet or more.
Part used—The roots.
Standard of strength—That of the U. S. Pharmacopœia, 1890; 1 c.c.
representing 1 gram of the drug; or, practically, minim for grain.
Action and uses—Alterative, diuretic and diaphoretic. It has been
recommended in syphilis, pseudosyphilis, mercuriosyphilis and struma
in all its forms.

PREPARATIONS.

Syrup Sarsaparilla—Fl. ext. Sarsaparilla, Lilly, 4 fl. ozs.; Syrup, 12
fl. ozs.; Mix—Dose 2 to 4 fl. drs.

Decoction Sarsaparilla Comp., U. S.—Fl. ext. Sarsaparilla,
Lilly, 1½ fl. ozs.; Fl. exts. Sassafras, Guaiac wood and Licorice, Lilly, of
each, 2½ fl. drs.; Fl. ext. Mezereum, Lilly, 75 m.; Water, sufficient to
make one pint; Mix—Dose 2 to 4 fl. ozs.

FL. EXT. SARSAPARILLA COMP., U. S............. Dose 30 to 60 m.
Standard of strength—One pint represents Sarsaparilla, 12 troy
ounces; Licorice root, 2 troy ounces; Sassafras bark, 1¾ troy ounces;
Mezereum, ½ troy ounce.
Action and uses—Used as an alterative.

FL. EXT. SARSAPARILLA COMP., for Syrup......Dose 30 to 60 m.

Standard of strength—One pint represents Sarsaparilla, 12½ troy ounces; Senna, Licorice, of each, 1 troy ounce; Oils Anise, Sassafras and Wintergreen, of each, 3 m.

Action and uses—Used solely for preparing syrup sarsaparilla comp., U. S. We omit from the formula the guaiac wood, as nothing of medicinal value in this drug can be held in solution in the finished syrup.

PREPARATION.

Syrup Sarsaparilla Comp., U. S.—Fl. ext. Sarsaparilla comp., Lilly, 4 fl. oz.; Syrup, 12 fl. ozs.; Mix—Dose 2 to 4 fl. drs.

FL. EXT. SASSAFRAS BARK..................Dose 30 to 60 m.

Sassafras variifolium (Salisbury) O. Kuntze. Nat. Ord.—*Laurineæ*.

Synonyms—S. sassafras (Linn.) Karst., S. officinale Nees & Eberm., Laurus sassafras Linn., L. variifolia Salisbury.

Range—Ontario to Florida, westward to Kansas and Eastern Texas.

Habitat—Rich woodlands.

Part used—The root bark.

Standard of strength—That of the U. S. Pharmacopœia, 1890; 1 c.c. representing 1 gram of the drug; or, practically, minim for grain.

Action and uses—A warming stimulant and alterative, diaphoretic and diuretic.

PREPARATION.

Infusion Sassafras—Fl. ext. Sassafras, Lilly, 1 fl. oz.; Hot water, 15 fl. ozs.; Mix—Dose 1 to 2 fl. ozs.

FL. EXT. SAVIN, U. S...................Dose 3 to 8 m.

Juniperus Sabina Linn. Nat. Ord.—*Coniferæ*.

Synonym—J. Sabina var. procumbens Pursh.

Range—Siberia, Europe, Canada, Northern United States.

Habitat—Along lake shores, borders of swamps, rocky banks.

Part used—The young leafy branches—tops.

Standard of strength—That of the U. S. Pharmacopœia, 1890; 1 c.c. representing 1 gram of the drug; or, practically, minim for grain.

Action and uses—POISONOUS IN OVERDOSES. Emmenagogue, diuretic, diaphoretic and anthelmintic. It should never be given when general or local inflammation exists, and it should not be given during pregnancy on account of its tendency to cause abortion. In small doses it is said to be beneficial in amenorrhagia. The cerate is applied to blistered surfaces to maintain a constant discharge.

PREPARATIONS.

Tincture Savin—Fl. ext. Savin, Lilly, 2 fl. ozs.; Alcohol, 14 fl. ozs.; Mix—Dose ½ to 1 fl. dr.

Savin Cerate—Fl. ext. Savin, Lilly, 5 fl. ozs.; Resin cerate, 13 troy ounces; Melt the cerate on a water bath, add the fluid extract, heat until the alcohol is expelled and stir till cold.

Infusion Savin—Fl. ext. Savin, Lilly, 1 fl. oz.; Hot water, 15 fl. ozs.; Mix—Dose 1 to 2 fl. drs.

FL. EXT. SAW PALMETTO BERRIES...........Dose 30 to 60 m.

Serenoa serrulata (R. & S.) Hooker f. Nat. Ord.—*Palmæ*.

Synonyms—Sabal serrulata R. & S., Serenoa serrulata Benth. & Hooker.

Range—South Carolina to Florida.

Habitat—Sandy soil in the lower districts near the coast.

Part used—The fruit—a drupe.

Standard of strength—That of the U. S. Pharmacopœia, 1890; 1 c.c. representing 1 gram of the drug; or, practically, minim for grain.

Action and uses—On account of its tonic and expectorant properties, Saw Palmetto is of service in phthisis pulmonalis. It is also valuable in atrophy of the mammae, testicles or uterus and exerts a beneficial influence upon the enlarged prostate. It has been used with success by many physicians in the treatment of enlargement of the prostate gland, and for dribbling urine when there seems to be want of power in the bladder. In cases of **irritation** of the bladder it has exerted its efficacy without **the** slightest inconvenience **or** impairment of **any** function.

FL. EXT. SAW PALMETTO COMP. . . . . **Dose 30 to 60 m.**

Standard of strength—One pint represents Saw Palmetto berries, 2½ troy ounces; Kola nut, 384 grains; **Parsley seed, Coca leaves**, of each, 192 grains, and aromatics.

Action and uses—On account of its tonic and expectorant properties, Saw Palmetto is of service in phthisis pulmonalis. It is also valuable in atrophy of the mammae, testicles or uterus and exerts a beneficial influence upon the enlarged prostate. It has been used with success by many physicians in the treatment of enlargement of the prostate gland, and for dribbling urine when there seems to be want of power in the bladder. In cases of irritation of the bladder it has exerted its efficacy without the slightest inconvenience or impairment of any function. To this is added the stimulating effect of the kola and coca so often required in such cases.

FL. EXT. SAXIFRAGE . . . . **Dose 30 to 60 m.**

Pimpinella Saxifraga Linn. **Nat. Ord.**—*Umbelliferæ*

Synonym—P. Saxifraga Linn. var. major Koch.

Range—Western Asia, Central Europe; naturalized in the United States, Delaware river to Easton Pennsylvania and Sycamore Ohio.

Habitat—Rocky banks **and** along roadsides, **dry soil.**

Part used—The root.

Standard of strength—That of the U. S. Pharmacopœia, 1890; 1 c.c. representing 1 gram of the drug; or, practically, minim for grain.

Action and uses—Aromatic, stomachic, diaphoretic and diuretic.

PREPARATION.

Infusion Saxifrage—Fl. ext. Saxifrage, Lilly, 1 fl. oz.; Hot water, 15 fl. ozs.; Mix—Dose 1 to 2 fl. ozs.

FL. EXT. SCULLCAP, U. S. . . . . **Dose 30 to 60 m.**

Scutellaria lateriflora Linn. **Nat. Ord.**—*Labiatæ.*

Synonyms—Scutellaria U. S., Hoodwort, Madweed, Mad-dog scull-cap.

Range—Canada to Florida, **New Mexico and northward** to Oregon and British Columbia.

Habitat—Wet banks, **borders of streams.**

Part used—The herb.

Standard of strength—That of the U. S. Pharmacopœia, 1890; 1 c.c. representing 1 gram of the drug; or, practically, minim for grain.

Action and uses—Tonic, nervine and antispasmodic. It has proved especially useful in chorea, convulsions, tremors, intermittent fever, neuralgia and all nervous affections. In delirium tremens, the infusion freely used will soon produce a calm sleep.

PREPARATIONS.

Tincture Scullcap—Fl. ext. Scullcap, Lilly, 2 fl. ozs.; Diluted alcohol, 14 fl. ozs.; Mix—Dose 2 to 4 fl. drs.

Infusion Scullcap—Fl. ext. Scullcap, Lilly, 1 fl. oz.; Hot water, 15 fl. ozs.; Mix—Dose 1 to 2 fl. ozs.

FL. EXT. SCULLCAP COMP. ....**Dose 30 to 60 m.**

Standard of strength—One pint represents Scullcap, 8 troy ounces; Ladies slipper, 4 troy ounces; Hops and Lettuce, of each, 2 troy ounces.

Action and uses—Tonic, nervine and antispasmodic.

PREPARATION.

Infusion Scullcap Comp.—Fl. ext. Scullcap comp., Lilly, 1 fl. oz.; Hot water, 15 fl. ozs.; Mix—Dose 1 to 2 fl. ozs.

FL. EXT. SENECIO ....   Dose 30 to 60 m.

Senecio gracilis Pursh.   **Nat. Ord.**—*Compositæ.*

Note.—A slender or depauperate form of *S. aureus* Linn., not now given specific rank, though specified and demanded by the profession.

Synonyms—Unkum, Female regulator, Life root.

Range—Newfoundland to Florida, Texas and to British **Columbia and** the Sierra Nevada, California.

Habitat—Swamps and wet banks; usually in shaded ground.

Part used—The herb.

Standard of strength—That of the U. S. Pharmacopœia, 1890; 1 c.c. representing 1 gram of the **drug**; or, practically, minim for grain.

Action and uses—Diuretic, tonic, pectoral and diaphoretic. It exerts peculiar influence upon the female generative organs; promotes the menstrual flow. It is also valuable in dysmenorrhea, and in combination with astringents useful in menorrhagia.

PREPARATION.

Infusion Senecio—Fl. ext. Senecio, Lilly, 1 fl. oz.; Hot water, 15 fl. ozs.; Mix—Dose 1 to 2 fl. ozs.

FL. EXT. SENEKA, U. S. ....**Dose 5 to 10 m.**

Polygala Senega Linn.   **Nat. Ord.**—*Polygaleæ.*

Synonyms—Seneka snakeroot.

Range—Nearly all parts of the United States east of the Rocky Mountains.

Habitat—Rocky soil.

Part used—The root.

Standard of strength—That of the U. S. Pharmacopœia, 1890; 1 c.c. representing 1 gram of the drug; or, practically, minim for grain.

Action and uses—Expectorant, diaphoretic and diuretic. It stimulates the mucous membrane of the bronchial tubes, and facilitates the expulsion of their contents. Of great service in the chronic conditions of pneumonia and bronchitis, helping the patient to get rid of large quantities of secretion frequently accumulated in the lungs. It is contraindicated in acute pulmonary affections, but is of real value in the latter stages of bronchitis, and those cases occurring among the very young or old.

PREPARATION.

Syrup Senega, U. S.—Fl. ext. Senega, Lilly, 3½ fl. ozs.; Aqua ammonia, 48 m.; Syrup, 12½ fl. ozs.; Mix—Dose 30 to 60

FL. EXT. SENNA, U. S. ....**Dose 60 to 240 m.**

Cassia acutifolia Delile and *C. angustifolia* Vahl.

         Nat. Ord.—*Leguminosæ.*

Synonyms—C. acutifolia or Alexandria senna=C. lanceolata Nectoux; C. angustifolia Vahl or India senna=C. elongata Lem., C. lanceolata Wright et Arnott.

Range—C. acutifolia—Northeastern Africa; C. angustifolia—India; cultivated.

Habitat—Barren ground, deserts.

Part used—The leaflets.

Standard of strength—That of the U. S. Pharmacopœia, 1890; 1 c.c. representing 1 gram of the drug; or, practically, minim for grain.

Action and uses—Senna irritates the small intestines, causing copious thin, yellow evacuations, stimulating the peristaltic action of the bowels. It may be prescribed in simple constipation, and wherever rapid and effectual unloading of the bowels is required. It is seldom prescribed alone, as it is apt to cause irregular contraction of the intestines and griping. The syrup of senna is a good purgative for children.

PREPARATIONS.

Syrup Senna—Fl. ext. Senna, Lilly, 4 fl. ozs.; Oil coriander, 36 m.; Syrup, 12 fl. ozs.; Mix—Dose ½ to 1 fl. oz.

Infusion Senna—Fl. ext. Senna, Lilly, 1 fl. oz.; Fl. ext. Coriander, Lilly, 1 fl. dr.; Hot water, 15 fl. ozs.; Mix—Dose 4 fl. ozs.

Infusion Senna Comp., U. S.—Fl. ext. Senna, Lilly, 1 fl. oz.; Fl. ext. Fennel seed, Lilly, 2½ fl. drs.; Magnesium sulphate, Manna, of each, 880 grains; Water, sufficient to make one pint; Dissolve the magnesium sulphate and manna in the water, add the fluid extracts and strain—Dose 2 to 4 fl. ozs.

FL. EXT. SENNA COMP. . . . . Dose 30 to 60 m.

Standard of strength—One pint represents Senna, 8 troy ounces; Jalap, 4 troy ounces; Fennel and Coriander, of each, 2 troy ounces.

Action and uses—Laxative and cathartic.

PREPARATION.

Syrup Senna Comp.—Fl. ext. Senna comp., Lilly, 4 fl. ozs.; Syrup, 12 fl. ozs.; Mix—Dose 2 to 4 fl. drs.

FL. EXT. SENNA DEODORIZED (Aqueous fluid extract of Senna.)
Dose 60 to 240 m.

Cassia acutifolia Delile and *C. angustifolia* Vahl.

Nat. Ord.—*Leguminosæ.*

Synonyms—C. acutifolia or Alexandria senna=C. lanceolata Nectoux; C. angustifolia Vahl or India senna=C. elongata Lem., C. lanceolata Wright et Arnott.

Range—C. acutifolia—Northeastern Africa; C. angustifolia—India; cultivated.

Habitat—Barren ground, deserts.

Part used—The leaflets.

Standard of strength—That of the U. S. Pharmacopœia, 1890, 1 c.c. representing 1 gram of the drug, or, practically, minim for grain.

Action and uses—Laxative and cathartic. Prepared from senna leaves after treatment with alcohol which removes the griping principle.

PREPARATION.

Syrup Senna Deodorized—Fl. ext. Senna deodorized, Lilly, 4 fl. ozs.; Syrup, 12 fl. ozs.; Mix—Dose ½ to 2 fl. ozs.

FL. EXT. SENNA AND JALAP   Dose 30 to 60 m.

Standard of strength—One pint represents Senna, 10 troy ounces; Jalap, 6 troy ounces; Potassium carbonate, 160 grains and aromatics.

Action and uses—Laxative and cathartic.

PREPARATION.

Syrup Senna and Jalap—Fl. ext. Senna, Lilly, 4 fl. ozs.; Syrup, 12 fl. ozs.; Mix—Dose 2 to 4 fl. drs.

FL. EXT. SERPENTARIA...... . ...Dose 10 to 30 m.
Aristolochia Serpentaria Linn., and *A. reticulata* Nutt.
Nat. Ord.—*Aristolochiaceæ.*

Synonyms—Virginia snakeroot, Snagrel, Snakeweed. A. reticulata is called Texan or Red River snakeroot.

Range—A. Serpentaria—United States; Connecticut to Florida, west to Michigan and Missouri; A. reticulata—Southwestern States.

Habitat—Rich woods.

Part used—The rhizome and roots.

Standard of strength—That of the U. S. Pharmacopœia, 1890; 1 c.c. representing 1 gram of the drug; or, practically, minim for grain.

Action and uses—Stimulant, tonic and diaphoretic. In small doses it promotes the appetite and gives tone to the organs of digestion, and is useful in cases of enfeebled stomach following exhausting diseases. In full doses it stimulates the system, producing increased arterial action and diaphoresis.

PREPARATIONS.

Tincture Serpentaria, U. S.—Fl. ext. Serpentaria, Lilly, 1½ fl. ozs.; Alcohol, 10½ fl. ozs.; Water, 3½ fl. ozs.; Mix—Dose 1 to 2 fl. drs.

Syrup Serpentaria—Fl. ext. Serpentaria, Lilly, 2 fl. ozs.; Syrup, 14 fl. ozs.; Mix—Dose 1 to 2 fl. drs.

FL. EXT. SHEEP LAUREL..... .... Dose 10 to 40 m.
Kalmia angustifolia Linn.   Nat. Ord.—*Ericaceæ.*

Synonyms—Lambkill, Wicky.

Range—Newfoundland to Michigan, south to Northern Georgia; common.

Habitat—Hillsides, among rocks.

Part used—The leaves.

Standard of strength—That of the U. S. Pharmacopœia, 1890; 1 c.c. representing 1 gram of the drug; or, practically, minim for grain.

Action and uses—Antisyphilitic, sedative and astringent. Valuable in primary and secondary syphilis, febrile and inflammatory diseases; in active hemorrhages, diarrhea and flux. This remedy should always be used with prudence, and the dose diminished or suspended if unfavorable symptoms occur.

PREPARATIONS.

Tincture Sheep **Laurel**—Fl. ext. Sheep laurel, Lilly, 2 fl. ozs.; Diluted alcohol, 14 fl. ozs.; Mix—Dose 1 to 4 fl. drs.

Infusion Sheep Laurel—Fl. ext. Sheep laurel, Lilly, 1 fl. oz.; Hot water, 15 fl. ozs.; Mix—Dose 2 to 4 fl. drs.

FL. EXT. SHEEP SORREL..... .... Dose 30 to 120 m.
Rumex Acetosella Linn.   Nat. Ord.—*Polygonaceæ.*

Range—Europe, naturalized in the United States; common.

Habitat—Along roadsides, and in waste places as a weed.

Part used—The herb.

Standard of strength—That of the U. S. Pharmacopœia, 1890; 1 c.c. representing 1 gram of the drug; or, practically, minim for grain.

Action and uses—Refrigerant and diuretic. Used in febrile inflammatory and scorbutic diseases.

FL. EXT. SHEPHERD'S PURSE, (from green drug,) Dose 30 to 60 m.
Capsella Bursa-Pastoris Mœnch.   Nat. Ord.—*Cruciferæ.*

Synonyms—Bursa Bursa-Pastoris (Linn.) Weber, Thlaspi Bursa-Pastoris Linn.,—Pickpocket, Toywort.

Range—Europe, naturalized in the United States; common.

Habitat—Along roadsides, borders of fields and in waste places as a weed.

Part used—The herb.

Standard of strength—That of the U. S. Pharmacopœia, 1890; 1 c.c. representing 1 gram of the drug; or, practically, minim for grain.

Action and uses—Mildly stimulant, astringent and diuretic. Valuable in urinary derangements of renal or cystic origin, and in hematuria. It has been used with some success as an expectorant, and to promote the catamenial flow in cases of simple amenorrhea.

PREPARATIONS.

Tincture Shepherd's Purse—Fl. ext. Shepherd's purse, Lilly, 4 fl. ozs.; Alcohol, 8 fl. ozs.; Water, 4 fl. ozs.; Mix the alcohol and water and add the fluid extract—Dose 2 to 4 fl. drs.

Infusion Shepherd's Purse—Fl. ext. Shepherd's purse, Lilly, 1 fl. oz.; Hot water, 15 fl. ozs.; Mix—Dose 1 to 2 fl. ozs.

FL. EXT. SILKWEED .... Dose 30 to 60 m.

Asclepias Syriaca Linn.   **Nat. Ord.**—*Asclepiadaceæ*.

Synonyms—A. Syriaca **var. Illinoensis** Pers., A. Cornuti Decaisne,— Milkweed, Swallowwort.

Range—Canada, New England to North Carolina, west to Nebraska and Minnesota.

Habitat—Rich soil, everywhere.

Part used—The root.

Standard of strength—That of the U. S. Pharmacopœia, 1890; 1 c.c. representing 1 gram of the drug; or, practically, minim for grain.

Action and uses—Tonic, diuretic, alterative, emmenagogue, purgative and emetic. It has been found useful in amenorrhœa, dropsy, retention of urine, asthma, dyspnœa, constipation, etc.

FL. EXT. SIMARUBA BARK .... Dose 30 to 60 m.

Simaruba officinalis D. C.   **Nat. Ord.**—*Simarubeæ*.

Synonyms—Simarouba amara Aublet, Quassia Simaruba Linn. f.

Range—Guiana, Venzuela and Northern Brazil.

Habitat—On hillsides in damp sandy ground.

Part used—The bark of the root.

Standard of strength—That of the U. S. Pharmacopœia, 1890; 1 c.c. representing 1 gram of the drug; or, practically, minim for grain.

Action and uses—Bitter tonic and febrifuge.

FL. EXT. SKUNK CABBAGE .... Dose 30 to 60 m.

Symplocarpus fœtidus Nutt.   **Nat. Ord.**—*Araceæ*.

Synonyms—Spathyema fœtida (Linn.) Raf., Dracontium fœtidum Linn., Polecatweed, Skunkweed.

Range—Nova Scotia to North Carolina, west to Minnesota and Iowa.

Habitat—Bogs and moist ground.

Part used—The root stock.

Standard of strength—That of the U. S. Pharmacopœia, 1890; 1 c.c. representing 1 gram of the drug; or, practically, minim for grain.

Action and uses—Stimulant, expectorant, powerful antispasmodic, slightly narcotic. Used successfully in asthma, whooping cough, nervousness, irritability, hysteria and convulsions during pregnancy and labor; also in chronic catarrh, pulmonary and bronchial affections.

PREPARATIONS.

Tincture Skunk Cabbage—Fl. ext. Skunk cabbage, Lilly, 4 fl. ozs.; Diluted alcohol, 12 fl. ozs.; Mix—Dose 2 to 4 fl. drs.

Syrup Skunk Cabbage—Fl. ext. Skunk cabbage, Lilly, 4 fl. ozs.; Syrup, 12 fl. ozs.; Mix—Dose 2 to 4 fl. drs.

FL. EXT. SOAP TREE BARK.

Quillaja Saponaria Molina.   **Nat. Ord.—*Rosaceæ.***

Synonym—Quillaja Lins.

Range—Chili and Peru; cultivated in Northern Hindoostan.

Part used—The inner bark.

Standard of strength—That of the U. S. Pharmacopœia, 1890; 1 c.c. representing 1 gram of the drug; or, practically, minim for grain.

Action and uses—Used in the form of tincture for preparing emulsions; also in toilet preparations for cleansing the teeth and hair and as a detergent for laces, etc. It is not without use as a medicine however, being proposed in form of a syrup as a substitute for senega.

PREPARATIONS.

Tincture Soap Tree Bark, U. S.—Fl. ext. Soap tree bark, Lilly, 3½ fl. ozs.; Alcohol, 4½ fl. ozs.; Water, 8½ fl. ozs.; Mix the alcohol and water and add the fluid extract.

Syrup Soap Tree Bark—Fl. ext. Soap tree bark, Lilly, 2 fl. ozs.; Syrup, 14 fl. ozs.; Mix—Dose ½ to 1 fl. dr.

FL. EXT. SOAPWORT....................................Dose 60 to 120 m.

Saponaria officinalis Linn.   **Nat. Ord.—*Caryophyllaceæ.***

Synonym—Bouncing Bet.

Range—Central and Southern Europe; naturalized in the United States.

Habitat—Roadsides and waste places.

Part used—The herb.

Standard of strength—That of the U. S. Pharmacopœia, 1890; 1 c.c. representing 1 gram of the drug; or, practically, minim for grain.

Action and uses—Tonic, diaphoretic and alterative. A valuable remedy in the treatment of syphilitic, scrofulous and cutaneous diseases; also in jaundice, liver affections, rheumatism and gonorrhea.

PREPARATION.

Infusion Soapwort—Fl. ext. Soapwort, Lilly, 1 fl. ounce; Hot water, 15 fl. ozs.; Mix—Dose 2 to 4 fl. ozs.

FL. EXT. SOLIDAGO CANADENSIS...............Dose 30 to 60 m.

Solidago Canadensis Linn.   **Nat. Ord.—*Compositæ.***

Synonyms—S. altissima Linn.,—Canada golden rod.

Range—New Brunswick to Florida, west to British Columbia and the mountains of Arizona.

Habitat—Moist or dry and shady ground.

Part used—The leaves and inflorescence.

Standard of strength—That of the U. S. Pharmacopœia, 1890; 1 c.c. representing 1 gram of the drug; or, practically, minim for grain.

Action and uses—Astringent, styptic. Used in affections of the throat, both locally as a gargle and for its constitutional effect.

PREPARATION.

Infusion Solidago Canadensis—Fl. ext. Solidago Canadensis, Lilly, 2 fl. ozs.; Hot water, 14 fl. ozs.; Mix—Dose ½ to 1 fl. oz. as a diaphoretic or, may be used as a gargle with chlorate of potash in sore throat.

FL. EXT. SOURWOOD LEAVES................Dose 30 to 120 m.

Oxydendron arboreum (Linn.) D. C.   **Nat. Ord.—*Ericaceæ.***

Synonyms—Andromeda arborea Linn.,—Sorrel tree.

Range—Pennsylvania, west to Indiana and southward, mostly along the Alleghanies, to Florida.

Habitat—Rich woodlands.

Part used—The leaves.

Standard of strength—That of the U. S. Pharmacopœia, 1890; 1 c.c. representing 1 gram of the drug; or, practically, minim for grain.

Action and uses—Tonic, refrigerant and diuretic. Used in dropsy.

PREPARATION.

Infusion Sourwood Leaves—Fl. ext. Sourwood leaves, Lilly, 1 fl. oz.; Hot water, 15 fl. ozs.; Mix—Dose 1 to 2 fl. ozs.

WHEN ORDERING OR PRESCRIBING.

FL. EXT. SPEARMINT........ ....Dose 30 to 60 m.
Mentha viridis Linn.   **Nat. Ord.**—*Labiatæ.*
Synonyms—M. spicata Linn., M. spicata var. viridis Linn.
Range—Europe, naturalized in the United States; cultivated, common.
Habitat—Wet ground in cultivated districts.
Part used—The leaves and inflorescence.
Standard of strength—That of the U. S. Pharmacopœia, 1890; 1 c.c. representing 1 gram of the drug; or, practically, minim for grain.
Action and uses—Aromatic, stimulant and carminative. It allays nausea and expels flatus.

PREPARATIONS.

Tincture Spearmint—Fl. ext. Spearmint, Lilly, 2 fl. ozs.; Alcohol, 10½ fl. ozs.; Water, 3½ fl. ozs.; Mix—Dose 2 to 4 fl. drs.

Infusion Spearmint—Fl. ext. Spearmint, Lilly, 1 fl. oz.; Hot water, 15 fl. ozs.; Mix—Dose 1 to 2 fl. ozs.

FL. EXT. SPEEDWELL ... .Dose 30 to 60 m.
Veronica officinalis Linn.   **Nat. Ord.**—*Scrophulariaceæ.*
Synonyms—Paul's betony, Ground heel.
Range—Europe, Asia; In United States from New England to Michigan and southward to the mountains of North Carolina and Tennessee.
Habitat—Dry hills and open woods.
Part used—The herb.
Standard of strength—That of the U. S. Pharmacopœia, 1890; 1 c.c. representing 1 gram of the drug; or, practically, minim for grain.
Action and uses—Expectorant, alterative tonic and diuretic. Used in scrofula, skin diseases and urinary disorders.

PREPARATION.

Infusion Speedwell—Fl. ext. Speedwell, Lilly, 2 fl. ozs.; Hot water, 14 fl. ozs. Mix—Dose 1 to 2 fl. ozs.

FL. EXT. SPIKENARD........ .. .. Dose 30 to 60 m.
Aralia racemosa Linn.   **Nat. Ord.**—*Araliaceæ*
Synonym—Spignet.
Range—New Brunswick to Minnesota, south to the mountains of Georgia.
Habitat—Rich woodlands.
Part used—The root.
Standard of strength—That of the U. S. Pharmacopœia, 1890; 1 c.c. representing 1 gram of the drug; or, practically, minim for grain.
Action and uses—Aromatic and alterative. Used principally in pulmonary diseases.

PREPARATIONS.

Syrup Spikenard—Fl. ext. Spikenard, Lilly, 4 fl. ozs.; Syrup, 12 fl. ozs.; Mix—Dose 2 to 4 fl. drs.

Infusion Spikenard—Fl. ext. Spikenard, Lilly, 2 fl. ozs.; Hot water, 14 fl. ozs.; Mix—Dose 1 to 2 fl. ozs.

FL. EXT. SQUAW VINE .. ..Dose 30 to 60 m.

Mitchella repens Linn. **Nat. Ord.—*Rubiaceæ*.**

Synonyms—Partridgeberry, **Winterclover,** Checkerberry.

Range—Mexico, Japan; Nova Scotia and Canada, south to Florida and Texas.

Habitat—Dry woodlands, creeping about the foot of trees, especially in coniferous forests.

Part used—The herb.

Standard of strength—That of the U. S. Pharmacopœia, 1890; 1 **c.c.** representing 1 gram of the drug; or, practically, minim for grain.

Action and uses—Parturient, diuretic and astringent. Exerts a powerful tonic and alterative influence upon the uterus; found valuable in some forms of dysmenorrhea, menorrhagia, chronic congestion of the uterus; also useful in dropsy, suppression of urine and diarrhea.

PREPARATION.

Infusion Squaw Vine—Fl. ext. Squaw vine, Lilly, 1 fl. oz.; Hot water, 15 fl. ozs.; Mix—Dose 1 to 2 fl. ozs.

FL. EXT. SQUAW VINE COMP. ... ..Dose 30 **to 60 m.**

Standard of strength—One pint represents Squaw vine, 8 troy ounces; False unicorn, Cramp bark and Blue cohosh, of each, 2¼ troy ounces; Sassafras, ½ troy ounce.

Action and uses—Used principally for preparing syrup squaw vine comp. or mother's cordial.

It is a uterine tonic and antispasmodic; useful in all cases where the functions of the internal reproductive organs are deranged, as in amenorrhea, dysmenorrhea, menorrhagia, leucorrhea, and to overcome the tendency to habitual abortion. Especially valuable to pregnant women of delicate or nervous system. One or two doses daily for several weeks before parturition imparts tone to the uterus, facilitates labor and removes the cramps to which some females are liable during the latter weeks of uterogestation.

PREPARATION.

Syrup Squaw Vine Comp. (Mother's Cordial.)—Fl. ext. Squaw vine comp., Lilly, 3 fl. ozs.; Diluted alcohol, 4 fl. **ozs.;** Syrup, 9 fl. ozs.; Mix—Dose 1 to 2 fl. ozs. or more as occasion requires.

FL. EXT. SQUILL. U. S. .... **Dose 2 to 3 m.**

Urginea maritima (Linn.) Baker **Nat. Ord.—*Liliaceæ*.**

Synonym—Scilla maritima Linn.

Range—Basin of the Mediterranean **Sea.**

Habitat—Frequently in dry sandy soil **near the coast.**

Part used—The bulb.

Standard of strength—That of the U. S. Pharmacopœia, 1890; 1 **c.c.** representing 1 gram of the drug; or, practically, minim for grain.

Action and uses—Expectorant, diaphoretic and emetic. Stimulates the bronchial mucous membrane and increases the urinary secretions. It is one of the most universal additions to prescriptions for the relief of various chronic lung affections, **as** bronchitis, also whooping cough.

PREPARATIONS.

Tincture Squill. U. S.—Fl. ext. Squill, Lilly, 2½ fl. ozs.; Alcohol, 9 fl. ozs.; Water, 4½ fl. **ozs.;** Mix—Dose 10 to 20 m.

Syrup Squill, U. S.—Fl. ext. Squill, Lilly, 6 fl. drs.; Acetic acid, 10 fl. drs.; Syrup, sufficient to make 16 fl. **ozs.;** Mix—Dose ½ to 1 fl. dr.

Vinegar Squill, U. S.—Fl. ext. Squill, Lilly, 1⅔ fl. ozs.; Diluted acetic acid, 14½ fl. ozs.; Mix—Dose 20 to 30 m.

FL. EXT. SQUILL COMP..................................Dose 2 to 3 m.

Standard of strength—One pint represents Squill and Senega, of each, 8 troy ounces.

Action and uses—Used almost exclusively for the preparation of syrup of squill comp., U. S. (Hive syrup).

PREPARATION.

Syrup Squill Comp., U. S. (Hive Syrup)—Fl. ext. Squill comp., Lilly, 2½ fl. ozs.; Syrup, 12½ fl. ozs.; Hot water, 1 fl. oz.; Tartar emetic, 14 grains; Dissolve the tartar emetic in the hot water, then add the syrup and the fluid extract—Dose for children 10 to 30 m.

FL. EXT. STAR ANISE ....Dose 10 to 30 m.

Illicium verum Hook. f.   **Nat. Ord.**—*Magnoliaceæ.*

Synonyms—I. anisatum Linn.,—Chinese anise.

Range—Northern Anam; cultivated.

Part used—The fruit.

Standard of strength—That of the U. S. Pharmacopœia, 1890; 1 c.c. representing 1 gram of the drug; or, practically, minim for grain.

Action and uses—Stimulant, carminative, aromatic. Removes flatulent colic of infants, nausea and griping. Is supposed to have the property of increasing the secretion of milk.

PREPARATION.

Infusion Star Anise—Fl. ext. Star anise, Lilly, 1 fl. oz.; Hot water, 15 fl. ozs.; Mix—Dose 1 to 2 fl. ozs.

FL. EXT. STAVESACRE SEED.

Delphinium staphisagria Linn.   **Nat. Ord.**—*Ranunculaceæ.*

Synonyms—Staphisagria macrocarpa Spach.,—Staphisagria, U. S.

Range—Basin of the Mediterranean Sea.

Habitat—Dry bushy places.

Part used—The seed.

Standard of strength—That of the U. S. Pharmacopœia, 1890; 1 c.c. representing 1 gram of the drug; or, practically, minim for grain.

Action and uses—A VIOLENT POISON and should never be given internally. Its action resembles that of aconite. The tincture and the ointment are used to destroy lice and the itch mite. Even externally it should not be used where the skin is abraded. The tincture is used as an embrocation in rheumatism.

PREPARATIONS.

Tincture Stavesacre Seed—Fl. ext. Stavesacre seed, Lilly, 2 fl. ozs.; Alcohol, 14 fl. ozs.; Mix—Use externally.

Ointment Stavesacre Seed—Fl. ext. Stavesacre seed, Lilly, 2 fl. ozs.; Simple ointment, 14 troy ounces; Melt the ointment, add the fluid extract and stir till cold.

FL. EXT. STILLINGIA, U. S. ....Dose 15 to 45 m.

Stillingia sylvatica Linn.   **Nat. Ord.**—*Euphorbiaceæ.*

Synonyms—Queen's root, Queen's delight.

Range—Eastern United States, Virginia to Florida, westward to Texas.

Habitat—Dry sandy soil, pine barrens.

Part used—The root.

Standard of strength—That of the U. S. Pharmacopœia, 1890; 1 c.c. representing 1 gram of the drug; or, practically, minim for grain.

Action and uses—Highly esteemed as an alterative in syphilis, skin diseases and scrofula. It has been found beneficial in chronic laryngeal and bronchial affections, and in leucorrhea. An important ingredient in STILLIX ALTERANS, Lilly

PREPARATIONS.

Tincture Stillingia—Fl. ext. Stillingia, Lilly, 2 fl. ozs.; Alcohol, dilute, 14 fl. ozs.; Mix—Dose 1 to 2 drs.

Infusion Stillingia—Fl. ext. Stillingia, Lilly, 2 fl. ozs.; Hot water, 14 fl. ozs.; Mix—Dose 1 to 2 fl. drs.

FL. EXT. STILLINGIA COMP.......   ...Dose 15 to 45 m.

Standard of strength—One pint represents Stillingia, 6½ troy ounces; Blue flag, 2 troy ounces; Anise, Prickly ash berries, Coriander, of each, 1 troy ounce; Blood root, ½ troy ounce.

Action and uses—Used in all syphilitic, scrofulous, osseous, mercurial, hepatic and glandular diseases, or in every case where an alterative is needed. It is commonly given with an ounce of iodide of potassium added to each pint of the syrup. The dose is a fluid drachm three or four times a day in a gill of water, but where the iodide is omitted the dose may be gradually increased to a fluid ounce three times a day in water. For the purpose named however, it is inferior to STILLIX ALTERANS, Lilly.

PREPARATION.

Syrup Stillingia Comp.—Fl. ext. Stillingia comp., Lilly, 4 fl. ozs.; Syrup, 10 fl. ozs.; Alcohol, 2 fl. ozs.; Mix the alcohol and syrup, and add the fluid extract—Dose 1 to 4 fl. drs.

FL. EXT. STONE ROOT. (from the green root) ....Dose 5 to 20 m.
Collinsonia Canadensis Linn.   **Nat. Ord.**—*Labiatæ.*

Synonyms—Horseweed, Richweed.

Range—Canada to Wisconsin and south to Florida.

Habitat—Rich woodlands.

Part used—The rhizome.

Standard of strength—That of the U. S. Pharmacopœia, 1890; 1 c.c. representing 1 gram of the drug; or, practically, minim for grain.

Action and uses—Collinsonia seems to exert an influence upon the mucous tissues, and is used with benefit in chronic catarrh of the bladder, fluor albus and debility of the stomach. As a stimulant it has been used in infusion in colic, headache, cramp, dropsical affections, etc. It is gently tonic and diuretic and is valuable in lithic acid gravel and and other urinary affections. It is highly recommended as a stimulant in atonic dyspepsia and in chronic diseases with feeble digestion; it relieves pulmonary irritation in chronic diseases of the respiratory apparatus and acts as a stimulant expectorant. In irritation of the pneumogastric nerve, heart disease, and in that distressing asthma simulating and sometimes attending phthisis, its quieting influence has been observed, giving increased strength and regularity to the heart's action. It will be found very efficacious **in** chronic laryngitis and clergymen's sore throat.

PREPARATIONS.

Tincture Stone Root—Fl. ext. Stone root, Lilly, 2 fl. ozs.; Alcohol, 10½ fl. ozs.; Water, 3½ fl. ozs.; Mix—Dose ½ to 2 fl. drs.

Syrup Stone Root—Fl. ext. Stone root, Lilly, 2 fl. ozs.; Syrup, 14 fl. ozs.; Mix—Dose ½ to 2 fl. drs.

FL. EXT. STRAMONIUM LEAVES.................. ....Dose 1 to 2 m.
Datura Stramonium Linn.   **Nat. Ord.**—*Solanaceæ.*

Synonyms—Thornapple, Jamestownweed, Jimsonweed, Apple Peru.

Range—Asia, Europe; naturalized in the United States, abundant.

Habitat—Waste grounds, along roadsides, common weed.

Part used—The leaves.

Standard of strength—0.3 per cent of alkaloid, estimated by titration with acid.

Action and uses—NARCOTIC POISON. In medicinal doses, anodyne and antispasmodic, without causing constipation; its action is similar to hyoscyamus and belladonna; it is much prized in asthma.

Antidotes—In poisoning by this drug tannic acid and emetics should be used, then morphine, physostigmine or pilocarpine for the nervous disturbance. Caustic alkalies are incompatible.

PREPARATION.

Tincture Stramonium Leaves—Fl. ext. Stramonium leaves, Lilly, 2½ fl. ozs.; Alcohol, 6¼ fl. ozs.; Water, 6¼ fl. ozs.; Mix—Dose 5 to 15 m.

FL. EXT. STRAMONIUM SEED, U. S. . . . . Dose 1 to 2 m.

Datura Stramonium Linn.   **Nat. Ord.**—*Solanaceæ.*

Synonyms—Thornapple, Jamestownweed, Jimsonweed, Apple Peru.

Range—Asia, Europe; naturalized in the United States, abundant.

Habitat—Waste grounds, along roadsides, common weed.

Part used—The seed.

Standard of strength—0.3 per cent. of alkaloid, estimated by titration with acid.

Action and uses—NARCOTIC POISON. In medicinal doses, anodyne and antispasmodic, without causing constipation; its action is similar to hyoscyamus and belladonna; it is much prized in asthma.

Antidotes—In poisoning by this drug tannic acid and emetics should be used, then morphine, physostigmine or pilocarpine for the nervous disturbance. Caustic alkalies are incompatible.

PREPARATION.

Tincture Stramonium Seed, U. S.—Fl. ext. Stramonium seed, Lilly, 2½ fl. ozs.; Alcohol, 6¼ fl. ozs.; Water, 6¼ fl. ozs.; Mix—Dose 5 to 15 m.

FL. EXT. STYLOSANTHES . . . . Dose 10 to 20 m.

Stylosanthes biflora (Linn.) B. S. P.   **Nat. Ord.**—*Leguminosæ.*

Synonyms—Trifolium biflorum Linn., S. elatior Swartz.

Range—Long Island, New Jersey to Florida, west to Southern Indiana, Kansas and Arkansas.

Habitat—Sandy soil, pine barrens.

Part used—The herb.

Standard of strength—That of the U. S. Pharmacopœia, 1890; 1 c.c. representing 1 gram of the drug; or, practically, minim for grain.

Action and uses—Said to have a peculiar effect upon the uterus, acting as a uterine sedative.

FL. EXT. SUMACH BARK . . . . Dose 20 to 30 m.

Rhus glabra Linn.   **Nat. Ord.**—*Anacardiaceæ.*

Synonyms—Smooth sumach, Upland sumach.

Range—Common over nearly all parts of the continent.

Habitat—Rocky or barren soil.

Part used—The bark.

Standard of strength—That of the U. S. Pharmacopœia, 1890; 1 c.c. representing 1 gram of the drug; or, practically, minim for grain.

Action and uses—Sumach is tonic, astringent, antiseptic. Valuable in gonorrhea, leucorrhea, diarrhea, dysentery. An infusion of the bark may be used as an injection in prolapsus uteri and ani.

PREPARATION.

Gargle Sumach Bark—Fl. ext. Sumach bark, Lilly, 2 fl. ozs.; Hot water, 8 fl. ozs.; Mix—Useful in quinsy and ulceration of the mouth and throat.

FL. EXT. SUMACH BERRIES, U. S. .... **Dose 20 to 30 m.**
Rhus glabra Linn. **Nat. Ord.—*Anacardiaceæ.***
Synonyms—Smooth sumach, Upland sumach.
Range—Common over nearly all parts of the continent.
Habitat—Rocky or barren soil.
Part used—The fruit.
Standard of strength—That of the U. S. Pharmacopœia, 1890; 1 **c.c.**
representing 1 gram of the drug; or, practically, minim for grain.
Action and uses—Refrigerant, diuretic and astringent. The infusion
may be used in diabetes, strangury, bowel complaints, febrile diseases
and as a gargle in quinsy and ulcerations of the mouth and throat and
as a wash for ringworm, tetter, ulcers, etc.

PREPARATION.

Infusion Sumach Berries—Fl. ext. Sumach berries, Lilly, 1 fl. oz.;
Hot water, 15 fl. ozs.; Mix.—Dose ½ to 1 fl. oz.

FL. EXT. SUNDEW .... **Dose 30 to 60 m.**
Drosera rotundifolia Linn. **Nat. Ord.—*Droseraceæ.***
Synonyms—Youthwort, Roundleaved sundew.
Range—Europe; in North America from Labrador to Minnesota, Indiana and southward; common.
Habitat—Boggy places.
Part used—The herb.
Standard of strength—That of the U. S. Pharmacopœia, 1890; 1 c.c.
representing 1 gram of the drug; or, practically, minim for grain.
Action and uses—Exerts a peculiar action upon the respiratory apparatus and has been found useful in pertussis, asthma, incipient phthisis, chronic bronchitis, with dry spasmodic cough, whether from pulmonary, cardiac or gastric diseases. Two fluid drams of the fluid extract may be added to four fluid ounces of water or wine, of which a teaspoonful may be given every three or four hours.

PREPARATION.

Infusion Sundew—Fl. ext. Sundew, Lilly, 1 fl. oz.; Hot water, 15 fl ozs.; Mix.—Dose 1 to 4 fl. ozs.

FL. EXT SUNFLOWER SEED .... **Dose 30 to 120 m.**
Helianthus annuus Linn. **Nat. Ord.—*Compositæ.***
Range—Saskatchewan to Texas, and west to the Pacific coast; cultivated.
Habitat—Plains and alluvial grounds.
Part used—The akenes.
Standard of strength—That of the U. S. Pharmacopœia, 1890; 1 c.c.
representing 1 gram of the drug; or, practically, minim for grain.
Action and uses—Diuretic and expectorant; has been used in pulmonary affections with considerable benefit.

PREPARATION.

Infusion Sunflower Seed—Fl. ext. Sunflower seed, Lilly, 4 fl. ozs.; Hot water, 12 fl. ozs.; Mix.—Dose 1 to 2 fl. ozs.

FL. EXT. SWEET GUM BARK .... **Dose 15 to 60 m.**
Liquidambar Styraciflua Linn. **Nat. Ord.—*Hamamelidaceæ.***
Range—Connecticut to Southern Illinois and south to Florida and Texas; Mexico and Central America.
Habitat—Moist woodlands.
Part used—The inner bark.

Standard of strength—That of the U. S. Pharmacopœia, 1890; 1 c.c. representing 1 gram of the drug; or, practically, minim for grain.

Action and uses—Astringent; has been used advantageously in diarrhea and dysentery, especially in children. Used principally in form of the syrup.

PREPARATION.

Syrup Sweet Gum Bark—Fl. ext. Sweet gum bark, Lilly, 4 fl. ozs.; Syrup, 12 fl. ozs.; Mix—Dose ½ to 1 fl. oz.

FL. EXT. TAG ALDER ....Dose 30 to 60 m.

Alnus serrulata Willd.　　　　　　**Nat. Ord.**—*Cupuliferæ.*

Synonyms—A. rugosa (Ehrh.) Koch, Betula rugosa Ehrh.,—Swamp alder.

Range—Massachusetts to Florida, west to Southeastern Minnesota and Texas; common.

Habitat—Borders of streams and swamps.

Part used—The bark.

Standard of strength—That of the U. S. Pharmacopœia, 1890; 1 c.c. representing 1 gram of the drug; or, practically, minim for grain.

Action and uses—Alterative, emetic and astringent. Used in scrofula and cutaneous diseases.

PREPARATION.

Infusion Tag Alder—Fl. ext. Tag alder, Lilly, 1 fl. oz.; Hot water, 15 fl. ozs.; Mix—Dose 1 to 2 fl. ozs.

FL. EXT. TAMARAC BARK ....Dose 30 to 60 m.

Larix laricina (Duroi) Koch.　　　　**Nat. Ord.**—*Coniferæ.*

Synonyms—L. Americana Michx., Pinus laricina Duroi, P. pendula Ait.,—Larch, Hackmatac, Black larch.

Range—Northern Pennsylvania to Northern Indiana and Central Minnesota and far northward.

Habitat—Chiefly in cold swamps.

Part used—The inner bark.

Standard of strength—That of the U. S. Pharmacopœia, 1890; 1 c. representing 1 gram of the drug; or, practically, minim for grain.

Action and uses—Laxative, tonic, diuretic and alterative. Recommended in obstructions of the liver, rheumatism and some cutaneous diseases.

PREPARATION.

Infusion Tamarac Bark—Fl. ext. Tamarac bark, Lilly, 1 fl. oz.; Hot water, 15 fl. ozs.; Mix—Dose 1 to 2 fl. ozs.

FL. EXT. TANSY ....Dose 30 to 60 m.

Tanacetum vulgare Linn.　　　　**Nat. Ord.**—*Compositæ.*

Range—Asia and Europe; naturalized in the Eastern United States and Canada; cultivated.

Habitat—Escaped from gardens, along roadsides and in waste places.

Part used—The leaves and inflorescence.

Standard of strength—That of the U. S. Pharmacopœia, 1890; 1 c.c. representing 1 gram of the drug; or, practically, minim for grain.

Action and uses—Tansy is tonic, emmenagogue and diaphoretic. The infusion has been found beneficial in intermittent fever, suppressed menstruation, tardy labor pains, and as a preventive of the paroxysms of gout.

PREPARATION.

Infusion Tansy—Fl. ext. Tansy, Lilly, 1 fl. oz.; Hot water, 15 fl. ozs.; Mix—Dose 1 to 2 fl. ozs.

FL. EXT. TAR, SOLUBLE, (for Syrup, U. S.).

This is a concentrated solution made from the best quality of washed pine tar and is intended for use in the extemporaneous preparation of the official syrup.

PREPARATION.

Syrup Tar, U. S.—Fl. ext. Tar, soluble, Lilly, 2 fl. ozs.; Syrup, 14 fl. ozs.; Mix—Dose ½ to 1 fl. oz.

FL. EXT. TEA .... Dose 15 to 30 m.

Thea Chinensis Linn.   **Nat. Ord.**—*Ternstræmiaceæ.*

Synonyms—T. sinensis Linn., Camellia Thea Link.

Range—Upper Assam; cultivated in China, Japan, several parts of India and to a small extent in Southern United States.

Habitat—Often in hedge rows around rice and corn fields; rich sandy loam of lower hillsides near a stream is regarded as the best soil for its cultivation.

Part used—The leaves.

Standard of strength—That of the U. S. Pharmacopœia, 1890; 1 c.c. representing 1 gram of the drug; or, practically, minim for grain.

Action and uses—Mildly stimulant and astringent. A valuable remedy for nervous headache and also moderates the copious sweats of hectic conditions. It is useful as an antidote in opium poisoning.

PREPARATION.

Infusion Tea—Fl. ext. Tea, Lilly, 1 fl. oz.; Hot water, 15 fl. ozs.; Mix—Dose 1 to 2 fl. ozs.

FL. EXT. TOLU, SOLUBLE, (for Syrup, U. S.).

Toluifera Balsamum Linn.   **Nat. Ord.**—*Leguminosæ.*

Synonyms—Myrospermum toluiferum A. Rich., Myroxylon Toluifera Kunth.,—Balsam of Tolu.

Range—Venezuela and New Granada.

Habitat—High rolling ground.

Part used—An exudation from fresh incisions upon the trunk of the tree.

Standard of strength—That of the U. S. Pharmacopœia, 1890; 1 c.c. representing 1 gram of the drug; or, practically, minim for grain.

Action and uses—The preparation is a concentrated solution of those principles in balsam tolu soluble in syrup. The syrup made from this preparation will, therefore, duplicate, in every respect the official article, making a clear mixture with syrup.

PREPARATION.

Syrup Tolu, U. S.—Fl. ext. Tolu, soluble, Lilly, 1 fl. oz.; Syrup, 15 fl. ozs.; Mix—Dose 2 to 4 fl. drs.; Chiefly used to impart its agreeable flavor to mixtures.

FL. EXT. TONKA BEAN.

Dipterix odorata (Aub.) Willd.   **Nat. Ord.**—*Leguminosæ.*

Synonyms—D. oppositifolia Willd., Coumarouma odorata Aublet,—Tonco, Tonguin or Tonga bean.

Range—Guiana and Cayenne.

Habitat—In forests.

Part used—The seeds.

Standard of strength—That of the U. S. Pharmacopœia, 1890; 1 c.c. representing 1 gram of the drug; or, practically, minim for grain.

Action and uses—Aromatic. Used for flavoring.

WHEN ORDERING OR PRESCRIBING.

FL. EXT. TRIFOLIUM COMP. (for Syrup).

Standard of strength—One pint represents Red clover, 4½ troy
ounces; Stillingia, Burdock root, Poke root, Berberis aquifolium, Cascara
amarga, of each, 2¼ troy ounces; Prickly ash bark, 150 grains, Potassium
iodide, 512 grains.

Action and uses—Alterative. Used principally for preparing syrup
trifolium comp.

PREPARATION.

Syrup Trifolium Comp.—Fl. ext. Trifolium comp., Lilly, 4 fl. ozs.;
Syrup, 12 fl. ozs.; Mix—Dose 2 to 4 fl. drs.

FL. EXT. TULIP TREE BARK.................Dose 30 to 60 m.

Liriodendron Tulipifera Linn.   **Nat. Ord.**—*Magnoliaceæ.*

Synonyms—Whitewood, Lyre tree, Tulip poplar.

Range—Southern New England to Michigan, Wisconsin and southward.

Habitat—Rich woodlands.

Part used—The bark of the branches.

Standard of strength—That of the U. S. Pharmacopœia, 1890; 1 c.c.
representing 1 gram of the drug; or, practically, minim for grain.

Action and uses—Antiperiodic, vermifuge, sudorific and diuretic.

PREPARATIONS.

Tincture Tulip Tree Bark—Fl. ext. Tulip tree bark, Lilly, 4 fl.
ozs.; Alcohol, 8 fl. ozs.; Water, 4 fl. ozs.; Mix the alcohol and water and
add the fluid extract—Dose 1 to 2 fl. drs.

Infusion Tulip Tree Bark—Fl. ext. Tulip tree bark, Lilly, 1 fl.
oz.; Hot water, 15 fl. ozs.; Mix—Dose ½ to 1 fl. oz.

FL. EXT. TURKEY CORN.................Dose 30 to 60 m.

Dicentra Canadensis D. C.   **Nat. Ord.**—*Papaveraceæ.*

Synonyms—Diclytra Canadensis D. C., Corydalis Canadensis Goldie,
Bicuculla Canadensis (Goldie) Millsp.

Range—Canada and the United States, south to Kentucky.

Habitat—Rich woodlands.

Part used—The tubers.

Standard of strength—That of the U. S. Pharmacopœia, 1890; 1 c.c.
representing 1 gram of the drug; or, practically, minim for grain.

Action and uses—Tonic, diuretic and alterative.

PREPARATIONS.

Tincture Turkey Corn—Fl. ext. Turkey corn, Lilly, 2 fl. ozs.;
Diluted alcohol, 14 fl. ozs.; Mix—Dose 2 to 4 fl. drs.

Syrup Turkey Corn—Fl. ext. Turkey corn, Lilly, 4 fl. ozs.; Syrup,
12 fl. ozs.; Mix—Dose 1 to 2 fl. drs.

FL. EXT. TURMERIC.

Curcuma longa Linn.   **Nat. Ord.**—*Zingiberaceæ.*

Synonyms—C. rotunda Linn., Amomum Curcuma Jacq.—Curcuma.

Range—India, Ceylon, many of the East Indian Islands and the Fijis;
cultivated.

Part used—The rhizome.

Standard of strength—That of the U. S. Pharmacopœia, 1890; 1 c.c.
representing 1 gram of the drug; or, practically, minim for grain.

Action and uses—Used as a coloring.

FL. EXT. UNICORN ROOT................ ....Dose 5 to 20 m.
Aletris farinosa Linn.   **Nat. Ord.**—*Hæmodoraceæ.*
Synonym—Stargrass.
Range—Massachusetts to Florida, west to Minnesota and Illinois.
Habitat—Grassy or sandy woods.
Part used—The rhizome.
Standard of strength—That of the U. S. Pharmacopœia, 1890; 1 c.c.
representing 1 gram of the drug; or, practically, minim for gram.
Action and uses—A valuable bitter tonic, used with advantage in
flatulent colic, hysteria, and to increase the tone of the stomach. Its
most valuable property is the tonic influence it exerts upon the female
generative organs, giving a normal energy to the uterus, and proving
useful where there is a tendency to habitual miscarriage; in chlorosis,
amenorrhea, dysmenorrhea and engorged conditions of the uterus, as
well as in prolapsus uteri, it is one of our most valuable agents.

PREPARATION.

Syrup Unicorn Root—Fl. ext. Unicorn root, Lilly, 4 fl. ozs.; Syrup
12 fl. ozs.; Mix—Dose ½ to 1 fl. dr.

FL. EXT. USTILAGO MAYDIS.................. ...Dose 60 to 120 m.
Ustilago Maydis Leveille.   *Fungi;* **Class**—*Ascomycetes;*
                             Nat. Ord.—*Ustilagineæ.*
Synonyms—Corn smut, Corn ergot.
Range—That of corn—Tropical and Temperate America; cultivated.
Habitat—Upon all parts of corn (*Zea Mays* Linn.), most frequently
upon the inflorescence.
Part used—The entire fungus growth collected when the spores are
fully developed.
Standard of strength—That of the U. S. Pharmacopœia, 1890; 1 c.c.
representing 1 gram of the drug; or, practically, minim for gram.
Action and uses—It has been recommended as a safe and successful
substitute for ergot; also used in ovarian irritation, ovaritis, amenorrhea,
dysmenorrhea, premature menstruation, and other menstrual derangements.

PREPARATIONS.

Tincture Ustilago Maydis—Fl. ext. Ustilago Maydis, Lilly, 4 fl.
ozs.; Alcohol, 4 fl. ozs.; Water, 8 fl. ozs.; Mix the alcohol and water and
add the fluid extract—Dose 2 to 4 fl. drs.

Syrup Ustilago Maydis—Fl. ext. Ustilago Maydis, Lilly, 2 fl. ozs.;
Syrup, 14 fl. ozs.; Mix—Dose ½ to 1 fl. oz.

Infusion Ustilago Maydis—Fl. ext. Ustilago Maydis, Lilly, 1 fl.
oz.; Hot water, 15 fl. ozs.; Mix—Dose 1 to 2 fl. ozs.

Wine Ustilago Maydis—Fl. ext. Ustilago Maydis, Lilly, 4 fl. ozs.;
White wine, 10½ fl. ozs.; Alcohol, 1½ fl. ozs.; Mix—Dose 2 to 4 fl. drs.

FL. EXT. UVA URSI, U. S....................Dose 30 to 60 m.
Arctostaphylus Uva Ursi (Linn.) Sprengel. **Nat. Ord.**—*Ericaceæ.*
Synonyms—Arbutus Uva Ursi Linn.,—Bearberry.
Range—Europe and Asia, United States; New Jersey and Pennsylvania
to Missouri and far north and westward.
Habitat—Rocks and bare hills.
Part used—The leaves.
Standard of strength—That of the U. S. Pharmacopœia, 1890; 1 c.c.
representing 1 gram of the drug; or, practically, minim for grain.
Action and uses—Uva Ursi is astringent and tonic, with special direction to the urinary organs; much used in gravel; it is recommended
in chronic nephritis, and where there is reason to conjecture the exist-
ence of ulceration in the kidneys, bladder or urinary passages; also serviceable in diabetes, catarrh of the bladder, incontinence of urine, gleet,
leucorrhea and menorrhagia.

PREPARATIONS.

Syrup Uva Ursi Comp.—Fl. exts. Uva Ursi, Buchu, Cubeb, Gravel plant, and Lovage, Lilly, of each, 1 fl. oz.; Syrup, 16 fl. ozs.; Mix—Dose 2 to 4 fl. drs.; Used in strangury or gravel.

Infusion Uva Ursi—Fl. ext. Uva Ursi, Lilly, 1 fl. oz.; Hot water, 15 fl. ozs.; Mix—Dose 1 to 2 fl. ozs.

FL. EXT. VALERIAN, U. S...... ....Dose 30 to 60 m.
Valeriana officinalis Linn.   **Nat. Ord.**— *Valerianeæ.*

Synonyms—V. angustifolia Tausch., V. sambucifolia Mikan.

Range—Europe and northern Asia; naturalized and cultivated in New England.

Habitat—Moist and dry localities, often on chalky soil.

Part used—The rhizome and roots.

Standard of strength—That of the U. S. Pharmacopœia, 1890; 1 c.c. representing 1 gram of the drug; or, practically, minim for grain.

Action and uses—Valerian is gently stimulant, with an especial direction to the nervous system, but without narcotic effects. It is probably used more largely in hysteria than any other remedy. In the state of unrest familiarly known as nervousness, by soothing and quieting the patient, it will often indirectly procure sleep. The ammoniated tincture is valuable in nervous headache.

PREPARATIONS.

Tincture Valerian, U. S.—Fl. ext. Valerian, Lilly, 3¼ **fl. ozs.**; Alcohol, 1½ fl. ozs.; Water, 3¼ fl. ozs.; Mix—Dose 1 to 2 fl. drs.

Tincture Valerian, Ammoniated, U. S.—Fl. ext. Valerian, Lilly, 3½ fl. ozs.; Aromatic spirit of ammonia, 12¼ fl. ozs.; Mix—Dose 1 to 2 fl. drs. in milk or sweetened water.

FL. EXT. VERATRUM VIRIDE, U. S.................Dose 1 to 3 m.
Veratrum viride Ait.   **Nat. Ord.**—*Liliaceæ.*

Synonyms—V. album var. viride Baker, Helonias viride Ker.,—Swamp hellebore.

Range—Canada and in the United States as far south as Georgia.

Habitat—In swampy places and in the borders of damp thickets.

Part used—The rhizome and rootlets.

Standard of Strength—1 per cent of total alkaloids, estimated gravimetrically.

Action and uses—ACRONARCOTIC POISON. Similar in its action to aconite. Veratrum viride in small doses lessens the frequency and force of the pulse, reducing it sometimes to even thirty-five a minute. Severe nausea or vomiting frequently accompany or follow the reduction of the pulse rate. Wood says: "In the early stages of sthenic pneumonia, it offers, I believe, the best known method of reducing the pulse rate and the temperature and of ameliorating the disease." It should be administered in gradually increasing doses until its physiological action is manifested. Vomiting is to be avoided as far as possible; to prevent this, 5 to 10 drops of laudanum should be exhibited fifteen minutes before each dose of Veratrum viride; an hour is generally the best interval between doses.

Antidotes—Recumbent posture absolute. Stomach pump, stimulants, heat to extremities, artificial respiration if necessary. Caffeine hypodermically or by the mouth. Atropine, morphine, ammonia, ether and amyl nitrite have been used. Dry heat applied to the body. Caustic alkalies are incompatible.

PREPARATIONS.

Tincture Veratrum Viride, U. S.—Fl. ext. Veratrum viride, Lilly, 6¼ fl. ozs.; Alcohol, 9¼ fl. ozs.; Mix—Dose 3 to 7 m.

Norwood's Tincture Veratrum Viride—Fl. ext. Veratrum viride, Lilly, 8 fl. ozs.; Syrup, 8 fl. ozs.; Mix—Dose 3 to 6 m.

FL. EXT. VERVAIN ....**Dose 30 to 60 m.**
Verbena hastata Linn. **Nat. Ord.—** *Verbenaceæ.*
Synonyms—V. paniculata Lam.,—Wild hyssop, Simpler's joy.
Range—Canada and Saskatchewan, south to Florida and New Mexico.
Habitat—Waste grounds and roadsides.
Part used—The leaves and inflorescence.
Standard of strength—That of the U. S. Pharmacopœia, 1890; 1 c.c.
representing 1 gram of the drug; or, practically, minim for grain.
Action and uses—Tonic, emetic, expectorant and sudorific. Used as
an emetic and sudorific in intermittent fever, in colds and suppressed
menstruation.

PREPARATION.

Infusion Vervain—Fl. ext. Vervain, Lilly, 2 fl. ozs.; Hot water, 14
fl. ozs.; Mix—Dose ½ to 1 fl. oz.

FL. EXT. VIBURNUM COMP......... ....**Dose 30 to** 120 m.
Standard of strength—One pint represents Cramp bark, 3 troy
ounces; Scullcap, Wild yam, of each, 1½ troy ounces, and aromatics.
Action and uses—Nervine and antispasmodic. Used as a remedy for
cramps, colic, spasms and in the treatment of hysteria and asthma;
quickly relieves dysmenorrhœa when not due to organic lesion or mal-
formation. It should be given in half a wineglassful of sweetened
hot water **or** milk and repeated **every** fifteen minutes until relief is
obtained.

FL. EXT. VIOLET HERB .... .. Dose 30 to 60 m.
Viola pedata Linn. **Nat. Ord.—** *Violaceæ.*
Synonyms—Sweet violet, Birdsfoot violet.
Range—New England to Minnesota and southward.
Habitat—Sandy or gravelly soil.
Part used—The herb.
Standard of strength—That of the U. S. Pharmacopœia, 1890; 1 c.c.
representing 1 gram of the drug; or, practically, minim for grain.
Action and uses—Laxative. In large doses cathartic and emetic.

PREPARATION.

Syrup Violet Herb—Fl. ext. Violet herb, Lilly, 2 fl. ozs.; Alcohol,
2 fl. ozs.; Syrup, 12 fl. ozs. Mix the alcohol with the syrup and add the
fluid extract; Dose ½ to 1 fl. oz.

FL. EXT. VIRGINIA STONE **CROP** .. .. Dose 30 to 60 m.
Penthorum sedoides Linn. **Nat. Ord.—** *Crassulaceæ.*
Synonym—Ditch stone crop.
Range—New Brunswick to Florida, west to Minnesota, Eastern Kansas
and Texas.
Habitat—Open wet places.
Part used—The herb.
Standard of strength—That of the U. S. Pharmacopœia, 1890; **1 c.c.**
representing 1 gram of the drug; or, practically, minim for grain.
Action and uses—Diuretic, demulcent, laxative and slightly astringent. This drug has been recommended both as a constitutional and
local remedy for catarrh, catarrhal laryngitis, pharyngitis, chronic
bronchitis and catarrhal affections of the stomach and bowels. In large
doses it causes a disagreeable fullness of the head, and excessive dream-
ing during sleep.

PREPARATIONS.

Tincture Virginia Stone Crop—Fl. ext. Virginia stone crop,
Lilly, 8 fl. ozs.; Alcohol, 6 fl. ozs.; Water, 2 fl. ozs. Mix—Dose 1 to 2 fl. drs.

Infusion Virginia Stone Crop—Fl. ext. Virginia stone crop,
Lilly, 1 fl. oz.; Hot water, 15 fl. ozs.; Mix—Dose 1 to 2 fl. ozs.

FL. EXT. WAFER ASH .... Dose 10 to 30 m.
Ptelea trifoliata Linn.   **Nat. Ord.**—*Rutaceæ.*

Synonyms—Wing seed, Shrubby trefoil, Hop-tree.

Range—Long Island to Minnesota and southward.

Habitat—Rocky places.

Part used—The root bark.

Standard of strength—That of the U. S. Pharmacopœia, 1890; 1 c.c. representing 1 gram of the drug; or, practically, minim for grain.

Action and uses—Wafer ash is a pure unirritating tonic, employed advantageously in convalescence after fevers and in debility connected with gastro-enteric irritation. It promotes the appetite, gives tone to the stomach, and will be tolerated when other tonics are rejected. It is also said to be valuable in intermittent fevers.

PREPARATIONS.

Tincture Wafer Ash—Fl. ext. Wafer ash, Lilly, 4 fl. ozs.; Alcohol, 12 fl. ozs.; Mix—Dose 1 to 2 fl. drs.

Infusion Wafer Ash—Fl. ext. Wafer ash, Lilly, 2 fl. ozs.; Hot water, 14 fl. ozs.; Mix—Dose 2 to 4 fl. drs.

FL. EXT. WAHOO ROOT BARK .... Dose 30 to 60 **m.**
Euonymus atropurpureus Jacq.   **Nat. Ord.**—*Celastrineæ.*

Synonyms—Indian arrow, Burning bush, Spindle-tree.

Range—Northern and Western United States.

Habitat—In woodlands along moist banks of streams.

Part used—The root bark.

Standard of strength—That of the U. S. Pharmacopœia, 1890; 1 c.c. representing 1 gram of the drug; or, practically, minim for grain.

Action and uses—Wahoo is tonic, laxative, alterative and diuretic. It has been highly recommended as a hepatic stimulant and in hepatic dyspepsia or biliousness. Its effects are felt most about forty-eight hours after taking.

PREPARATION.

Syrup Wahoo Root Bark—Fl. ext. Wahoo root bark, Lilly, 4 fl. ozs.; Syrup, 12 fl. ozs.; Mix—Dose 2 to 4 fl. drs.

FL. EXT. WATER AVENS ROOT.................... Dose 30 to 60 m.
Geum rivale Linn.   **Nat. Ord.**—*Rosaceæ.*

Synonyms—Purple avens, Chocolate root.

Range—Europe, North America; Newfoundland to New Jersey, west to Minnesota and Missouri.

Habitat—Bogs and wet meadows.

Part used—The root.

Standard of strength—That of the U. S. Pharmacopœia, 1890; 1 c.c. representing 1 gram of the drug; or, practically, minim for grain.

Action and uses—Tonic and powerfully astringent. Used with success in hemorrhages, chronic diarrhœa and dysentery, leucorrhœa, etc.

PREPARATION.

Infusion Water Avens Root—Fl. ext. Water avens root, Lilly, 2 fl. ozs.; Hot water, 14 fl. ozs.; Mix—Dose ½ to 1 fl. oz.

FL. EXT. WATER ERYNGO .... Dose 20 to 60 m.
Eryngium aquaticum Linn.   **Nat. Ord.**—*Umbelliferæ.*

Synonym—E. yuccæfolium Michx.

Range—New Jersey to Minnesota, south to Florida and Texas.

Habitat—Dry or damp soil, often in pine barrens or on prairies.

Part used—The rhizome.

Standard of strength—That of the U. S. Pharmacopœia, 1890; 1 c.c. representing 1 gram of the drug; or, practically, minim for grain.

Action and uses—Diuretic, stimulant, diaphoretic, expectorant and, in large doses, emetic. Useful in dropsy, nephritic and calculous affections; also in scrofula and syphilis; as a diaphoretic and expectorant in pulmonary diseases, and of value in chronic laryngitis and bronchitis.

PREPARATION.

Infusion Water Eryngo—Fl. ext. Water eryngo, Lilly, 1 fl. oz.; Hot water, 15 fl. ozs.; Mix—Dose 1 to 2 fl. ozs.

FL. EXT. WATER HEMLOCK........................**Dose 1 to 5 m.**
Cicuta maculata Linn.   **Nat. Ord.**—*Umbelliferæ.*
Synonyms—C. virosa var. maculata Coult. and Rose,—Spotted hemlock, Spotted parsley.
Range—Throughout the United States.
Habitat—Around marshes and in wet ground.
Part used—The leaves.
Standard of strength—That of the U. S. Pharmacopœia, 1890; 1 c.c. representing 1 gram of the drug; or, practically, minim for gram.
Action and uses—Narcotic and sedative, possessing also properties similar to belladonna. Of benefit in all affections attended with an excited state of the nervous and vascular systems.
Antidotes—In poisoning by this drug tannic acid and emetics should be used, then morphine, physostigmine or pilocarpine for the nervous disturbance. Caustic alkalies are incompatible.

FL. EXT. WATERMELON SEED....................Dose 30 to 60 m.
Citrullus vulgaris Schrader.   **Nat. Ord.**—*Cucurbitaceæ.*
Synonym—Cucumis citrullus Seringe.
Range—Southern Asia; cultivated in nearly all parts of the temperate and warm temperate zones.
Habitat—Rich sandy soil.
Part used—The seed.
Standard of strength—That of the U. S. Pharmacopœia, 1890; 1 c.c. representing 1 gram of the drug; or, practically, minim for gram.
Action and uses—Diuretic, refrigerant and tenifuge.

PREPARATION.

Infusion Watermelon Seed—Fl. ext. Watermelon seed, Lilly, 2 fl. ozs.; Hot water, 14 fl. ozs.; Mix—Dose 1 to 2 fl. ozs.

FL. EXT. WATER PEPPER....   .....Dose 30 to **60 m.**
Polygonum punctatum Ell.   **Nat. Ord.**—*Polygonaceæ.*
Synonyms—P. acre H. B. K., P. Hydropiper Michx., P. hydropiperoides Pursh., smart weed, Hydropiper.
Range—Ontario; New England to Florida, west to Minnesota, the Dakotas, Missouri and Arkansas.
Habitat—Shallow water and wet ground.
Part used—The herb.
Standard of strength—That of the U. S. Pharmacopœia, 1890; 1 c.c. representing 1 gram of the drug; or, practically, minim for gram.
Action and uses—Stimulant, diuretic, emmenagogue, antiseptic and diaphoretic. It has been found very efficacious in amenorrhea; doses repeated every four or five hours.

PREPARATION.

Infusion Water Pepper—Fl. ext. Water pepper, Lilly, 1 fl. oz.; Hot water, 15 fl. ozs.; Mix—Dose 1 to 2 fl. ozs.

FL. EXT. WHITE BRYONY...... ... ... .Dose 10 to 15 m.
Bryonia alba Linn. **Nat. Ord.**—*Cucurbitaceæ.*
Synonyms—Bryonia U. S.,—Wild bryony, Wild hops, Tetter berry.
Range—Central and Southern Europe.
Habitat—In thickets and hedges.
Part used—The root.
Standard of strength—That of the U. S. Pharmacopœia, 1890; 1 c.c. representing 1 gram of the drug; or, practically, minim for grain.
Action and uses—An active hydragogue cathartic, similar to jalap.

PREPARATIONS.

Tincture White Bryony, U. S.—Fl. ext. White bryony, Lilly, 1½ fl. ozs., Alcohol, 7½ fl. ozs.; Water,7½ fl. ozs.; Mix—Dose 1 to 2 fl. drs

Infusion White Bryony—Fl. ext. White bryony, Lilly, 1 fl. oz.; Hot water, 15 fl. ozs.; Mix—Dose 1 to 2 fl. ozs.

FL. EXT. WHITE CLOVER ....Dose 30 to 60 m.
Trifolium repens Linn. **Nat. Ord.**—*Leguminosæ.*
Synonym—Shamrock.
Range—Europe; probably indigenous in Northeastern United States; widely distributed.
Habitat—Fields and copses, along roadsides.
Part used—The inflorescence.
Standard of strength—That of the U. S. Pharmacopœia, 1890; 1 c.c. representing 1 gram of the drug; or, practically, minim for grain.
Action and uses—Detergent.

PREPARATION.

Infusion White Clover—Fl. ext. White clover, Lilly, 2 fl. ozs.; Hot water, 14 fl. ozs.; Mix—Dose 1 to 2 fl. ozs.

FL. EXT. WHITE COHOSH...... .... Dose 5 to 20 m.
Actæa alba (Linn.) Mill. **Nat. Ord.**—*Ranunculaceæ.*
Synonyms—Actæa spicata var. alba Linn.,—White baneberry.
Range—Europe, North America; common.
Habitat—Rich woodlands.
Part used—The rhizome.
Standard of strength—That of the U. S. Pharmacopœia, 1890; 1 c.c. representing 1 gram of the drug; or, practically, minim for grain.
Action and uses—Purgative and emetic.

PREPARATION.

Infusion White Cohosh—Fl. ext. White cohosh, Lilly, 1 fl. oz.; Hot water, 15 fl. ozs.; Mix—Dose 2 to 4 fl. drs.

FL. EXT. WHITE INDIAN HEMP. .... Dose 5 to 15 m.
Asclepias incarnata Linn. **Nat. Ord.**—*Asclepiadaceæ.*
Synonyms—Flesh-colored asclepias, Swamp milkweed.
Range—New Brunswick to Georgia and Louisiana, west to Manitoba, Dakota, Nebraska and Texas.
Habitat—Swamps, wet grounds.
Part used—The rhizome.
Standard of strength—That of the U. S. Pharmacopœia, 1890; 1 c.c. representing 1 gram of the drug; or, practically, minim for grain.
Action and uses—Anthelmintic, cathartic and emetic.

PREPARATIONS.

Tincture White Indian Hemp—Fl. ext. White Indian hemp, Lilly, 2 fl. ozs.; Diluted alcohol, 14 fl. ozs., Mix—Dose ½ to 2 fl. drs.

Syrup White Indian Hemp—Fl. ext. White Indian hemp, Lilly, 4 fl. ozs.; Syrup, 12 fl. ozs.; Mix—Dose 20 to 60 m.

FL. EXT. WHITE OAK BARK...... ....**Dose, diluted, 10 to 20 m.**
Quercus alba Linn.   **Nat. Ord.**—*Cupuliferæ.*
Range—Maine to Southeastern Minnesota, Eastern Kansas and south to
the Gulf.
Habitat—In all soils.
Part used—The inner bark.
Standard of strength—That of the U. S. Pharmacopœia, 1890; 1 c.c.
representing 1 gram of the drug; or, practically, minim for grain.
Action and uses—Slightly tonic, powerfully astringent and antiseptic.
Used internally in chronic diarrhœa, chronic mucous discharges, passive
hemorrhages. In the form of a gargle it is an excellent application in
relaxed uvula and sore throat; also makes a good stimulating astringent
lotion for ulcers with spongy granulation, and an astringent injection for
leucorrhœa, prolapsus ani and hemorrhoids.

FL. EXT. WHITE PINE BARK .. .. **Dose 10 to 20 m.**
Pinus strobus Linn.   **Nat. Ord.**—*Coniferæ.*
Range—Newfoundland to Pennsylvania, along the mountains to Georgia,
west to Minnesota and Eastern Iowa.
Habitat—Dry soil.
Part used—The bark.
Standard of strength—That of the U. S. Pharmacopœia, 1890; 1 c.c.
representing 1 gram of the drug; or, practically, minim for grain.
Action and uses—Expectorant.

PREPARATION.

Syrup White Pine Bark—Fl. ext. White pine bark, Lilly, 2 fl.
ozs.; Syrup, 14 fl. ozs.; Mix—Dose 2 to 4 fl. drs.

FL. EXT. WHITE PINE COMP.

Designed for the extemporaneous preparation of syrup white pine compound.
Standard of strength—Each fluid ounce represents White pine
bark, 120 grs.; Cherry bark, 120 grs.; Sanguinaria, 14 grs.; Balm of Gilead
buds, 16 grs.; Spikenard, 16 grs.; Sassafras, 16 grs.; Morphine acetate,
¼ gr.; Chloroform, 16 m.
Action and uses—Intended only for preparing syrup white pine
comp., a very popular and valuable remedy in bronchial and pulmonary
diseases.
PREPARATION.

Syrup White Pine Comp.—Fl. ext. White pine comp., Lilly,
4 fl. ozs.; Syrup, 12 fl. ozs. Mix.—Dose, ½ to 2 fl. drs.

FL. EXT. WHITE POND LILY.. ... Dose 30 to 60 m.
Nymphæa odorata Aiton.   **Nat. Ord.**—*Nymphæaceæ.*
Synonyms—Castalia odorata (Dryand.) Woodv. Wood.—Sweet-scented
water lily.
Range—Nova Scotia to Florida, west to Manitoba, Minnesota and
Arkansas; common.
Habitat—Ponds and still or slow-flowing water.
Part used—The rootstock.
Standard of strength—That of the U. S. Pharmacopœia, 1890; 1 c.c.
representing 1 gram of the drug; or, practically, minim for grain.
Action and uses—Astringent, demulcent, anodyne and antiscrofu-
lous. Used in dysentery, diarrhœa, gonorrhœa, leucorrhœa and scrofula.
PREPARATION.

Infusion White Pond Lily—Fl. ext. White pond lily, Lilly, 2 fl.
ozs.; Hot water, 14 fl. ozs.; Mix—Dose ½ to 1 fl. oz.

FL. EXT. WHITE POPLAR BARK .... Dose 30 to 60 m.

Populus tremuloides Michx.   **Nat Ord.**—*Salicaceæ.*

Synonyms—Aspen, Quaking asp.

Range—Maine to the mountains of Pennsylvania, Northern Kentucky, Minnesota and far north and westward.

Habitat—Hillsides and open forests.

Part used—The bark of the branches.

Standard of strength—That of the U. S. Pharmacopœia, 1890; 1 c.c. representing 1 gram of the drug; or, practically, minim for grain.

Action and uses—Tonic, febrifuge and diuretic. Used in intermittent fever, impaired digestion, chronic diarrhea, urinary affections, gonorrhea and gleet.

FL. EXT. WHITE WILLOW BARK .... Dose 30 to 60 m.

Salix alba Linn.   **Nat. Ord.**—*Salicaceæ.*

Range—Europe; introduced in the United States; common, cultivated.

Habitat—Moist places, along streams, etc.

Part used—The bark of the branches of several years growth.

Standard of strength—That of the U. S. Pharmacopœia, 1890; 1 c.c. representing 1 gram of the drug; or, practically, minim for grain.

Action and uses—Febrifuge and antiperiodic.

FL. EXT. WILD BERGAMOT .... Dose 30 to 60 m.

Monarda fistulosa Linn.   **Nat. Ord.**—*Labiatæ.*

Synonyms—M. Mollis Linn., M. fistulosa var. Mollis Benth.

NOTE—This species is polymorphous and many varieties have been described.

Range—Canada, Vermont, Eastern Massachusetts to Florida and far westward.

Habitat—Dry soil.

Part used—The leaves and inflorescence.

Standard of strength—That of the U. S. Pharmacopœia, 1890; 1 c.c. representing 1 gram of the drug; or, practically, minim for grain.

Action and uses—Aromatic and stomachic.

PREPARATION.

Infusion Wild Bergamot—Fl. ext. Wild bergamot, Lilly, 1 fl. oz.; Hot water, 15 fl. ozs.; Mix—Dose 1 to 2 fl. ozs.

FL. EXT. WILD INDIGO.........   Dose 15 to 30 m.

Baptisia tinctoria (Linn.) R. Brown.   **Nat. Ord.**—*Leguminosæ.*

Synonyms—Sophora tinctoria Linn.,—Horsefly weed.

Range—New England to Florida, west to Minnesota and Louisiana.

Habitat—Dry sandy soil.

Part used—The root.

Standard of strength—That of the U. S. Pharmacopœia, 1890; 1 c.c. representing 1 gram of the drug; or, practically, minim for grain.

Action and uses—Purgative, emetic, astringent and antiseptic.

PREPARATION.

Tincture Wild Indigo—Fl. ext. Wild indigo, Lilly, 2 fl. ozs.; Diluted alcohol, 14 fl. ozs.; Mix—Dose 1 to 2 fl. drs.

FL. EXT. WILD YAM .... Dose 20 to 40 m.

Dioscorea villosa Linn.   **Nat. Ord.**—*Dioscoreaceæ.*

Synonym—Colic root.

Range—Southern New England to Florida, west to Minnesota, Kansas and Texas.

Habitat—In thickets and along fences, climbing.

Part used—The rhizome.

Standard of strength—That of the U. S. Pharmacopœia, 1890; 1 c.c. representing 1 gram of the drug; or, practically, minim for grain.

Action and uses—Almost a specific in bilious colic. It has also proved valuable in painful cholera morbus, attended with cramps; in neuralgic affections; in irritable conditions of the nervous system, especially when attended with pain or spasms.

PREPARATION.

Infusion Wild Yam—Fl. ext. Wild yam, Lilly, 2 fl. ozs.; Hot water, 14 fl. ozs.; Mix—Dose ½ to 1 fl. oz.

FL. EXT. WILLOW HERB .... **Dose 60 to 120 m.**
Epilobium angustifolium Linn. **Nat. Ord.—***Onagraceæ.*

Synonyms—E. spicatum Lam., Chamænerion angustifolium (Linn.) Scop.,—Rosebay.

Range—Europe, Asia, North America; New England to North Carolina, west to Minnesota and Eastern Kansas, far north and westward.

Habitat—Low grounds, especially in newly cleared land.

Part used—The leaves, inflorescence and smaller branches of the stem.

Standard of strength—That of the U. S. Pharmacopœia, 1890; 1 c.c. representing 1 gram of the drug; or, practically, minim for grain.

Action and uses—Tonic, astringent, demulcent and emollient. The infusion is beneficial in chronic diarrhea, dysentery, leucorrhea, menorrhagia and uterine hemorrhage.

PREPARATION.

Infusion Willow Herb—Fl. ext. Willow herb, Lilly, 2 fl. ozs.; Hot water, 14 fl. ozs.; Mix—Dose 1 to 2 fl. ozs.

FL. EXT. WINTERGREEN .... **Dose 60 to 120 m.**
Gaultheria procumbens Linn. **Nat. Ord.—***Ericaceæ.*

Synonyms—Mountain tea, Deerberry, Checkerberry.

Range—United States; Maine to Minnesota and southward.

Habitat—Cool damp woods.

Part used—The leaves.

Standard of strength—That of the U. S. Pharmacopœia, 1890; 1 c.c. representing 1 gram of the drug; or, practically, minim for grain.

Action and uses—Stimulant, aromatic and astringent. The infusion is used as an astringent in chronic mucous discharges; as a diuretic in dysury; as an emmenagogue and as a stimulant in cases of debility.

PREPARATION.

Infusion Wintergreen—Fl. ext. Wintergreen, Lilly, 1 fl. oz.; Hot water, 15 fl. ozs.; Mix—Dose 2 to 4 fl. ozs.

FL. EXT. WITCH HAZEL, U. S. .... **Dose 30 to 60 m.**
Hamamelis Virginiana Linn. **Nat. Ord.—***Hamamelidaceæ.*

Synonyms—Winter bloom, Snapping hazel, Spotted alder.

Range—New England to Minnesota, southward to Louisiana.

Habitat—Damp woods, along streams and on hillsides.

Part used—The leaves.

Standard of strength—That of the U. S. Pharmacopœia, 1890; 1 c.c. representing 1 gram of the drug; or, practically, minim for grain.

Action and uses—Tonic, astringent and said to be sedative. Recommended in hemorrhage of the lungs and stomach.

PREPARATION.

Infusion Witch Hazel—Fl. ext. Witch hazel, Lilly, 2 fl. ozs.; Hot water, 14 fl. ozs.; Mix—Dose ½ to 1 fl. oz.

WHEN ORDERING OR PRESCRIBING.

FL. EXT. WOOD BETONY .... Dose 30 to 60 m.

Betonica officinalis Linn.   **Nat. Ord.**—*Labiatæ.*

Synonym—Stachys Betonica Benth.

Range—Europe, introduced into the United States; has been found in thickets in Massachusetts escaped from gardens.

Part used—The leaves and inflorescence.

Standard of strength—That of the U. S. Pharmacopœia, 1890; 1 c.c. representing 1 gram of the drug; or, practically, minim for grain.

Action and uses—Nervine, tonic, discutient. Useful in headache, nervousness and hysteria.

PREPARATION.

Infusion Wood Betony—Fl. ext. Wood betony, Lilly, 2 fl. ozs.; Hot water, 14 fl. ozs.; Mix—Dose ½ to 1 fl. oz.

FL. EXT. WORMWOOD .... Dose 30 to 60 m.

Artemisia Absinthium Linn.   **Nat. Ord.**—*Compositæ.*

Range—Northern Asia, Europe and Northern Africa, naturalized in North America; Newfoundland to New England and westward, escaped from cultivation.

Habitat—Along roadsides, in waste places, on dry soil.

Part used—The leaves and inflorescence.

Standard of strength—That of the U. S. Pharmacopœia, 1890; 1 c.c. representing 1 gram of the drug; or, practically, minim for grain.

Action and uses—Bitter tonic and anthelmintic.

PREPARATION.

Infusion Wormwood—Fl. ext. Wormwood, Lilly, 1 fl. oz.; Hot water, 15 fl. ozs.; Mix—Dose 1 to 2 fl. ozs.

FL. EXT. YARROW .... Dose 30 to 60 m.

Achillea Millefolium Linn.   **Nat. Ord.**—*Compositæ.*

Synonyms—Nosebleed, Milfoil.

Range—The northern hemisphere; North America, Greenland to Alaska, south to Florida, Texas and Mexico; common.

Habitat—Fields and hills, edges of woods and shores of lakes.

Part used—The leaves and inflorescence.

Standard of strength—That of the U. S. Pharmacopœia, 1890; 1 c.c. representing 1 gram of the drug; or, practically, minim for grain.

Action and uses—Tonic and astringent; said to be diuretic and alterative. Recommended in chronic diseases of the urinary organs. It exerts a tonic influence upon the venous system as well as mucous membranes. Useful in dysentery.

PREPARATION.

Infusion Yarrow—Fl. ext. Yarrow, Lilly, 1 fl. oz.; Hot water, 15 fl. ozs.; Mix—Dose 1 to 2 fl. ozs.

FL. EXT. YELLOW DOCK, U. S. .... Dose 30 to 60 m

Rumex crispus Linn. and some other species of *Rumex.*

          Nat. Ord.—*Polygonaceæ.*

NOTE—*R. obtusifolius* Linn. and *R. sanguineus* Linn., resembling and having about the same range and habitat as *R. crispus,* are probably the other species collected.

Synonyms—Curled dock, Narrow dock.

Range—Europe, naturalized in North America; common and widely distributed over the United States.

Habitat—Along roadsides, in grassy places and in cultivated fields.

Part used—The root.

Standard of strength—That of the U. S. Pharmacopœia, 1890; 1 c.c. representing 1 gram of the drug; or, practically, minim for grain.

Action and uses—Alterative, tonic and mildly astringent. Useful in scorbutic, cutaneous, scrofulous, scirrhous and syphilitic affections.

PREPARATION.

Syrup Yellow Dock—Fl. ext. Yellow dock, Lilly, 4 fl. ozs.; Syrup, 12 fl. ozs.; Mix—Dose 2 to 4 fl. drs.

FL. EXT. YELLOW PARILLA, **U. S.** ....Dose 30 to 60 m.

Menispermum Canadense Linn. **Nat. Ord.**—*Menispermaceæ.*

Synonyms—M. Virginicum Linn.,—Texas sarsaparilla. Vine maple, Moonseed.

Range—Quebec to **New England** and **North** Carolina, **west to the** Dakotas and Arkansas.

Habitat—Moist rich woods and thickets; climbing.

Part used—The rhizome and roots.

Standard of strength—That of the U. S. Pharmacopœia, 1890; 1 c.c. representing 1 gram of the drug; or, practically, minim for grain.

Action and uses—Tonic, laxative, alterative and diuretic. It is much esteemed as a remedy in scrofulous, cutaneous, arthritic, rheumatic, syphilitic and mercurial diseases.

PREPARATIONS.

Syrup Yellow Parilla—Fl. ext. Yellow parilla, Lilly, 4 fl. ozs.; Syrup, 12 fl. ozs.; Mix—Dose 2 to 4 fl. drs.

Infusion Yellow Parilla—Fl. ext. Yellow parilla, Lilly, 1 fl. oz.; Hot water, 15 fl. ozs.; Mix—Dose 1 to 2 fl. ozs.

FL. EXT. YERBA BUENA......................**Dose 30 to 120 m.**

Micromeria Douglassii Benth. **Nat. Ord.**— *Labiatæ.*

Synonyms—M. barbata Fisch. & Meyer, Thymus Douglassii Benth.

Range—Vancouver's **Island to** Los Angeles Co., California.

Habitat—Woodlands, in sandy soil.

Part used—The herb.

Standard of strength—That of the U. S. Pharmacopœia, 1890; 1 c.c. representing 1 gram of the drug; or, practically, minim for grain.

Action and uses—Carminative, febrifuge, anthelmintic and emmenagogue. Given as a hot infusion it allays nausea, spasmodic pains in the stomach, reduces the frequency and force of the pulse, causing mild perspiration and gradually inducing a refreshing sleep.

PREPARATIONS.

Tincture Yerba Buena—Fl. ext. Yerba buena, **Lilly, 4 fl. ozs.;** Diluted alcohol, 12 fl. ozs.; Mix—Dose 2 to 4 fl. drs.

Infusion Yerba Buena—Fl. ext. Yerba buena, Lilly, 1 fl. oz.; Hot water, 15 fl. ozs.; Mix—Dose 1 to 2 fl. ozs.

FL. EXT. YERBA REUMA ....**Dose 10 to 20 m.**

Frankenia grandifolia Cham. et Schlecht.

Nat. Ord.—*Frankeniaceæ.*

Range—Western United States, sea shore from San Francisco to San Diego, southward and eastward in the desert to Arizona and southern Nevada.

Habitat—Dry soil.

Part used—The herbaceous portions of the plant.

WHEN ORDERING OR PRESCRIBING.

Standard of strength—That of the U. S. Pharmacopœia, 1890; 1 c.c. representing 1 gram of the drug; or, practically, minim for grain.

Action and uses—Recommended as a mild astringent, acting favorably upon diseased mucous membranes and serviceable in diarrhœa, dysentery, vaginal leucorrhea, gonorrhea, gleet and catarrh.

PREPARATION.

Infusion Yerba Reuma—Fl. ext. Yerba reuma, Lilly, 2 fl. ozs.; Hot water, 14 fl. ozs.; Mix—Applied locally by injection or spray.

FL. EXT. YERBA SANTA, U. S................. ....**Dose 20 to 60 m.**
Eriodyction glutinosum Benth.   **Nat. Ord.**—*Hydrophyllaceæ.*

Synonyms—Wigandia Californica Hook. & Arn.,—Mountain balm, Consumptive's weed.

Range—Western and Southern California.

Habitat—Dry hills among rocks.

Part used—The leaves.

Standard of strength—That of the U. S. Pharmacopœia, 1890; 1 c.c. representing 1 gram of the drug; or, practically, minim for grain.

Action and uses—Yerba santa has been recommended in the treatment of laryngeal and bronchial affections, and in chronic pulmonary difficulties generally; also used in the treatment of hemorrhoids and chronic catarrh of the bladder.

PREPARATION.

Tincture Yerba Santa—Fl. ext. Yerba santa, Lilly, 4 fl. ozs.; Alcohol, 9 fl. ozs ; Water, 3 fl. ozs ; Mix—Dose 2 to 4 fl. drs.

FL. EXT. YERBA SANTA, AROMATIC, for Syrup.

Standard of strength—One pint represents Yerba santa, 15¼ troy ounces and aromatics.

Action and uses—Used in the form of syrup for the purpose of disguising the bitter taste of quinine and as an adjuvant. For these purposes it is, however, inferior to YERBAZIN, Lilly.

PREPARATION.

Syrup Yerba Santa, Aromatic—Fl. ext. Yerba santa, for syrup, Lilly, 4 fl. ozs.; Syrup, 12 fl. ozs.; Mix.

FL. EXT. ZEDOARY...............................**Dose 10 to 30 m.**
Curcuma Zedoaria Rosc.   **Nat. Ord.**—*Scitamineæ.*

Synonym—Round zedoary.

Range—India and some of the East Indian Islands.

Part used—The rhizome.

Standard of strength—That of the U. S. Pharmacopœia, 1890; 1 c.c. representing 1 gram of the drug; or, practically, minim for grain.

Action and uses—Stimulant and carminative. Used to promote digestion and in flatulency.

PREPARATION.

Infusion Zedoary—Fl. ext. Zedoary, Lilly, 1 fl. oz.; Hot water, 15 fl. ozs.; Mix—Dose ¼ to 1 fl. oz.

Eli Lilly & Company's

Gelatin Coated and Sugar Coated

PILLS.

The requirements for the production of a complete and satisfactory line of Gelatin Coated and Sugar Coated Pills, it may well be imagined, are of the most comprehensive and exacting character. The range of remedies used in the pill form cover nearly the entire field of Materia Medica, comprising materials of the most varied and often the most refractory physical and chemical qualities.

The practical consideration and manipulation of these materials in connection with their presentation in the pill form in such a way that each pill shall be the exact counterpart of all others of the same kind, that it shall keep indefinitely, unchanged, under all reasonable condions and that it shall be readily soluble as well as active in its constituents, so as to promptly serve its remedial purpose, have been the exacting problems completely solved in the many years of experience in the laboratory of Eli Lilly & Company.

In addition to the general line we prepare to special order from private formulas, pills either round, oval or capsule shaped, coated in any color. Formulas may be submitted in confidence and when possible sample should accompany requests for quotations.

Gelatin Coated Pills we make in lots of one thousand or more.

Sugar Coated Pills we make in lots of three thousand or more.

We are prepared to promptly execute contracts for pills of any coating in lots of one million or more, guaranteeing, of course, satisfaction in every detail.

ELI LILLY & COMPANY'S
GELATIN COATED AND SUGAR COATED
PILLS AND GRANULES.

PIL. ACETANILID; **2** grs., **4** grs., **5** grs.

Action and uses—Acetanilid is analgesic, hypnotic, antispasmodic and antipyretic. It lessens reflex action of the spinal cord and inhibits the sensibility of the sensory nerves. It raises arterial tension in a degree and correspondingly slows the heart, producing quiet sleep. Used in phthisis and typhoid fever for the hyperexia. For the pains of locomotor ataxia, rheumatism, sciatica and lumbago it is very efficient, as it is also in acute rheumatism, influenza, scarlet fever and acute bronchitis. With children it should be used with caution both as to dose and repetition.

Dose, from 2 to 10 grains.—If the desired effect is not produced in thirty minutes the dose should be repeated, but not to exceed thirty grains should be given in the twenty four hours. As an antipyretic four grains may be given every fifteen or thirty minutes until twelve or sixteen grains have been administered, which will usually be sufficient.

PIL. ACONITINE, CRYSTALS; 1-500 gr., 1-200 gr.

Action and uses—Similar to Fl. Ext. Aconite root, see pages 6 and 7.
Dose, 1-500 to 1-100 of a grain.

PIL. AGARICIN **1-6** gr.

Action and uses—Agaricin, from Polyporus officinalis. Antihidrotic. Useful in night sweats from phthisis, also in sweating from acetanilid and allied compounds, resorcin and salicylates. It also decreases the secretions of the bronchi and mamma.
Dose, 1-6 grain to 1 grain.

PIL. ALOES, U. S., Pil. Aloetic.

Formula—Each pill contains: Purified aloes, Soap, of each, 2 grs.
Action and uses—A convenient laxative in habitual constipation. A single pill daily, after dinner or at bed time, is the usual dose. In larger doses, as a cathartic, it is less desirable than other aloetic preparations.
Dose, 1 to 5 pills.

PIL. ALOES AND ASAFETIDA, U. S.

Formula—Each pill contains: Purified aloes, Asafetida, Soap, of each, 1½ grs.
Action and uses—Replaces the simple Aloetic pill in constipation with flatulence, especially in nervous or hysterical persons.
Dose, 2 to 3 pills.

PIL. ALOES AND IRON.

Formula—Each pill contains: Purified aloes, ½ gr.; Iron sulph. oxsic., 1 gr.; Ext. Conium seed, ½ gr.; Ginger, 1 gr.
Action and uses—Used in the the treatment of amenorrhea associated with anemia and constipation. It should be used habitually in the smaller doses and in the larger ones at the menstrual epoch.
Dose, 2 to 3 pills.

PIL. ALOES AND IRON, U. S.

Formula—Each pill contains: Purified aloes, Iron sulph. exsic., Aromatic powder, of each, 1 gr.; Confection rose, q. s.
Action and uses—Used in the treatment of amenorrhea, associated

with anemia and constipation. It should be used habitually in the smaller doses, and in the larger one at the menstrual epoch.
Dose, 2 to 3 pills.

PIL. ALOES AND MASTICH, U. S., Lady Webster's **Dinner Pills.**
Formula—Each pill contains: Purified aloes, 2 grs.; Mastich, 3-5 gr.; Red rose, ½ gr.
Action and uses—Used to quicken defecation. Being slowly soluble the action is principally upon the large intestine.
Dose, 1 pill before or after dinner.

PIL. ALOES AND MYRRH, U. S.
Formula—Each pill contains: Purified aloes, 2 grs.; Myrrh, 1 gr.; Aromatic powder, 3-5 gr.
Action and uses—Principally used in amenorrhea, uterine catarrh, etc. In such cases one or two pills at bed time for a week or more should be given.
Dose, as a laxative, 1 to 2 pills; as a purgative, 3 to 6 pills.

PIL. ALOES, MYRRH AND IRON.
Formula—Each pill contains: Purified aloes, 2 grs.; Myrrh, iron sulph. exsic., of each, 1 gr.
Action and uses—The addition of Iron to the Pil. Aloes and Myrrh is advantageous in cases of amenorrhea in which anemia is a factor.
Dose, 2 to 3 **pills.**

PIL. ALOES AND NUX VOMICA.
Formula—Each pill contains: Purified aloes, 1½ grs.; Ext. Nux vomica, ½ gr.
Action and uses—An excellent laxative and tonic.
Dose, 1 to 2 pills.

PIL. ALOES, **NUX VOMICA AND BELLADONNA.**
Formula—Each pill contains: Purified aloes, 1½ grs.; Ext. Nux vomica, ¾ gr.; Ext. Belladonna, ⅛ gr.
Action and uses—Valuable in constipation; the griping tendency of the aloes being overcome by the Ext. Belladonna which also exerts a tonic influence on the muscular structure of the intestines. The Ext. Nux vomica increases the peristaltic action.
Dose, 1 to 2 pills.

PIL. ALOETIC, See Pil. Aloes, U. S.

PIL. ALOIN, 1-10 gr., 1-8 gr., **1-5** gr., 1-4 gr., 1-2 gr., 1 gr.
Action and uses—Aloin may be used in all cases where aloes is admissible, the advantage in its use being the smallness of the dose and its freedom from the griping tendency found in Aloes.
Dose, 1-10 gr. to 2 grs.

PIL. ALOIN COMP.
Formula—Each pill contains: Aloin, Podophyllin, of each, ⅛ gr.; Ext. Belladonna, ⅛ gr.
Action and uses—An excellent laxative and cathartic.
Dose, 1 to 2 pills.

PIL. ALOIN COMP. AND STRYCHNINE; see Pil. Anticonstipation, special.

PIL. ALOIN AND NUX VOMICA.
Formula—Each pill contains: Aloin, ¼ gr.; Ext. Nux vomica, ⅛ gr.
Action and uses—An excellent laxative and tonic.
Dose, 1 to 2 pills.

PIL. ALOIN, NUX VOMICA AND BELLADONNA.

Formula—Each pill contains: Aloin, 1-5 gr.; Ext. Nux vomica, ½ gr.
Ext. Belladonna, ⅛ gr.

Action and uses—See Pil. Aloes, Nux vomica and Belladonna.

Dose, 1 to 2 pills.

PIL. ALOIN AND STRYCHNINE.

Formula—Each pill contains: Aloin, 1-5 gr.; Strychnine, 1-60 gr.

Action and uses—Tonic and laxative.

Dose, 1 to 2 pills.

PIL. ALOIN, STRYCHNINE AND BELLADONNA, NO. 1.

Formula—Each pill contains: Aloin, 1-5 gr.; Strychnine, 1-60 gr.; Ext.
Belladonna, ½ gr.

Action and uses—See Pil. Aloes, Nux vomica and Belladonna.

Dose, 1 to 2 pills.

PIL. ALOIN, STRYCHNINE AND BELLADONNA, NO. 2.

Formula—Each pill contains: Aloin, 1-10 gr.; Strychnine, 1-50 gr.; Ext.
Belladonna, 1-6 gr.

Action and uses—See Pil. Aloes, Nux vomica and Belladonna.

Dose, 1 to 2 pills.

PIL. ALOIN, STRYCHNINE AND BELLADONNA, NO. 3.

Formula—Each pill contains: Aloin, 1-5 gr.; Strychnine, 1-120 gr.; Ext.
Belladonna, ⅛ gr.

Action and uses—See Pil. Aloes, Nux vomica and Belladonna.

Dose, 1 to 2 pills.

PIL. ALOIN, STRYCHNINE AND BELLADONNA, COMP.

Formula—Each pill contains: Aloin, 1-5 gr.; Strychnine, 1-60 gr.; Ext.
Belladonna, ⅛ gr.; Ext. Cascara sagrada, ½ gr.

Action and uses—An excellent pill in chronic constipation.

Dose, 1 to 2 pills.

PIL. A. S. B. AND I., Lilly.

Formula—Each pill contains: Aloin, ¼ gr.; Strychnine, 1-60 gr.; Ext.
Belladonna, ⅛ gr.; Ipecac, 1-10 gr.

Action and Uses—This formula is very popular as a tonic laxative in
chronic constipation and atonic dyspepsia. It is free from griping
tendency, increases peristalsis, overcomes atony of the bowels, has
decided cholagogue action and increases the gastric secretions.

Dose, 1 to 3 pills.

PIL. ALOIN, STRYCHNINE, BELLADONNA AND PODOPHYLLIN.

Formula—Each pill contains: Aloin, 1-5 gr.; Strychnine, 1-60 gr.; Ext.
Belladonna, Podophyllin, of each, ⅛ gr.

Action and uses—A valuable combination in chronic constipation.
Decidedly cathartic in the larger dose.

Dose, 1 to 3 pills.

PIL. ALTERATIVE.

Formula—Each pill contains: Blue mass, 1 gr.; Ipecac, Powd. Opium,
of each, ⅛ gr.

Action and uses—A mercurial alterative with a decided tendency to
to the liver without action on the bowels.

Dose, 1 to 3 pills.

PIL. AMMONIUM VALERIANATE, 1 gr., 2 grs.

Action and uses—Similar to Fl. Ext. Valerian. See page 120.

Dose, 1 to 6 grs., repeated as required.

効6

PIL. ANODYNE.
Formula—Each pill contains: Camphor, Ext. Hyoscyamus, of each, 1 gr.; Morphine acetate, Oil Capsicum, of each, 1-20 gr.
Dose, 1 to 2 pills.

PIL. ANTIBILIOUS.
Formula—Each pill contains: Ext. Colocynth comp., 2½ grs.; Podophyllin, ¼ gr.
Dose, 1 to 2 pills.

PIL. ANTICHILL.
Formula—Each pill contains: Chinoidin, Iron ferrocyanide, Oil Black pepper, of each, 1 gr.; Arsenous acid, 1-20 gr.
Action and uses—An excellent antiperiodic in chills and fever.
Dose, 1 to 2 pills.

PIL. ANTICHILL, HALF STRENGTH.
Formula—Each pill contains: Chinoidin, Iron ferrocyanide, Oil Black pepper, of each, ½ gr.; Arsenous acid, 1-40 gr.
Action and uses—See Pil. Antichill.

PIL. ANTICONSTIPATION, BRUNDAGE.
Formula—Each pill contains: Podophyllin, Ext. Belladonna, of each, 1-10 gr.; Ext. Nux vomica, Ext. Hyoscyamus, Capsicum, of each, ⅛ gr.
Action and uses—A most valuable pill in habitual constipation, especially in women.
Dose, 1 pill at bed time, repeated nightly for one week, then alternate nights until natural evacuations are produced.

PIL. ANTICONSTIPATION, CARSON.
Formula—Each pill contains: Ext. Cascara sagrada, Ext. Rhubarb, of each, 1 gr.; Aloin, ⅓ gr.; Ext. Nux vomica, ¼ gr.
Action and uses—An excellent tonic laxative and cathartic.
Dose, 1 to 2 pills.

PIL. ANTICONSTIPATION, FOTHERGILL.
Formula—Each pill contains: Strychnine, 1-24 gr.; Purified aloes, Black pepper, of each, 1¼ grs.; Ext. Cascara sagrada, 1⅔ grs.
Dose, 1 to 2 pills.

PIL. ANTICONSTIPATION, GOSS.
Formula—Each pill contains: Podophyllin, Ext. Colocynth, Ext. Cascara sagrada, Ext. Gentian, of each, ¼ gr.; Ext. Nux vomica, Ext. Hyoscyamus, of each, ⅛ gr.; Ext. Butternut, Black Indian hemp, of each, ½ gr.
Dose, 1 to 2 pills.

PIL. ANTICONSTIPATION, PALMER.
Formula—Each pill contains: Purified aloes, Ext. Hyoscyamus, of each, 1 gr.; Ext. Nux vomica, ⅓ gr.; Ipecac, 1-10 gr.
Dose, 1 to 2 pills.

PIL. ANTICONSTIPATION, SPECIAL.
Formula—Each pill contains: Aloin, Podophyllin, Ext. Belladonna, of each, ⅛ gr.; Strychnine, 1-80 gr.; Oleoresin Capsicum, 1-10 gr.
Dose, 1 to 2 pills.

PIL. ANTIDYSPEPSIA, FOTHERGILL.
Formula—Each pill contains: Strychnine, 1-20 gr.; Ipecac, ⅔ gr.; Black pepper, 1½ grs.; Ext. Gentian, 1 gr.

Action and uses—A valuable combination in atonic and chronic catarrhal dyspepsia.
Dose, 1 to 2 pills.

PIL. ANTIDYSPEPSIA, FOTHERGILL, MODIFIED.

Formula—Each pill contains: Strychnine, 1-50 gr.; Ipecac, ⅔ gr.; Black pepper, ¼ gr.; Ext. Gentian, 1 gr.; Oil Cloves, 1-20 gr.
Dose, 1 to 2 pills.

PIL. ANTIDYSPEPTIC.

Formula—Each pill contains: Strychnine, 1-40 gr.; Ext. Belladonna, Ipecac, of each, 1-10 gr., Blue mass, Ext. Colocynth comp., of each, 2 grs.
Action and uses—Useful in dyspepsia attended with constipation and torpidity of the liver.
Dose, 1 to 2 pills.

PIL. ANTI-EPILEPTIC.

Formula—Each pill contains: Iron ferrocyanide, Zinc valerianate, of each, ½ gr.; Quinine valerianate, Ext. Valerian, of each, 1 gr.
Action and uses—Especially useful in cases of epilepsy of malarial origin.
Dose, 1 to 2 pills.

PIL. ANTIMALARIAL, HARPER.

Formula—Each pill contains: Quinine sulph., 1½ grs.; Iron by hydrogen ⅔ gr.; Arsenous acid, 1-30 gr.; Strychnine, 1-60 gr.; Ammonium picrate, 1-3 gr., Ext. Colocynth comp., ¼ gr.
Action and uses—An excellent pill in chronic malaria, especially where anemia and splenic enlargement are present and in malarial neuralgia.
Dose, 1 to 2 pills.

PIL. ANTIMALARIAL, MADDIN, MILDER.

Formula—Each pill contains: Strychnine, 1-40 gr.; Arsenous acid, 1-24 gr.; Iron by hydrogen, Quinine sulphate, of each, 1 gr.; Purified aloes, 1-6 gr.
Action and uses—It may be said of this and kindred combinations that the general effect is to overcome periodicity of the attack, diminish splenic engorgement and to remove the anemia usually present in cases of chronic malaria. The treatment in severe cases should be extended over a considerable time and where constipation is a persistent factor the condition should be relieved by occasional doses of ELIXIR PURGANS, (Lilly).
Dose, 1 to 2 pills.

PIL. ANTIMALARIAL, MADDIN, MILDER, WITHOUT ALOES.

Formula—Each pill contains: Strychnine, 1-40 gr.; Arsenous acid, 1-24 gr.; Iron by hydrogen, Quinine sulphate, of each, 1 gr.
Dose, 1 to 2 pills.

PIL. ANTIMALARIAL, MADDIN, STRONGER.

Formula—Each pill contains: Strychnine, 3-100 gr.; Arsenous acid, 1-20 gr.; Iron by hydrogen, Quinine sulphate, of each, 1 1-5 grs.; Purified aloes, 1-5 gr.
Dose, 1 to 2 pills.

PIL. ANTIMALARIAL, MADDIN, STRONGER, WITHOUT ALOES.

Formula—Each pill contains: Strychnine, 3-100 gr.; Arsenous acid, 1-20 gr.; Iron by hydrogen, Quinine sulphate, of each, 1 1-5 grs.
Dose, 1 to 2 pills.

PIL. ANTIMALARIAL, MADDIN, WITH PHOSPHORUS, MILDER.

Formula—Each pill contains: Phosphorus, 1-120 gr.; Strychnine, 1-40 gr.; Arsenous acid, 1-24 gr.; Iron by hydrogen, Quinine sulphate, of each, 1 gr.; Purified aloes, 1-6 gr.

Dose, 1 to 2 pills.

PIL. ANTIMALARIAL, **MADDIN, WITH PHOSPHORUS, STRONGER.**

Formula— Each pill contains: Phosphorus, 1-100 gr.; Strychnine, 3-100 gr.; Arsenous acid, 1-20 gr.; Iron by hydrogen, Quinine sulphate, of each, 1½ grs.; Purified aloes, 1-5 gr.

Dose, 1 to 2 pills.

PIL. ANTIMALARIAL, McCAW.

Formula— Each pill contains: Quinine sulphate, 1 gr.; Iron sulphate exsic., Gelsemin, of each, ⅛ gr.; Podophyllin, ⅛ gr.; Oil Black pepper, 1-16 gr.; Arsenous acid, 1-80 gr.

Dose, 1 to 2 pills.

PIL. ANTIMONY COMP., **U. S.; Plummer's Pills; Pil. Calomel Comp.**

Formula— Each pill contains: Calomel, Antimony sulphurated, of each, 5-5 gr.; Resin guaiac, 1½ grs.

Action and uses— Adapted to the treatment of chronic rheumatism and of scaly and other eruptions of the skin.

Dose, 1 to 2 pills twice a **day.**

PIL. ANTINERVOUS.

Formula— Each pill contains: Zinc oxide, Ext. Valerian, Ext. Hyoscyamus, of each, ⅔ gr.

Action and uses— A nerve sedative valuable in hysteria and especially in cases of hysterical dyspepsia.

Dose, 1 to 3 pills.

PIL. ANTIPERIODIC.

Formula— Each pill contains: Cinchonidine sulphate, 1 gr.; Iron sulph. exsic., ½ gr.; Podophyllin, Gelsemin, of each, 1-20 gr.; Strychnine sulphate, 1-32 gr.; Oleoresin Capsicum, 1-10 gr.

Dose, 1 to 2 pills.

PIL. ANTIRHEUMATIC.

Formula—Each pill contains: Ext. Cascara sagrada, ½ gr.; Sodium salicylate, 2½ grs.

Action and uses—Said to be especially valuable in acute rheumatism.

Dose, 1 to 4 pills.

PIL. ANTISEPTIC.

Formula— Each pill contains: Sodium sulphate, Salicylic acid, of each, 1 gr.; Ext. Nux vomica, ⅛ gr.

Action and uses—Used in cases of dyspepsia attended with acidity of the stomach.

Dose, 1 to 2 pills.

PIL. ANTISEPTIC COMP.

Formula—Each pill contains: Sodium sulphite, Salicylic acid, Pepsin, of each, 1 gr.; Ext. Nux vomica, ½ gr.; Capsicum, 1-10 gr.

Action and uses—Used in dyspepsia and indigestion.

Dose, 1 to 2 pills.

PIL. ANTISEPTIC, INTESTINAL.

Formula—Each pill contains: Mercury protiodide, ⅛ gr.; Podophyllin, Aloin, Ext. Nux vomica, Ext. Hyoscyamus, of each, 1-16 gr.

Dose, 1 to 2 pills.

PIL. ANTISPASMODIC.

Formula—Each pill contains: Morphine acetate, 1-10 gr.; Ext. Hyoscyamus, Camphor monobrom., Capsicum, of each, ½ gr.

Dose, 1 to 2 pills.

PIL. ANTISYPHILITIC; See Pil. Syphilitic.

PIL. APERIENT.

Formula—Each pill contains: Ext. Colocynth comp., 2 grs.; Ext. Hyoscyamus, ½ gr.; Ext. Nux vomica, ⅓ gr.

Dose, 1 to 2 pills.

PIL. APERIENT, BAUER.

Formula—Each pill contains: Ext. Hyoscyamus, ½ gr.; Ext. Aloes, Ext. Colocynth comp., of each, 1 gr.; Potassium and sodium tartrate, 1½ grs.

Dose, 1 to 2 pills.

PIL. APERIENT, DRYSDALE.

Formula—Each pill contains: Rhubarb, Purified aloes, of each, 1¼ grs.; Nux vomica, ½ gr.; Ipecac 5-12 gr.

Dose, 1 to 2 pills.

PIL. APERIENT, IMPROVED.

Formula—Each pill contains: Aloin, Irisin, Podophyllin, Ext. Belladonna, Ext. Nux vomica, of each, ½ gr.; Oil Capsicum, 1-16 gr.

Dose, 1 to 2 pills.

PIL. APERIENT, MILD.

Formula—Each pill contains: Ext. Colocynth comp., ½ gr.; Ext. Hyoscyamus, 5-6 gr.; Rhubarb, 2 grs.; Oil Caraway, 1-20 gr.

Dose, 1 to 2 pills.

PIL. APHRODISIACA, Lilly ; See page 324.

Formula—Each pill contains: Ext. Turnera **Aph.**, 2 grs.; Ext. Nux vomica, ½ gr.; Phosphorus, 1-100 gr.

Action and uses—Used with the greatest **success** in the treatment of diseases consequent on nervous breakdown **from** whatever cause, but principally in cases of sexual debility, impotency and mental over work. It is decidedly beneficial in nocturnal emissions, the result of excesses, mental apathy or indifference and in an enfeebled condition of the general system, gradually removing abnormal conditions, at the same time imparting tone and vigor. It is of value also in leucorrhea, amenorrhea, dysmenorrhea and to remove the tendency to repeated miscarriage.

Dose, 1 to 2 pills daily, with food.

PIL. APOCYNIN COMP.

Formula—Each pill contains: Apocynin, Leptandrin, of each, ¼ gr.; Podophyllin, ½ gr.; Ampelopsin, Oil Capsicum, of each, 1-16 gr.

Dose, 1 to 3 pills.

PIL. APOCYNUM EXT., 2 grs.

Action and uses—See Fluid Ext. Black Indian Hemp, U. S., page 22.

Dose, 2 to 4 grs.

PIL. ARTHROSIA.

Formula—Each pill contains: Salicylic acid, Quinine sulphate, of each, 1 gr.; Podophyllin, 1-10 gr.; Capsicum, Ext. Colchicum root, of each, ¼ gr.; Ext. Poke root, ½ gr.

Action and uses—Valuable in rheumatism, and especially in rheumatic gout.

Dose, 1 to 2 pills.

PIL. ARSENIC IODIDE, 1-50 gr., 1-35 gr.

Action and uses—Alterative. Thought to retard formation of scirrhous tumors of the breast in feeble and cachectic patients. Used generally in cutaneous diseases.

Dose from 1-50 to 1-10 gr.

PIL. ARSENIC SULPHIDE, 1-100 gr., 1-60 gr.

Action and uses—Alterative.

Dose, 1-100 to 1-10 gr.

PIL. ARSENOUS ACID, 1-100 gr., 1-60 gr., 1-50 gr., 1-40 gr., 1-30 gr., 1-20 gr., 1-12 gr.

Action and uses—Antiperiodic, antiseptic and alterative. Used in malarial fevers, skin diseases, chorea, neuralgia, gastralgia, uterine disorders, diabetes, bronchitis. See Pil. Asiatic.

Dose, 1-100 to 1-12 gr. The effects should be carefully watched and the dose decreased or suspended for a time if necessary. For antidotes to poisonous doses see "Poisons and Antidotes," page 286.

PIL. ARSENOUS ACID AND STRYCHNINE.

Formula—Each pill contains: Arsenous acid, 1-40 gr.; Strychnine, 1-60 gr.

Action and uses—Antiperiodic, antiseptic, alterative, nerve stimulant.

Dose, 1 to 2 pills.

PIL. ASAFETIDA, 1 gr., 2 grs., 3 grs., 4 grs., 5 grs., 6 grs.

Action and uses—Asafetida is a powerful antispasmodic and stimulant to the brain and nervous system. Very valuable in hysteria and hypochondriasis with indigestion and flatulence. Recently praised in the treatment of habitual abortion.

Dose, 2 to 12 grs.

PIL. ASAFETIDA, U. S.

Formula—Each pill contains: Asafetida, 3 grs.; Soap, 1 gr.

Action and uses—See Pil. Asafetida.

Dose, 1 to 4 pills.

PIL. ASAFETIDA COMP.

Formula—Each pill contains: Asafetida, 2 grs.; Iron sulph. exsic., 1 gr.

Action and uses—Antispasmodic and tonic. Especially valuable in chronic mucous catarrh, leucorrhœa, gleet, etc.

Dose, 1 to 2 pills.

PIL. ASAFETIDA AND IRON: See Pil. Asafetida comp.

PIL. ASAFETIDA AND NUX VOMICA.

Formula—Each pill contains: Asafetida, 3 grs.; Ext. Nux vomica, ¼ gr.

Action and uses—Antispasmodic and tonic.

Dose, 2 to 4 pills.

PIL. ASIATIC NO. 1.

Formula—Each pill contains: Arsenous acid, 1-16 gr.; Black pepper, ½ gr.

Action and uses—Antiperiodic, antiseptic and alterative. The presence of Black pepper in this pill modifies the effect of arsenous acid to the extent that gastric disorder is not liable to be produced. See Pil. Arsenous acid.

Dose, 1 pill.

PIL. ASIATIC NO. 2.

Formula—Each pill contains: Arsenous acid, 1-32 gr.; Black pepper, ¼ gr.

Action and uses—See Pil. Asiatic No. 1.

Dose, 1 to 2 pills.

PIL. ASIATIC NO. 3.

Formula—Each pill contains: Arsenous acid, 1-64 gr.; Black pepper, ⅛ gr.

Action and uses—See Pil. Asiatic No. 1.

Dose, 1 to 4 pills.

PIL. ASTRINGENT.

Formula—Each pill contains: Ext. Cranesbill, 2 grs.; Powd. Opium, ¼ gr.; Oil Peppermint, Oleoresin Ginger, of each, 1-20 gtt.

Action and uses—A very serviceable pill in diarrhea and chronic dysentery.

Dose, 1 to 2 pills.

PIL. ATROPINE, 1-300 gr., 1-200 gr., 1-120 gr., 1-100 gr., 1-60 gr.

Action and uses—From Atropa Belladonna. See Fluid Ext. Belladonna, page 17. Atropine has the advantage over belladonna of quicker action. Especially useful in poisoning by Opium, Calabar bean and Hydrocyanic acid; in ptyalism from pregnancy, in the sweats of phthisis and in sudden cardiac failure. In opium poisoning it should be given in very small doses, repeated, to avoid superinducing belladonna narcosis upon the opium narcosis.

Dose, 1-300 to 1-60 gr.

PIL. BELLADONNA EXT., 1-20 gr., 1-8 gr., 1-4 gr., 1-2 gr.

Action and uses—See Fluid Ext. Belladonna, page 17. The pill form retards the action of Belladonna.

Dose, 1-20 to 1-2 gr.

PIL. BERBERINE AND PODOPHYLLIN; See Pil. Podophyllin and Hydrastin.

PIL. BERBERIS COMP.; See Pil. Cascara comp.

PIL. BLACK HAW, EXT. 3 grs.

Action and uses—See Fluid Ext. Black Haw, page 21.

Dose, 3 to 12 grs.

PIL. BLADDERWRACK, EXT. 3 grs.

Action and uses—See Fl. Ext. Bladderwrack, page 23.

Dose, 3 to 12 grs.

PIL. BLAUD; See Pil. Ferruginous, Blaud.

PIL. BLUE MASS, 1-2 gr., 1 gr., 2 grs., 3 grs., 5 grs.

Action and uses—Blue mass acts more mildly than calomel or other mercurials.

Dose, as an alterative, 1-2 to 3 grs.; as a purgative, 5 to 20 grs. When administered as an alterative it may be given every night or every other night followed by a dose of ELIXIR PURGANS (Lilly) in the morning if the bowels have not moved.

PIL. BLUE MASS AND IRON.

Formula—Each pill contains: Blue mass, 2 grs.; Iron sulph. exsic., 1 gr.

Action and uses—Alterative and tonic.

Dose, 1 to 3 pills.

PIL. CALCIUM SULPHIDE, 1-20 gr., 1-12 gr., 1-10 gr., 1-8 gr., 1-6 gr., 1-5 gr., 1-4 gr., 1-2 gr., 1 gr., 2 grs., 2 1-2 grs., 3 grs.

Action and uses—DR. SIDNEY RINGER, in his "Hand Book of Therapeutics," speaks in the highest terms of calcium sulphide. Where inflammation threatens to end in suppuration, it is especially valuable. In scrofulous glandular enlargements in children, or in enlargement of the glands behind the angle of the jaw, in scarlet fever or measles, 1-10 gr. every hour or two. In boils and carbuncles, 1-10 gr. every two or three hours generally prevents the formation of fresh boils, lessens the inflammation, and liquifies the core of existing boils so that the separation is more speedy. It is valuable in mammary abscesses, rarely producing temporary pain, but as a rule the pain is speedily mitigated and a rapid cure is effected. It improves the general health, removing the debility associated with these eruptions. It is also beneficial in scrofulous sores often seen upon children. Treatment should be continued several weeks; the dose may be increased to 3 grains.

Dose, 1-20 to 3 grs.

PIL. CALOMEL, 1-20 gr., 1-16 gr., 1-10 gr., 1-8 gr., 1-4 gr., 1-2 gr., 1 gr., 2 grs., 3 grs., 5 grs.

Action and uses—Purgative and alterative.

Dose, as an alterative 1-2 grain to 1 grain every night or every other night followed, if the bowels do not act, by a dose of ELIXIR PURGANS Lilly, in the morning. The purgative dose of calomel is from 3 to 15 grains.

PIL. CALOMEL COMP.; See Pil. Antimony comp., U. S.

PIL. CALOMEL, EXT. COLOCYNTH COMP. AND HYOSCYAMUS.

Formula—Each pill contains: Calomel, Ext. Hyoscyamus, of each, 1 gr.; Ext. Colocynth comp., 3 grs.

Action and uses—Cathartic and hepatic stimulant.

Dose, 1 to 2 pills.

PIL. CALOMEL AND SODA.

Formula—Each pill contains: Calomel, Sodium bicarbonate, of each, 1 gr.

Action and Uses—Efficient in irritable stomach with obstinate vomiting.

Dose, 1 to 2 pills.

PIL. CAMPHOR AND HYOSCYAMUS.

Formula—Each pill contains: Camphor, Ext. Hyoscyamus, of each, 1 gr.

Action and uses—Antispasmodic and sedative.

Dose, 1 to 2 pills.

PIL. CAMPHOR, HYOSCYAMUS AND VALERIAN.

Formula—Each pill contains: Camphor, Ext. Hyoscyamus, of each, 1 gr.; Ext. Valerian, 2 gr.

Action and uses—Antispasmodic and nervine. Useful in all derangements of the nervous functions.

Dose, 1 to 2 pills.

PIL. CAMPHOR MONOBROMATED, 1 gr., 2 grs., 3 grs., 5 grs.

Action and uses—Nerve sedative and hypnotic. Used with benefit in delirium tremens, hysteria and epilepsy. It is also recommended in spermatorrhea.

Dose, 1 to 10 grs.

PIL. CAMPHOR AND OPIUM.

Formula—Each pill contains: Camphor, 2 grs.; Opium, 1 gr.

Action and uses—Anodyne and sedative.

Dose, 1 pill.

PIL. CAMPHOR, OPIUM AND HYOSCYAMUS.

Formula—Each pill contains: Camphor, Ext. Hyoscyamus, of each, 1 gr.; Powd. Opium, ½ gr.
Action and uses—Anodyne and sedative.
Dose, 1 pill.

PIL. CAMPHOR, OPIUM AND LEAD ACETATE.

Formula—Each pill contains: Camphor, Opium, Lead acetate, of each, 1 gr.
Action and uses—Anodyne and astringent.
Dose, 1 pill.

PIL. CAMPHOR, OPIUM AND TANNIN.

Formula—Each pill contains: Camphor, 1 gr.; Opium, ¼ gr.; Tannin, 2 grs.
Action and uses—Anodyne and astringent.
Dose, 1 to 2 pills.

PIL. CANNABIS INDICA EXT., 1-4 gr., 1-3 gr., 1-2 gr., 1 gr.

Action and uses—See Fl. Ext. Cannabis Indica, page 52.
Dose, 1-4 to 1 gr. In extreme cases the dose may be very greatly increased without danger.

PIL. CARMINATIVE; See Pil. Antidyspepsia, Fothergill.

PIL. CARMINATIVE MODIFIED; See Pil. Antidyspepsia, Fothergill, modified.

PIL. CASCARA SAGRADA EXT., 1 gr., 2 grs., 3 grs., 4 gr., 5 grs.

Action and uses—Recommended in habitual constipation. Its specific action is upon the lower bowel.
Dose, 1 to 10 grs.

PIL. CASCARA COMP.

Formula—Each pill contains: Ext. Cascara sagrada, 1 gr.; Ext. Berberis aquifolium, 2 grs.
Action and uses—Laxative and cathartic.
Dose, 1 to 3 pills.

PIL. CASCARA COMP., D'ARY.

Formula—Each pill contains: Ext. Cascara sagrada, Xanthoxylin, of each, 4-15 gr.; Ext. Nux vomica, 1-30 gr.; Ext. Belladonna, 1-60 gr.; Euonymin, 1-5 gr.; Oleoresin capsicum, 1-20 gr.
Action and uses—Recommended in habitual constipation.
Dose, 1 to 3 pills.

PIL. CASCARA AND NUX VOMICA.

Formula—Each pill contains: Ext. Cascara sagrada, 2 grs.; Ext. Nux vomica, 1-5 gr.
Action and uses—Cathartic, laxative.
Dose, 1 to 2 pills.

PIL. CASCARA, NUX VOMICA AND BELLADONNA.

Formula—Each pill contains: Ext. Cascara sagrada, 2 grs.; Ext. Nux vomica, ½ gr.; Ext. Belladonna, 1-16 gr.
Action and uses—Tonic, laxative and cathartic.
Dose, 1 to 2 pills.

PIL. CASCARA AND PODOPHYLLIN.

Formula—Each pill contains: Ext. Cascara sagrada, 3 grs.; Podophyllin, ¼ gr.
Action and uses—Cathartic.
Dose, 1 to 2 pills.

PIL. CATHARTIC COMP., U. S.

Formula—Each pill contains: Ext. Colocynth comp., 1¼ grs.; Calomel, 1 gr.; Ext. Jalap, ½ gr.; Gamboge, ¼ gr.
Action and uses—Cathartic.
Dose, 2 to 4 pills.

PIL. CATHARTIC COMP., ACTIVE.

Formula—Each pill contains: Purified aloes, 1¼ grs.; Gamboge, 3-16 gr.; Podophyllin, Capsicum, of each, ¼ gr.; Croton Oil, 1-30 gr.
Action and uses—Cathartic.
Dose, 2 to 4 pills.

PIL. CATHARTIC COMP., MODIFIED.

Formula—Each pill contains: Ext. Colocynth comp., 1 gr.; Ext. Jalap, Calomel, of each, ¾ gr.; Gamboge, 1-6 gr.; Rhubarb, ½ gr.; Ginger, ¼ gr.
Action and uses—Cathartic.
Dose, 2 to 4 pills.

PIL. CATHARTIC COMP., PHYSIOMEDICAL, HASTY.

Formula—Each pill contains: Gamboge, Podophyllum, Sanguinaria, Purified aloes, of each, ½ gr.; Lobelia seed, ¼ gr; Capsicum, ⅜ gr.; Oil Peppermint, 1-32 gr.; Ext. Juglans, ¼ gr.
Action and uses—Cathartic.
Dose, 2 to 4 pills.

PIL. CATHARTIC COMP., VEGETABLE.

Formula—Each pill contains: Ext. Colocynth, Resin Scammony, of each, ¼ gr.; Podophyllin, ¼ gr.; Purified aloes, 1¼ grs.; Cardamom, Soap, of each, ½ gr.
Action and uses—Cathartic.
Dose, 1 to 3 pills.

PIL. CATHARTIC COMP., VEGETABLE GRANULES.

Formula—Each pill contains: Jalapin, 1-16 gr.; Aloin, ¾ gr.; Podophyllin, ¼ gr.; Leptandrin, 1-16 gr.; Gamboge, 1-22 gr.; Ext. Hyoscyamus, ¼ gr.; Soap, 1-16 gr.; Capsicum, 1-84 gr.; Oil Peppermint, 1-128 gr.
Action and uses—Cathartic, laxative.
Dose, 1 to 4 pills.

PIL. CATHARTIC GRANULES.

Formula—Each pill contains: Aloin, Jalapin, of each, 1-16 gr.; Podophyllin, 1-5 gr.; Ext. Hyoscyamus, Ext. Nux vomica, Oleoresin Capsicum, of each, 1-20 gr.
Action and uses—Cathartic.
Dose, 1 to 4 pills.

PIL. CATHARTIC, IMPROVED.

Formula—Each pill contains: Ext. Colocynth comp., 1 gr.; Ext. Jalap, Ext. Gentian, of each, ½ gr.; Podophyllin, Leptandrin, Ext. Hyoscyamus, of each, ¼ gr.; Oil Peppermint.
Action and uses—Cathartic.
Dose, 1 to 3 pills.

PIL. CATHARTIC, VEGETABLE.

Formula—Each pill contains: Ext. Colocynth comp., 1½ grs.; Podophyllin, ¾ gr.; Leptandrin, Jalap, of each, ⅛ gr.; Purified aloes, ½ gr., Ext. Hyoscyamus, ¼ gr.; Oil Peppermint.

Action and uses—Cathartic.

Dose, 1 to 3 pills.

PIL. CATHARTIC, VEGETABLE, U. S.

Formula—Each pill contains: Ext. Colocynth comp., 1 gr.; Ext. Hyoscyamus, Ext. Jalap, of each, ½ gr.; Ext. Culver's root, Podophyllin, of each, ¼ gr.; Oil Peppermint, ¼ gr.

Action and uses—Cathartic.

Dose, 1 to 3 pills.

PIL. CHALYBEATE; See Pil. Ferruginous, Blaud.

PIL. CHALYBEATE COMP.; See Pil. Ferruginous, Blaud, comp.

PIL. CHALYBEATE COMP., JARVIS.

Formula—Each pill contains: Ext. Nux vomica, 1-10 gr.; Iron sulph. exsic., Potassium carbonate, of each, 1½ grs.

Action and uses—Especially valuable in the treatment of anemia, chlorosis, phthisis, etc.

Dose, 1 to 3 pills.

PIL. CHINOIDIN, 1 gr., 2 grs., 3 grs.

Action and uses—Chinoidin is a cheap and excellent antiperiodic and tonic.

Dose, from 1 to 20 grs. The rule is to give it in about double the doses of quinine sulphate.

PIL. CHINOIDIN COMP.

Formula—Each pill contains: Chinoidin, 2 grs.; Iron sulph. exsic., 1 gr.; Piperin, ½ gr.

Action and uses—A valuable tonic and antiperiodic.

Dose, 1 to 3 pills.

PIL. CIMICIFUGIN, 1 gr.

Action and uses—See Fl. Ext. Black Cohosh, page 21.

Dose, 1 to 4 grs.

PIL. CINCHONIDINE SALICYLATE, 2 1-2 grs.

Action and uses—Highly recommended in neuralgic and rheumatic pains, and especially in intercostal neuralgia.

Dose, 2 1-2 to 10 grs.

PIL. CINCHONIDINE SULPHATE, 1 gr., 2 grs., 3 grs., 4 grs., 5 grs.

Action and uses—A reliable tonic and antiperiodic, apparently equal to quinine sulphate, in doses one-third larger.

Dose, 1 to 15 grs.

PIL. CINCHONIDINE, IRON, STRYCHNINE AND ARSENIC.

Formula—Each pill contains: Cinchonidine sulph., Iron by hydrogen, of each, 1 gr.; Strychnine, Arsenous acid, of each, 1-60 gr.

Action and uses—Tonic and antiperiodic.

Dose, 1 to 2 pills.

PIL. COCA EXTRACT, 1 gr., 2 grs.

Action and uses—See Fl. Ext. Coca leaves, U. S., page 42.

Dose, 1 to 6 grs.

PIL. COCA, PHOSPHORUS AND STRYCHNINE.

Formula—Each pill contains: Ext. Coca, 3 grs.; Phosphorus, 1-50 gr.; Strychnine, 1-60 gr.

Action and uses—Tonic and stimulant. Useful in insomnia dependent on cerebral anemia and exhaustion, wakefulness of the aged accompanied by muscular cramps, feebleness of memory, and trembling of the voluntary muscles on exertion, early decay of mental powers, paralysis, neuralgia and nervous breakdown from overwork.

Dose, 1 to 2 pills.

PIL. COCAINE HYDROCHLORATE, 1-10 gr., 1-8 gr.

Action and uses—Cerebral, cardiac respiratory and nerve stimulant and diuretic. See Fl. Ext. Coca, U. S., page 42.

Dose, 1-10 to 1-2 gr.

PIL. CODEINE, 1-16 gr., 1-8 gr., 1-5 gr., 1-4 gr., 1-2 gr., 1 gr.

Action and uses—Codeine (methylmorphine), motor paralyzant. It exalts the spinal cord more than morphine and affects the cerebrum less. Anodyne and analgesic especially in abdominal and pelvic pain. Hypnotic with less disturbance than produced by morphine. Especially useful in the pill form in diabetes. Abates the morphine habit.

Dose, 1-16 to 1 gr.

PIL. COLOCYNTH, COMP. EXT., 3 grs.

Action and uses—Cathartic. One of the best remedies in constipation due to torpor of the bowels.

Dose, 3 to 15 grs.

PIL. COLOCYNTH COMP. EXT. AND BLUE MASS, 3 grs.

Formula—Each pill contains: Ext. Colocynth comp., 2½ grs.; Blue mass, ½ gr.

Action and uses—Cathartic.

Dose, 1 to 4 pills.

PIL. COLOCYNTH COMP. EXT. AND BLUE MASS, 5 grs.

Formula—Each pill contains: Ext. Colocynth comp., Blue mass, of each, 2½ grs.

Action and uses—Cathartic.

Dose, 1 to 2 pills.

PIL. COLOCYNTH COMP. EXT. AND HYOSCYAMUS.

Formula—Each pill contains: Ext. Colocynth comp., 2½ grs.; Ext. Hyoscyamus, 1½ grs.

Action and uses—Gentle Laxative. The Hyoscyamus overcomes the tendency to gripe which is noticed in some cases where Ext. Colocynth comp. alone is used.

Dose, 1 to 2 pills.

PIL. COLOCYNTH COMP. EXT., IPECAC AND BLUE MASS.

Formula—Each pill contains: Ext. Colocynth comp., Blue mass, of each, 2 grs.; Ipecac, 1-4 gr.

Action and uses—Cholagogue, cathartic.

Dose, 1 to 3 pills.

PIL. COLOCYNTH COMP. EXT. AND PODOPHYLLIN; See Pil. Antibilious.

PIL. COLOCYNTH COMP. EXT., NUX VOMICA AND BELLADONNA.

Formula—Each pill contains: Ext. Colocynth comp., 2 grs.; Ext. Nux vomica, ½ gr.; Ext. Belladonna, 1-10 gr.

Action and uses—Laxative.

Dose, 1 to 2 pills.

PIL. COOK'S.

Formula—Each pill contains: Purified aloes, Rhubarb, of each, 1 gr.; Calomel, Soap, of each, ½ gr.

Action and uses—Cathartic.

Dose, 2 to 4 pills.

PIL. COPAIBA, 3 grs.

Action and uses—Of value in subacute and chronic inflammation of the genito-urinary mucous membrane. Chiefly used in gonorrhea. If given in beginning, before the inflammation has fully developed, it may abate the attack; if it fails, it may greatly aggravate the symptoms. It should not be used during the height of the inflammation, but is especially useful in the advanced stages of the disease.

Dose, 3 to 15 grs.

PIL. COPAIBA COMP., 3 grs.

Formula—Each pill contains: Mass Copaiba, 1½ grs.; Resin Guaiac, Iron citrate, of each, ¾ gr.; Oleoresin Cubeb, ⅓ gr.

Action and uses—Used in chronic inflammation of the genito-urinary mucous membrane.

Dose, 2 to 4 pills.

PIL. COPAIBA COMP., 4 grs.

Formula—Each pill contains: Mass Copaiba, 2 grs.; Resin Guaiac, Iron citrate, of each, ½ gr.; Oleoresin Cubeb, 1 gr.

Action and uses—See Pil. Copaiba, comp., 3 grs.

Dose, 1 to 3 pills.

PIL. COPAIBA COMP., 5 grs.

Formula—Each pill contains: Mass Copaiba, 2½ grs.; Resin Guaiac, Iron citrate, of each, ¾ gr.; Oleoresin Cubeb, 1½ grs.

Action and uses—See Pil. Copaiba comp., 3 grs.

Dose, 1 to 3 pills.

PIL. COPAIBA AND CUBEB, 3 grs.

Formula—Each pill contains: Mass Copaiba, 2 grs.; Oleoresin Cubeb, 1 gr.

Action and uses—The best effects in treatment of gonorrhea are frequently obtained by combining cubeb with copaiba. It is less liable to disturb digestion. See Pil. Copaiba, 3 grs.

Dose, 2 to 5 pills.

PIL. COPAIBA AND CUBEB, 4 grs.

Formula—Each pill contains: Mass Copaiba, 3 grs.; Oleoresin Cubeb, 1 gr.

Action and uses—See Pil. Copaiba and Cubeb, 3 grs.

Dose, 1 to 4 pills.

PIL. COPPER ARSENITE, 1-100 gr.

Action and uses—Exceedingly poisonous. Intestinal antiseptic, antispasmodic and sedative. Used in cholera morbus, enteric fever, Asiatic cholera, dysentery.

Dose, 1-100 grain every half hour till relieved then every hour.

Antidotes—See "Poisons and Antidotes," Index.

PIL. CORROSIVE SUBLIMATE, 1-100 gr., 1-60 gr., 1-50 gr., 1-40 gr., 1-32 gr., 1-30 gr., 1-20 gr., 1-16 gr., 1-12 gr., 1-10 gr. 1-8 gr., 1-6 gr., 1-4 gr.

Action and uses—Exceedingly poisonous. Alterative and tonic. Used principally in syphilis but is not applicable to the tertiary form of that disease.

Dose, 1-100 to 1-4 gr., not to exceed ½ grain per day although in some cases the dose has been pushed to 1 grain per day without salivation.

Antidotes—See "Poisons and Antidotes," Index.

PIL. CREOSOTE, BEECHWOOD, 1-4 gr., 1-2 gr., 3-4 gr., 1 gr., 2 grs.

Action and uses—Antitubercular, antiseptic, antipyretic. In chronic bronchitis, bronchorrhea, phthisis and in diabetes mellitus beechwood creosote has been given with marked benefit, it checks fermentation in the stomach and relieves nausea and diarrhea. Useful in seasickness and in the vomiting of pregnancy.

Dose, 1-4 to 2 grs. From 10 to 15 grains may be given daily.

PIL. DAMIANA EXT., 2 grs., 3 grs.

Action and uses—See Fl. Ext. Damiana, page 49.

Dose, 2 to 6 grs.

PIL. DANDELION EXT., 3 grs.

Action and uses—See Fl. Ext. Dandelion, page 49.

Dose, 3 to 15 grs.

PIL. DIGESTIVE.

Formula—Each pill contains: Pepsin, 1 gr.; Nux vomica, ¼ gr.; Gingerine, 1-16 gr.; Sulphur, ½ gr.

Action and uses—An efficient remedy in dyspepsia and to impart tone to the digestive apparatus.

Dose, 1 to 3 pills at meal time or when suffering pain from indigestion.

PIL. DIGITALIN, PURE, 1-100 gr., 1-60 gr.

Action and uses—See Fl. Ext. Digitalis, page 50.

Dose, 1-100 to 1-30 gr. Maximum dose, 1-15 gr. Not to exceed ⅓ gr. in 24 hours.

PIL. DIGITALIS COMP.

Formula—Each pill contains: Digitalis, Squill, of each, 1 gr.; Potassium nitrate, 2 grs.

Action and uses—Diuretic. Recommended in cardiac, acute and renal dropsy.

Dose, 1 pill 2 or 3 times a day.

PIL. DIGITALIS EXT., 1-2 gr.

Action and uses—See Fl. Ext. Digitalis, page 50.

Dose, 1-2 to 2 grs.

PIL. DINNER, LADY WEBSTER; See Pil. Aloes and Mastich.

PIL. DIPSOMANIA; See Pil. Strychnine nitrate.

PIL. DIURETIC.

Formula—Each pill contains: Ext. Buchu, Potassium nitrate, of each, 1 gr.; Squill, ½ gr.

Action and uses—Diuretic and antacid.

Dose, 2 to 3 pills.

PIL. DIURETIC COMP.

Formula—Each pill contains: Soap, Sodium carb, of each, 1½ grs.; Oil Juniper, 1-16 gr.

Action and uses—Diuretic and antacid.

Dose, 2 to 3 pills.

PIL. DOVER'S POWDER; See Pil. Ipecac and Opium.

PIL. ELATERIN, 1-20 gr.

Neutral principle from Elaterium.

Action and uses—POISONOUS. Powerful hydragogue cathartic, causing profuse watery stools, and when given in large doses, great prostration, gastro-intestinal irritation, nausea and vomiting. Used in ascites, anasarca, uremia and cerebral disorders. Should be used with caution.

Dose, 1-20 to 1-10 gr. See Pil. Elaterium, Clutterbuck.

PIL. ELATERIUM, CLUTTERBUCK, 1-16 gr., 1-12 gr., 1-10 gr., 1-8 gr., 1-4 gr.

Action and uses—A powerful hydragogue cathartic, considered one of the most efficient remedies in the treatment of dropsy.

Dose, 1-16 to 1-2 gr. See Pil. Elaterin.

PIL. EMMENAGOGUE, IMPROVED.

Formula—Each pill contains: Ergotin, Bonjean, Ext. Black Hellebore, Purified aloes, Iron sulph. exsic., of each, 1 gr.; Oil Savin, ½ gr.

Action and uses—An active emmenagogue and tonic.

Dose, 1 to 3 pills.

PIL. EMMENAGOGUE, IMPROVED, HALF STRENGTH.

Formula—Each pill contains: Ergotin, Bonjean, Ext. Black **Hellebore**, Purified aloes, Iron sulph. exsic., of each, ½ gr.; Oil Savin, ¼ **gr.**

Action and uses—See Pil Emmenagogue, Improved.

Dose, 1 to 6 pills.

PIL. EMMENAGOGUE, MUTTER.

Formula—Each pill contains: Iron sulph. exsic., Gum Turpentine, of each, 1½ grs.; Purified aloes, ½ gr.

Action and uses—Emmenagogue.

Dose, 1 to 3 pills.

PIL. EMMENAGOGUE, RIGAUD.

Formula—Each pill contains: Purified aloes, 1½ grs.; Rue, Saffron, Savin, of each, ¼ gr.

Action and uses—Emmenagogue.

Dose, 1 to 3 pills.

PIL. EMMENAGOGUE, WITH EXTRACT COTTON ROOT.

Formula—Each pill contains: Ergotin, Bonjean, Purified aloes, Ext. Cotton root, Iron sulph. exsic., of each, 1 gr.; Oil Savin, ½ gr.

Action and uses—Emmenagogue and tonic.

Dose, 1 to 3 pills.

PIL. ERGOTIN, BONJEAN, 1-4 gr., 1-2 gr., 1 gr., 2 grs., 3 grs., 5 grs.

Action and uses—See Fl. Ext. Ergot, page 52.

Dose, 3 to 10 grs.

PIL. ERGOTIN AND CANNABIS INDICA.

Formula—Each pill contains: Ergotin, Bonjean, 1 gr.; Ext. Cannabis Indica, ½ gr.

Action and uses—Used in that form of menorrhagia which occurs at the climacteric period. Arrests hemorrhage. A valuable remedy in the treatment of impotence.

Dose, 1 to 2 pills.

PIL. ERGOTIN COMP.

Formula—Each pill contains: Ergotin, Bonjean, 3 grs.; Ext. Cannabis Indica, 1-6 gr.; Strychnine, 1-60 gr.

Action and uses—Said to be especially valuable in functional impotence.

Dose, 1 to 2 pills.

PIL. EUCALYPTUS EXT., 2 grs.

Action and uses—See Fl. Ext. Eucalyptus, page 53.

Dose, 2 to 4 grs.

PIL. EUCALYPTUS COMP.

Formula—Each pill contains: Ext. Eucalyptus, 1 gr.; Ext. Apocynum, ½ gr.; Sanguinarin, ¼ gr.

Action and uses—Tonic, febrifuge and antiperiodic.

Dose, 1 to 2 pills.

PIL. EVACUANT; See Pil. A. S. B. and I., Lilly.

PIL. FEMALE, AMENORRHEA.

Formula—Each pill contains: Ext. Black Cohosh, Iron sulph. exsic., Ext. Cotton root, Purified aloes, of each, 1 gr.

Action and uses—A valuable emmenagogue. Useful in amenorrhea and dysmenorrhea.

Dose, 1 to 2 pills.

PIL. FEMALE, LEUCORRHEA.

Formula—Each pill contains: Hamamelin, 2 grs.; Senecin, Hydrastin, of each, ½ gr.

Dose, 1 to 2 pills.

PIL. FERRI CARBONATIS, U. S.; See Pil. Ferruginous, Blaud.

PIL. FERRUGINOUS, BLAUD, 3 grs., Pil. Ferri Carbonatis, U. S., Blaud's pills, Chalybeate pills, Pills of Ferrous carbonate.

Formula—Each pill contains: Iron sulphate, Potassium carbonate, of each, 1½ grs.

Action and uses—Antichlorotic. Valuable in chlorosis, amenorrhea, etc. In anemia, Niemeyer recommends three pills three times a day, an additional pill being added daily. These large doses of iron, while rarely deranging the stomach or producing headache, cure anemia with astonishing rapidity.

Dose, 1 to 5 pills.

PIL. FERRUGINOUS, BLAUD, 5 grs.

Formula—Each pill contains: Iron sulphate, Potassium carbonate, of each, 2½ grs.

Action and uses—See Pil. Ferruginous, Blaud, 3 grs.

Dose, 1 to 3 pills.

PIL. FERRUGINOUS, BLAUD, CASCARA AND NUX VOMICA.

Formula—Each pill contains: Iron sulphate, Potassium carbonate, of each, 2½ grs.; Ext. Cascara sagrada, 1 gr.; Ext. Nux vomica, ¼ gr.

Action and uses—Antichlorotic, tonic and laxative.

Dose, 1 to 2 pills.

PIL. FERRUGINOUS, BLAUD, COMP.

Formula—Each pill contains: Blaud's mass, 2 grs.; Ext. Nux vomica, 1-6 gr.

Action and uses—Antichlorotic.

Dose, 1 to 3 pills.

WHEN ORDERING OR PRESCRIBING.

PIL. FERRUGINOUS, BLAUD, COMP. WITH ARSENIC.

Formula—Each pill contains: Blaud's mass, 5 grs.; Ext. Nux vomica, 1-10 gr.; Arsenous acid, 1-50 gr.

Action and uses—Antichlorotic.

Dose, 1 to 2 pills.

PIL. FERRUGINOUS, BLAUD, IMPROVED.

Formula—Each pill contains: Blaud's mass, 3 grs.; Arsenous acid, 1-60 gr.

Action and uses—Antichlorotic.

Dose, 1 to 2 pills.

PIL. FERRUGINOUS, BLAUD, MODIFIED.

Formula—Each pill contains: Blaud's mass, 5 grs.; Arsenous acid, 1-40 gr.

Action and uses—Antichlorotic.

Dose, 1 to 2 pills.

PIL. GALBANUM COMP.

Formula—Each pill contains: Galbanum, Myrrh, of each, 1½ grs.; Asafetida, ½ gr.

Action and uses—Antispasmodic and emmenagogue. Useful in chlorosis and hysteria.

Dose, 2 to 4 pills.

PIL. GENTIAN COMP., 3 grs.

Formula—Each pill contains: Ext. Gentian, Purified aloes, of each, ⅔ gr.; Rhubarb, 1⅓ grs.; Oil Caraway, 1-5 gr.

Action and uses—Laxative, tonic.

Dose, 2 to 4 pills.

PIL. GLONOIN; See Pil. Nitroglycerin.

PIL. GOLD, CHORIDE, 1-30 gr., 1-20 gr.

Action and uses—See Pil. Gold and Sodium chloride.

Dose, 1-30 to 1-10 gr.

PIL. GOLD AND SODIUM CHLORIDE, 1-40 gr., 1-20 gr., 1-10 gr.

Action and uses—Poisonous. This is a more stable salt than gold chloride and is official. When administered internally it closely resembles the action of bichloride of mercury. In small doses it promotes appetite and digestion, and stimulates the functions of the brain. Continued, it seems to induce aphrodisiac effects in both sexes and in women increases the menstrual flow. Effects of a toxic dose are similar to those produced by corrosive sublimate. It is used in irritative dyspepsia, gastroduodenal catarrh, hypochondriasis, functional impotence, chronic metritis, habitual abortion and ovarian dropsy. Especially recommended in chronic albuminuria, sclerosis, granular and fibroid kidney, preventing hyperplasia of connective tissue.

Dose, 1-40 to 1-10 gr.

Antidotes—Same as corrosive sublimate. See Poisons and Antidotes, Index.

PIL. GONORRHEA, 3 grs.

Formula—Each pill contains: Cubeb, Mass Copaiba, of each, 1¼ grs.; Iron sulph. exsic., Venice Turpentine, of each, ¼ gr.

Action and uses—Tonic and alterative to the mucous membrane. An old and valuable prescription for obstinate gonorrhea and gleet.

Dose, 2 to 4 pills.

PIL. GONORRHEA, 4 grs.

Formula—Each pill contains: Cubeb, Mass Copaiba, of each, 1⅔ grs.; Iron sulph. exsic., Venice Turpentine, of each, ⅓ gr.

Action and uses—See Pil. Gonorrhea, 3 grs.

Dose, 2 to 3 pills.

PIL. HELONIAS COMP.

Formula—Each pill contains: Helonin, Viburnin, of each, ¼ gr., Caulophyllin, ½ gr.; Squaw vine, 1½ grs.

Action and uses—Uterine tonic and antispasmodic. Useful in amenorrhea, dysmenorrhea, menorrhagia, leucorrhea and to overcome the tendency to habitual abortion. Especially valuable to pregnant women when delicate or nervous. Should be given daily for several weeks before parturition.

Dose, 2 to 4 pills.

PIL. HENBANE EXT.; See Pil. Hyoscyamus Ext.

PIL. HEPATIC.

Formula—Each pill contains: Blue mass, 3 grs.; Ext. Colocynth comp., 2 grs.; Ext. Belladonna, ⅙ gr.

Action and uses—A mild purgative with special action on the liver.

Dose, 1 to 2 pills.

PIL. HEPATIC ECLECTIC.

Formula—Each pill contains: Leptandrin, ½ gr.; Podophyllin, Irisin, of each, ⅛ gr.; Ext. Nux vomica, 1-16 gr.; Capsicum, ⅕ gr.

Action and uses—A valuable cathartic and hepatic stimulant.

Dose, 1 to 3 pills.

PIL. HEPATICA.

Formula—Each pill contains: Blue mass, 2 grs.; Ext. Coloc comp., Ext. Hyoscyamus, of each, ½ gr.

Action and uses—Cathartic and hepatic stimulant.

Dose, 1 to 2 pills.

PIL. HOOPER'S, FEMALE.

Formula—Each pill contains: Aloes, purified, 1 gr.; Iron sulph. exsic., ½ gr.; Myrrh, Ext. Black Hellebore, of each, ¼ gr.; Ginger, Soap, Canella, of each, ⅛ gr.

Action and uses—Emmenagogue.

Dose, 1 to 3 pills.

PIL. HYOSCINE HYDROBROMATE, 1-400 gr.

Action and uses—Hyoscine is a derivative of hyoscyamine and is more powerful. Used in chronic mania and dementia, insomnia, asthma and sciatica. See Fl. Ext. Henbane, page 64.

Dose for the insane, 1-50 gr. very cautiously repeated till the effect is produced. In other cases the dose is from 1-400 to 1-100 grain.

PIL. HYOSCYAMINE CRYSTALS, 1-200 gr.

Action and uses—The alkaloid of hyoscyamus niger is isomeric with atropine and probably identical with daturine and duboisine. Used in acute and chronic mania, dementia, epilepsy, paralysis agitans and chorea. Eases the cough in consumption and asthma. See Fl. Ext. Henbane, page 64.

Dose, 1-200 to 1-100 gr. As a hypnotic for the insane, the dose may be increased to 1-25 grain or more and cautiously repeated.

PIL. HYOSCYAMUS EXT., 1-4 gr., 1-2 gr., 1 gr.

Action and uses—See Fl. Ext. Henbane, page 64.

Dose, 1-4 to 1 gr.

PIL. HYOSCYAMUS AND CAMPHOR MONOBROMATED.

Formula—Each pill contains: Ext. Hyoscyamus, Camphor monobromated, of each, 1 gr.
Action and uses—Nerve sedative, anodyne and hypnotic.
Dose, 1 pill.

PIL. ICHTHYOL, 1 1-2 grs., 2 1-2 grs.

Action and uses—Antiphlogistic, anodyne, alterative. Used in eczema, psoriasis and other skin diseases, rheumatism, scrofula, nephritis, gonorrhea.
Dose, 1 to 4 pills.

PIL. INTESTINAL ANTISEPTIC; See Pil. Antiseptic, Intestinal.

PIL. IODOFORM, 1 gr.

Action and uses—Alterative and tonic. It is said to check the activity of the bacillus of tuberculosis, also used in diabetes and in syphilis.
Dose, 1 to 3 pills.

PIL. IODOFORM AND IRON.

Formula—Each pill contains: Iodoform, 1 gr.; Iron by hydrogen, 1¼ grs.
Action and uses—Tonic and alterative. Valuable as a remedy in scrofula, anemia, neuralgia, chlorosis, phthisis, syphilis and cutaneous eruptions.
Dose, 1 to 3 pills.

PIL. IPECAC AND OPIUM, NO. 1.

Formula—Each pill contains: Powd. Opium, Ipecac, of each, ¼ gr. Equal to 2½ grs. Dover's powder.
Action and uses—Anodyne, soporific.
Dose, 1 to 6 pills.

PIL. IPECAC AND OPIUM, NO. 2.

Formula—Each pill contains: Powd. Opium, Ipecac, of each, ½ gr. Equal to 5 grs. Dover's powder.
Action and uses—Anodyne, soporific.
Dose, 1 to 3 pills.

PIL. IPECAC AND OPIUM, NO. 3.

Formula—Each pill contains: Ipecac, Powd. Opium, of each, 1 gr. Equal to 10 grs. Dover's powder
Action and uses—Anodyne, soporific.
Dose, 1 pill.

PIL. IRON ARSENATE, 1-20 gr., 1-8 gr., 1-4 gr.

Action and uses—Hematinic, alterative. Used in chronic skin diseases.
Dose, 1-20 to 1-4 gr.

PIL. IRON BY HYDROGEN, 1-4 gr., 1 gr. 2 grs., 3 grs.

Action and uses—Chalybeate tonic. Peculiarly well fitted to improve the quality of the blood when impoverished from any cause. Useful in diseases characterized by debility. Employed in chronic anemia or chlorosis, passive hemorrhages, neuralgia and dyspepsia when it depends upon deficient energy of the digestive organs; contra-indicated in all inflammatory diseases. It does not agree with epileptics, increasing the tendency to fits. Iron, as a rule, is best taken after meals, and the patient should avoid the use of tea near the time of taking the iron.
Dose, 1-4 to 6 grs.

PIL. IRON CARBONATE, VALLET, 2 grs., 3 grs., 5 grs.
 Action and uses—Chalybeate tonic. Especially indicated in pure anemic chlorosis and in all affections in which the red corpuscles of the blood are deficient.
 Dose, 2 to 5 grs.

PIL. IRON **CITRATE, 2 grs.**
 Action and **uses**—Tonic.
 Dose, 2 to 6 **grs.**

PIL. IRON CLAD; See Pil. Quinine comp. and Strychnine.

PIL. IRON IODIDE, U. S., 1 gr.
 Action and uses—Tonic, alterative, diuretic and emmenagogue. Employed in amenorrhea, leucorrhea and in secondary syphilis.
 Dose, 1 to 3 grs.

PIL. IRON PROTOCARBONATE; See Pil. Iron carbonate, Vallet.

PIL. IRON AND ALOES; Compare Pil. Aloes and Iron and Pil. Aloes and Iron, U. S.
 Formula—Each pill contains: Purified aloes, 2 grs.; Iron sulph. exsic., 1 gr.
 Action and uses—Used in amenorrhea associated with anemia and constipation.
 Dose, 1 to 3 pills.

PIL. IRON CITRATE AND STRYCHNINE.
 Formula—Each pill contains: Iron citrate, 2 grs.; Strychnine, 1-50 gr.
 Action and uses—Tonic and nerve stimulant.
 Dose, 1 to 2 pills.

PIL. IRON PHOSPHATE AND STRYCHNINE.
 Formula—Each pill **contains:** Iron phosphate, 2 grs.; Strychnine, 1-60 gr.
 Action and uses—Tonic and nerve stimulant.
 Dose, 1 to 2 pills.

PIL. IRON AND QUININE CITRATE, 1 gr., 2 grs., 3 grs., 5 grs.
 Action and uses—Tonic and antiperiodic.
 Dose, 1 to 5 grs.

PIL. IRON, QUININE AND **STRYCHNINE.**
 Formula—Each pill contains: Quinine sulphate, 1 gr.; Iron carbonate, Vallet, 2 grs.; Strychnine, 1-60 gr.
 Action and uses—Tonic and antiperiodic.
 Dose, 1 to 2 pills.

PIL. IRON, **QUININE AND** STRYCHNINE CITRATES.
 Formula—Each pill contains: Iron and Quinine citrate, 2 grs.; Strychnine citrate, 1-60 gr.
 Action and uses—Tonic and antiperiodic.
 Dose, 1 to 2 pills.

PIL. IRON, QUININE AND STRYCHNINE PHOSPHATES.
 Formula—Each pill contains: Iron phosphate, 2 grs.; Quinine phosphate, 1 gr.; Strychnine phosphate, 1-60 gr.
 Action and uses—Tonic and antiperiodic.
 Dose, 1 to 2 pills.

PIL. IRON AND STRYCHNINE.

Formula—Each pill contains: Iron by hydrogen, 2 grs.; Strychnine, 1-60 gr.

Action and uses—Tonic and nerve stimulant.

Dose, 1 to 2 pills.

PIL. IRON, STRYCHNINE AND ARSENIC.

Formula—Each pill contains: Iron by hydrogen, 1 gr.; Strychnine, 1-60 gr.; Arsenous acid, 1-100 gr.

Action and uses—Tonic and alterative.

Dose, 1 pill.

PIL. LAXATIVE.

Formula—Each pill contains: Purified aloes, 1 gr.; Sulphur, Podophyllin, of each, 1-5 gr.; Resin Guaiac, ½ gr.; Syrup Frangula, q. s.

Action and uses—Gentle purgative.

Dose, 1 to 2 pills.

PIL. LAXATIVE, COLE.

Formula—Each pill contains: Podophyllin, 1-10 gr.; Calomel, 1 gr.; Ext. Colocynth comp., 3 grs.

Action and uses—Laxative with tendency to the liver.

Dose, 1 to 2 pills.

PIL. LAXATIVE, SPECIAL, FORDYCE BARKER.

Formula—Each pill contains: Ext. Colocynth comp., 1¾ grs.; Ext. Hyoscyamus, 1¼ grs.; Purified aloes, 5-6 gr.; Ext. Nux vomica, 5-12 gr.; Podophyllin, Ipecac, of each, 1-12 gr.

Action and uses—Recommended by Dr. Barker in constipation of puerperal women where there is aversion to the use of enema. Two of the above pills in the morning before breakfast will act effectually and without pain.

PIL. LEPTANDRIN, 1-4 gr., 1-2 gr., 1 gr.

Action and uses—See Fl. Ext. Culver's Root, page 49.

Dose, 1-4 to 4 grs.

PIL. LEPTANDRIN COMP.

Formula—Each pill contains: Leptandrin, 1 gr.; Irisin, ¼ gr.; Podophyllin, ⅛ gr.

Action and uses—Cathartic and cholagogue.

Dose, 1 to 2 pills.

PIL. LIVER, GRANULES.

Formula—Each pill contains: Aloin, Jalapin, of each, 1-10 gr.; Podophyllin, 1-5 gr.; Ext. Hyoscyamus, Ext. Nux vomica, Oleoresin Capsicum, of each, 1-20 gr.

Action and uses—An efficient laxative.

Dose, 1 to 4 pills.

PIL. LIVER, IMPROVED VEGETABLE.

Formula—Each pill contains: Purified aloes, Jalap, of each, 1 gr.; Gamboge, Leptandrin, Podophyllin, of each, ½ gr.; Oil Capsicum, 1-48 gr., Tr. Veratrum viride, ½ gr.

Action and uses—Hepatic stimulant and cathartic.

Dose, 1 to 4 pills.

PIL. LOBELIA COMP., 3 grs.

Formula—Lobelia seed, Capsicum, Ladies' slipper, of each, 1 gr.; Ext. Boneset, q. s.

Action and uses—Nervine and antispasmodic.

Dose, 1 pill.

PIL. MANGANESE BINOXIDE, C. P., 1-2 gr., 1 gr., 2 grs., 3 grs.
  Action and uses—Emmenagogue. Especially recommended in membranous dysmenorrhœa, also in sudden suppression of the menses as a result of cold and when the menstrual discharge is scanty and irregular.
  Dose, 1-2 to 10 grs., twice or thrice daily.

PIL. MERCURIC IODIDE; See Pil. Mercury biniodide.

PIL. MERCUROUS IODIDE; See Pil. Mercury protiodide.

PIL. MERCURY BINIODIDE, 1-40 gr., 1-25 gr., 1-16 gr., 1-12 gr., 1-10 gr., 1-8 gr., 1-6 gr., 1-4 gr.
  Action and uses—Powerful irritant poison. Alterative. Used in syphilitic affections.
  Dose, 1-40 to 1-4 gr. The beginning dose should be very small and increased with great caution.
  Antidotes—See Poisons and Antidotes, Index.

PIL. MERCURY PROTIODIDE, 1-20 gr., 1-16 gr., 1-10 gr., 1-8 gr., 1-6 gr., 1-5 gr., 1-4 gr., 1-3 gr., 1-2 gr., 1 gr.
  Action and uses—Alterative. Used in syphilitic affections.
  Dose, 1-20 to 1 gr.

PIL. MERCURY PROTIODIDE AND HYOSCYAMUS.
  Formula—Each pill contains: Mercury protiodide, 1-6 gr.; Ext. Hyoscyamus, 1-20 gr.
  Action and uses—Alterative. Used in syphilitic affections.
  Dose, 1 to 3 pills.

PIL. MERCURY RED IODIDE; See Pil. Mercury biniodide.

PIL. MERCURY TANNATE, 1 gr.
  Action and uses—Alterative. Used in syphilitic affections.
  Dose, 1 pill.

PIL. MERCURY, YELLOW IODIDE; See Pil. Mercury protiodide.

PIL. MERCURY AND CHALK, NO. 1.
  Formula—Each pill contains: Mercury and Chalk, 1 gr.; Confection Rose, q. s.
  Action and uses—Alterative.
  Dose, 1 to 3 pills.

PIL. METALLORUM N. F.; See Pil. Quinine comp. and Strychnine.

PIL. MIGRAINE, NO. 1.
  Formula—Each pill contains: Acetanlid, 2 grs.; Camphor monobromated, ½ gr.
  Action and uses—Analgesic, hypnotic and antispasmodic.
  Dose, 1 to 3 pills.

PIL. MIGRAINE, NO. 2.
  Formula—Each pill contains: Acetanlid, 2 grs.; Camphorated monobromated, Caffeine citrate, of each, ½ gr.
  Action and uses—Analgesic, hypnotic and antispasmodic.
  Dose, 1 to 2 pills.

PIL. MORPHINE SULPHATE, 1-20 gr., 1-16 gr., 1-10 gr., 1-8 gr., 1-6 gr., 1-4 gr., 1-3 gr., 1-2 gr.

Action and uses—Narcotic poison. Antispasmodic, hypnotic, analgesic, narcotic. Relieves pain, produces sleep. Useful in diarrhea and dysentry. See Fl. Ext. Opium, concentrated, page 88.

Dose, 1-20 to 1-2 gr., the latter being the maximum dose in extreme cases and not more than 2 grains should be given per day.

PIL. MORPHINE VALERIANATE, 1-8 gr., 1-4 gr.

Action and uses—Sedative. Used in hysteria, nervousness, delirium tremens, etc.

Dose, 1-8 to 1-2 gr.

PIL. MORPHATROPIA, NO. 1.

Formula—Each pill contains: Morphine sulphate, 1-24 gr.; Atropine sulphate, 1-600 gr.

Action and uses—In small doses atropine increases the hypnotic power of morphine, causing a less disturbed and more normal sleep than morphine alone; the pain relieving power is increased by atropine, while the after headache, vertigo, nausea and depression of the heart's action, caused by morphine, are to a large extent, prevented by its combination with atropine.

Dose, 1 to 2 pills cautiously increased.

PIL. MORPHATROPIA, NO. 2.

Formula—Each pill contains: Morphine sulphate, 1-8 gr.; Atropine sulphate, 1-200 gr.

Action and uses—See Pil. Morphatropia, No. 1.

Dose, 1 pill cautiously increased.

PIL. MORPHATROPIA, NO. 3.

Formula—Each pill contains: Morphine sulphate, 1-4 gr.; Atropine sulphate, 1-150 gr.

Action and uses—See Pil. Morphatropia, No. 1.

Dose, 1 pill cautiously increased.

PIL. MORPHATROPIA, NO. 4.

Formula—Each pill contains: Morphine sulphate, ⅛ gr.; Atropine sulphate, 1-300 gr.

Action and uses—See Pil. Morphatropia, No. 1.

Dose, 1 to 2 pills cautiously increased.

PIL. MORPHATROPIA, NO. 5.

Formula—Each pill contains: Morphine sulphate, 1-6 gr.; Atropine sulphate, 1-150 gr.

Action and uses—See Pil. Morphatropia, No. 1.

Dose, 1 to 2 pills cautiously increased.

PIL. MORPHINE, HYOSCYAMUS AND CAMPHOR.

Formula—Each pill contains: Morphine sulphate, ¼ gr., Ext. Hyoscyamus, 2 grs., Camphor, 1 gr.

Action and uses—Anodyne and antispasmodic.

Dose, 1 to 2 pills.

PIL. NAPTHALIN, 3 grs.

Action and uses—Antiseptic, anthelmintic antipyretic. Used in chronic and acute intestinal inflammation, cholera, typhoid fever.

Dose, 3 to 15 grs. For tape worm, the full dose, followed some hours later by castor oil.

PIL. NEURALGIC, BROWN-SEQUARD.

Formula—Each pill contains: Ext. Hyoscyamus, Ext. Conium seed, of each, ⅔ gr.; Ext. Ignatia, Ext. Opium, of each, ½ gr.; Ext. Aconite leaves, ⅓ gr.; Ext. Cannabis indica, ¼ gr.; Ext. Stramonium, 1-5 gr.; Ext. Belladonna, 1-6 gr.

Action and uses—Anodyne.

Dose, 1 pill.

PIL. NEURALGIC, BROWN-SEQUARD, HALF STRENGTH.

Formula—Each pill contains Ext. Hyoscyamus, Ext. Conium seed, of each, ⅓ gr.; Ext. Ignatia, Ext. Opium, of each, ¼ gr.; Ext. Aconite leaves, 1-6 gr.; Ext. Cannabis indica, ⅛ gr.; Ext. Stramonium, 1-10 gr.; Ext. Belladonna, 1-12 gr.

Action and uses—Anodyne.

Dose, 1 to 2 pills.

PIL. NEURALGIC, GROSS.

Formula—Each pill contains: Quinine sulphate, 2 grs.; Morphine sulphate, 1-20 gr.; Strychnine, 1-30 gr.; Arsenous acid, 1-20 gr.; Ext. Aconite leaves, ½ gr.

Action and uses—Tonic, alterative and anodyne.

Dose, 1 to 2 pills.

PIL. NEURALGIC, GROSS, HALF STRENGTH.

Formula—Each pill contains: Quinine sulphate, 1 gr.; Morphine sulphate, 1-40 gr.; Strychnine, 1-60 gr.; Arsenous acid, 1-40 gr.; Ext. Aconite leaves, ¼ gr.

Action and uses—Tonic, alterative and anodyne.

Dose, 1 to 3 pills.

PIL. NEURALGIC, GROSS, WITHOUT MORPHINE.

Formula—Each pill contains: Quinine sulphate, 2 grs.; Strychnine, 1-30 gr.; Arsenous acid, 1-20 gr.; Ext. Aconite leaves, ½ gr.

Action and uses—Tonic, alterative and anodyne.

Dose, 1 to 2 pills.

PIL. NIGHT SWEAT.

Formula—Each pill contains: Zinc oxide, ½ gr.; Salicin, 1 gr.; Ext. Belladonna, 1-25 gr.; Hydrastin, 1 gr.; Pepsin, ½ gr.

Dose, 1 to 3 pills.

PIL. NITROGLYCERIN, Pil. Glonoin, Pil. Trinitrin, 1-200 gr., 1-150 gr., 1-100 gr., 1-50 gr., 1-33 gr.

Action and uses—It has the same physiological effects as nitrite of amyl, but the action is slower and more permanent. MURRELL praises it in typical angina and for breathlessness and pseudo-angina. Strychnine, belladonna and sclerotinic acid are its physiological antagonists.

Dose, 1-200 to 1-33 gr.

PIL. NUX VOMICA EXT., 1-8 gr., 1-4 gr., 1-2 gr.

Action and uses—See Fl. Ext. Nux vomica, page 87.

Dose, 1-8 to 1 gr.

PIL. NUX VOMICA AND BELLADONNA.

Formula—Each pill contains: Ext. Nux vomica, Ext. Belladonna, of each, ¼ gr.

Dose, 1 to 2 pills.

PIL. OPIUM, 1-4 gr., 1-2 gr., 1 gr.

Action and uses—Narcotic. See Fl. Ext. Opium, concentrated, page 88.

Dose, 1-4 to 2 grs.

PIL. OPIUM EXT., 1-4 gr., 1-2 gr., 1 gr.

Action and uses—Narcotic. See Fl. Ext. Opium, concentrated, page 88.

Dose, 1-4 to 1 gr.

PIL. OPIUM AND CAMPHOR; See Pil. Camphor and Opium.

PIL. OPIUM AND LEAD ACETATE, NO. 1.

Formula—Each pill contains: Powd. Opium, Lead acetate, of each, 1 gr.

Action and uses—Anodyne and astringent. Of great benefit in chronic dysentery, diarrhea and bronchitis.

Dose, 1 pill.

PIL. OPIUM AND LEAD ACETATE, NO. 2.

Formula—Each pill contains: Powd. Opium, ½ gr.; Lead acetate, 1½ grs.

Action and uses—See Pil. Opium and Lead acetate, No. 1.

Dose, 1 pill.

PIL. OPIUM AND SILVER NITRATE.

Formula—Each pill contains: Powd. Opium, 1 gr.; Silver nitrate, ¼ gr.

Action and uses—Useful in dysentery of chronic type, the diarrhea of phthisis and typhoid fever.

Dose, 1 pill.

PIL. OX GALL.

Formula—Each pill contains: Ox gall, 2 grs.; Ginger, 1 gr.

Action and uses—Recommended in habitual constipation depending on atony of the intestines; also in jaundice depending upon catarrh of the bile ducts.

Dose, 2 to 3 pills.

PIL. OX GALL COMP.

Formula—Each pill contains: Ox gall, 2 grs.; Purified aloes, 1-10 gr.; Ext. Stramonium seed, 1-6 gr.; Berberine hydrochlorate, 1-12 gr.

Action and uses—See Pil. Ox gall.

Dose, 2 to 3 pills.

PIL. OX GALL AND PEPSIN.

Formula—Each pill contains: Purified aloes, 1 gr.; Iron sulph. exsic., ½ gr.; Ext. Nux vomica, 1-12 gr.; Ox gall, 1½ grs.; Pepsin, 1 gr.

Action and uses—Tonic, laxative and antidyspeptic.

Dose, 2 to 3 pills.

PIL. PALMETOL.

Formula—Each pill represents 30 grs. Saw Palmetto berries.

Action and uses—For the treatment of diseases of the genito-urinary system. Especially indicated in presenility, prostrate troubles, irritation of the bladder and urethral inflammation. Send for pamphlet.

Dose, 1 to 2 pills.

PIL. PEPSIN, BISMUTH AND STRYCHNINE.

Formula—Each pill contains: Pepsin sacch., Bismuth subnitrate, of each, 2½ grs.; Strychnine, 1-30 gr.

Action and uses—A valuable tonic in dyspepsia and indigestion.

Dose, 1 pill.

PIL. PETROLEUM, CRUDE, 2 grs.

Action and uses—Used in pulmonary diseases.

Dose, 2 to 3 pills.

PIL. PHENACETINE, 2 grs., 4 grs., 5 grs.

Action and uses—A coal tar product analogous to acetanilid, slightly antipyretic and has some analgesic power. It is much more expensive, with no advantage over acetanilid.

Dose, 2 to 10 grs.

PIL. PHENACETINE AND CAFFEINE CIT.

Formula—Each pill contains: Phenacetine, 3 grs.; Caffeine cit., 1½ grs.

Dose, 1 to 3 pills.

PIL. PHENACETINE AND QUININE.

Formula—Each pill contains: Phenacetine, 3 grs.; Quinine sulphate, 2 grs.

Dose, 1 to 3 pills.

PIL. PHENACETINE AND QUININE COMP.

Formula—Each pill contains: Phenacetine, 3 grs.; Quinine sulphate, 2 grs.; Dover's powder, ½ gr.; Ext. Aconite, 1-12 gr.

Dose, 1 to 3 pills.

PIL. PHENACETINE AND SALOL.

Formula—Each pill contains: Phenacetine, Salol, of each, 2½ grs.

Dose, 1 to 3 pills.

PIL. PHOSPHORUS, 1-200 gr., 1-100 gr., 1-50 gr., 1-30 gr., 1-25 gr., 1-20 gr., 1-12 gr.

Note—The phosphorus in these pills is presented in a free state, thoroughly and accurately subdivided and perfectly protected from oxidation, thus insuring safety and absence from any cause of irritation to the stomach.

Action and uses—Nutritive and stimulant to the nervous system. Used in mania, melancholia, sexual exhaustion, cerebral softening, neuralgia, etc. As a rule phosphorus and its compounds should be administered with food.

Dose, 1-200 to 1-12 gr.

PIL. PHOSPHORUS COMP., NO. 1.

Formula—Each pill contains: Phosphorus, 1-100 gr.; Ext. Nux vomica, ¼ gr.

Action and uses—Nutritive, tonic and stimulant. Valuable in atonic dyspepsia, mental overwork and depression.

Dose, 1 pill.

PIL. PHOSPHORUS COMP., NO. 2.

Action and uses—Each pill contains: Phosphorus, 1-50 gr.; Ext. Nux vomica, ¼ gr.

Action and uses—See Pil. Phosphorus comp., No. 1.

Dose, 1 to 2 pills.

PIL. PHOSPHORUS COMP., NO. 3.

Formula—Each pill contains: Phosphorus, 1-50 gr.; Ext. Nux vomica, ⅛ gr.

Action and uses—See Pil. Phosphorus comp., No. 1.

Dose, 1 to 3 pills.

PIL. PHOSPHORUS COMP. AND IRON.

Formula—Each pill contains: Phosphorus, 1-100 gr.; Iron phosphate, ½ gr.; Ext. Nux vomica, ⅛ gr.

Action and uses—See Pil. Phosphorus comp., No. 1.

Dose, 1 to 2 pills.

PIL. PHOSPHORUS, IRON AND DAMIANA.

Formula—Each pill contains: Phosphorus, 1-100 gr.; Iron carbonate, Vallet, 1 gr.; Ext. Damiana, 2 grs.

Action and uses—Nutritive, tonic and aphrodisiac.

Dose, 1 to 2 pills.

PIL. PHOSPHORUS, IRON AND NUX VOMICA.

Formula—Each pill contains: Phosphorus, 1-100 gr.; Iron carbonate, Vallet, 1 gr.; Ext. Nux vomica, ¼ gr.

Action and uses—A powerful nervine and tonic. Especially valuable in consumption, scrofula, the scrofulous diseases, debilitated and anemic conditions of children and in anemia, chlorosis, sciatica and other forms of neuralgia. A good adjunct to a course of cod liver oil. For children, one pill twice a day.

Dose, 1 to 2 pills.

PIL. PHOSPHORUS, IRON, QUININE AND STRYCHNINE.

Formula—Each pill contains: Phosphorus, 1-100 gr.; Iron carbonate, Vallet, Quinine sulphate, of each, 1 gr.; Strychnine, 1-60 gr.

Action and uses—Nerve stimulant and tonic.

Dose, 1 to 2 pills.

PIL. PHOSPHORUS, IRON AND STRYCHNINE.

Formula—Each pill contains: Phosphorus, 1-100 gr.; Iron carbonate, Vallet, 1 gr.; Strychnine, 1-60 gr.

Action and uses—Nerve stimulant and tonic.

Dose, 1 to 2 pills.

PIL. PHOSPHORUS AND NUX VOMICA; See Pil. Phosphorus comp., No. 1.

PIL. PHOSPHORUS, NUX VOMICA AND CANTHARIDES.

Formula—Each pill contains: Phosphorus, 1-50 gr.; Nux vomica, Cantharides, of each, 1 gr.

Action and uses—Stimulating emmenagogue and diuretic. Recommended as a gentle stimulant to the genito-urinary organs, in incontinence and retention of urine, in premature loss of sexual power, and in some cases of amenorrhea and leucorrhea.

Dose, 1 to 2 pills.

PIL. PHOSPHORUS, NUX VOMICA AND DAMIANA; See Pil. Aphrodisiacs, Lilly, page 324

PIL. PHOSPHORUS AND STRYCHNINE.

Formula—Each pill contains: Phosphorus, 1-50 gr.; Strychnine, 1-60 gr.

Action and uses—Nerve tonic and stimulant.

Dose, 1 to 2 pills.

PIL. PHYSOSTIGMINE SALICYLATE, 1-100 gr.

Action and uses—Physostigmine, also known as eserine, the alkaloidal principle of Calabar bean, is efficient in constipation due to torpor of the bowels, in tetanus, progressive paralysis of the insane, writers' cramp, and locomotor ataxia, also in controlling night sweats of phthisis. See Fl. Ext. Calabar bean, page 59.

Dose, 1-100 to 1-25 gr.

PIL. PHYTOLLACIN, 1-2 gr.

Action and uses—See Fl. Ext. Poke root, page 95.

Dose, 1-2 to 2 grs.

PIL. PICROTOXIN, 1-60 gr.

Action and uses—The active principle of Cocculus indicus. Narcotic poison. In small doses it acts as a bitter tonic to the digestive tract and is therefore advised in atonic conditions of the stomach and intestinal indigestion, attended by torpor of the intestinal walls and constipation. Also in epilepsy, chorea, alcoholic tremor, paralysis agitans and functional nervous disorders.

MURRELL says that a pill of Picrotoxin, 1-60 grain at bed time, is of great value in controlling night sweating of phthisis. See Fl. Ext. Cocculus indicus, page 42.

Dose, 1-60 to 1-30 gr.

PIL. PILOCARPINE HYDROCHLORATE, 1-8 gr.

Action and uses—The alkaloidal principle of jaborandi. It is convenient as a diaphoretic in removing matters from the blood or to reduce temperature. Thus in acute erysipelas its action is prompt and effective. Used with great benefit in dropsies, especially the renal form, but it is contraindicated where from any cause there is a weak heart. Ptyalism is frequently relieved by minute doses, 1-30 grain.

Dose, 1-4 gr., not exceeding 3-4 gr. per day.

PIL. PLUMMER; See Pil. Antimony comp., U. S.

PIL. PODOPHYLLIN, 1-40 gr., 1-20 gr., **1-16 gr., 1-10 gr., 1-8 gr.,** 1-6 gr., 1-5 gr., 1-4 gr., 1-2 gr., 1 gr.

Action and uses—Cathartic, emetic, alterative, anthelmintic, hydragogue and sialagogue. One half to two grains generally operates as an active cathartic, leaving the bowels in a soluable condition. In doses of $\frac{1}{20}$ to $\frac{1}{4}$ grain it is gently aperient and alterative, from $\frac{1}{2}$ to 1 grain it is one of our most valuable cholagogue cathartics, operating mildly, yet effectually arousing the whole biliary and digestive apparatus to a normal action. See Fl. Ext Mandrake, page 81.

Dose, 1-40 to 1 gr.

PIL. PODOPHYLLIN AND BELLADONNA COMP.

Formula—Each pill contains: Podophyllin, $\frac{1}{4}$ gr.; Ext. Belladonna, $\frac{1}{8}$ gr.; Capsicum, $\frac{1}{2}$ gr.; Milk sugar, 1 gr.

Action and uses—Stimulating laxative and cathartic.

Dose, 1 to 3 pills.

PIL. PODOPHYLLIN AND BLUE MASS.

Formula—Each pill contains: Podophyllin, $\frac{1}{4}$ gr.; Blue mass, 2 grs.

Action and uses—Cathartic with special tendency to the liver.

Dose, 1 to 2 pills.

PIL. PODOPHYLLIN, COLOCYNTH, HYOSCYAMUS AND CALOMEL.

Formula—Each pill contains: Podophyllin, Ext. Colocynth comp., of each, $\frac{1}{4}$ gr; Ext. Hyoscyamus, Calomel, of each, 1 gr.

Action and uses—Cathartic with special action on the liver.

Dose, 1 to 2 pills.

PIL. PODOPHYLLIN COMP.

Formula—Each pill contains: Podophyllin, $\frac{1}{2}$ gr.; Ext. Hyoscyamus, $\frac{1}{4}$ gr.; Ext. Nux vomica, 1-16 gr.

Action and uses—An active cathartic deprived of its tendency to gripe by its combination with Ext. Hyoscyamus.

Dose, 1 to 2 pills.

PIL. PODOPHYLLIN COMP., ECLECTIC.

Formula—Each pill contains: Podophyllin, $\frac{1}{4}$ gr.; Juglandin, Leptandrin, of each, 1-16 gr.; Macrotin, Oil Capsicum, of each, 1-32 gr.

Action and uses—Laxative and cathartic.

Dose, 1 to 4 pills.

PIL. PODOPHYLLIN COMP., JANEWAY.

Formula—Each pill contains: Podophyllin, ½ gr.; Purified aloes, 1 gr.; Ext. Belladonna, Ext. Nux vomica, of each, ¼ gr.

Action and uses—An excellent combination in obstinate constipation.

Dose, 1 pill.

PIL. PODOPHYLLIN AND HYDRASTIA, SCUDDER.

Formula—Each pill contains: Podophyllin, 1-20 gr.; Hydrastia sulph., ¼ gr.

Action and uses—Valuable in habitual constipation.

Dose, 1 to 2 pills.

PIL. PODOPHYLLIN AND LEPTANDRIN.

Formula—Each pill contains: Podophyllin, ½ gr.; Leptandrin, 1 gr.

Action and uses—Cholagogue cathartic.

Dose, 1 to 2 pills.

PIL. POST PARTUM, FOYDYCE BARKER.

Formula—Each pill contains: Ext. Colocynth comp., Calomel, of each, 1½ grs.; Ext. Nux vomica, Purified aloes, Ipecac, of each, 1-6 gr.; Ext. Hyoscyamus, ½ gr.

Dose, 1 pill.

PIL. POTASSIUM IODIDE, 2 grs., 5 grs.

Action and uses—Alterative.

Dose, 2 to 10 grs.

PIL. POTASSIUM PERMANGANATE, 1-2 gr., 1 gr., 2 grs., 3 grs.

Action and uses—Emmenagogue and antizymotic. Valuable in amenorrhœa, dysmenorrhœa, peritonitis after labor, involution or atrophy of uterus, diptheria, zymotic diseases generally and in morphine poisoning.

Dose, 1-2 to 3 grs.

PIL. QUININE BISULPHATE, 1-2 gr., 1 gr., 2 grs., 3 grs., 4 grs., 5 grs.

Action and uses—Tonic and antiperiodic. Preferred by some to the sulphate on account of its greater solubility.

Dose, 1-2 to 10 grs.

PIL. QUININE SULPHATE, 1-2 gr., 1 gr., 2 grs., 3 grs., 4 grs., 5 grs.

Action and uses—Tonic and antiperiodic.

Dose, 1-2 to 10 grs.

PIL. QUININE VALERIANATE, 1-2 gr., 1 gr.

Action and uses—Tonic, nervine. Used in debility attended with nervous disorders and in hemicrania.

Dose 1-2 to 2 grs. three times per day.

PIL. QUININE AND ARSENIC.

Formula—Each pill contains: Quinine sulphate, 1 gr.; Arsenous acid, 1-30 gr.

Action and uses—Tonic, alterative.

Dose, 1 to 2 pills.

PIL. QUININE AND BLUE MASS.

Formula—Each pill contains: Quinine sulphate, 2 grs.; Blue mass, 1 gr.

Action and uses—Tonic, alterative.

Dose, 1 to 2 pills.

PIL. QUININE AND CAPSICUM, NO. 1.

Formula—Each pill contains: Quinine sulphate, 1 gr.; Capsicum, ¼ gr.
Action and uses—Tonic, antiperiodic and stimulant.
Dose, 1 to 4 pills.

PIL. QUININE AND CAPSICUM, NO. 2.

Formula—Each pill contains: Quinine sulphate, 2 grs.; Capsicum, ¼ gr.
Action and uses—Tonic, antiperiodic and stimulant.
Dose, 1 to 3 pills.

PIL. QUININE COMP., NO. 1

Formula—Each pill contains: Quinine sulphate, Iron by hydrogen, of each, 1 gr.; Arsenous acid, 1-32 gr.
Action and uses—Tonic, alterative and febrifuge.
Dose, 1 to 2 pills three times per day.

PIL. QUININE COMP., NO. 2.

Formula—Each pill contains: Quinine sulphate, Iron by hydrogen, of each, 1 gr.; Arsenous acid, 1-60 gr.
Action and uses—Tonic, alterative and febrifuge.
Dose, 1 to 2 pills.

PIL. QUININE COMP. WITH STRYCHNINE, Iron Clad Pills.

Formula—Each pill contains: Quinine sulphate, Iron by hydrogen, of each, 1 gr.; Arsenous acid, Strychnine, of each, 1-20 gr.
Action and uses—Tonic, antiperiodic and alterative. Valuable in chronic ague and persistent malarial attacks.
Dose, 1 pill three times per day.

PIL. QUININE, IRON AND NUX VOMICA.

Formula—Each pill contains: Quinine sulphate, 1 gr.; Iron carbonate, Vallet, 2 grs.; Ext. Nux vomica, ¼ gr.
Action and uses—Tonic and antiperiodic. A valuable general tonic, by some practitioners Ext. Nux vomica is considered preferable to strychnine in various dyspeptic conditions, and to improve the appetite.
Dose, 1 to 2 pills.

PIL. QUININE, IRON, STRYCHNINE AND ARSENIC, NO. 1.

Formula—Each pill contains: Quinine sulphate, 1 gr.; Iron by hydrogen, 1½ grs.; Strychnine, Arsenous acid, of each, 1-20 gr.
Action and uses—See Pil. Quinine comp. with Strychnine.
Dose, 1 to 2 pills.

PIL. QUININE, IRON, STRYCHNINE AND ARSENIC, NO. 2.

Formula—Each pill contains: Quinine sulphate, 1 gr.; Iron by hydrogen, 1½ grs.; Strychnine, 1-30 gr.; Arsenous acid, 1-30 gr.
Action and uses—See Pil. Quinine comp. with Strychnine.
Dose, 1 to 2 pills.

PIL. QUININE, IRON BY HYDROGEN AND STRYCHNINE.

Formula—Each pill contains: Quinine sulphate, Iron by hydrogen, of each, 1 gr.; Strychnine sulphate, 1-60 gr.
Action and uses—See Pil. Quinine, Iron and Nux vomica.
Dose, 1 to 2 pills.

PIL. QUININE, IRON AND STRYCHNINE VALERIANATES.

Formula—Each pill contains: Quinine valerianate, Iron valerianate, of each, 1 gr.; Strychnine valerianate, 1-60 gr.
Action and uses—Tonic and nervine. Useful in nervous debility and hysterical disorders.
Dose, 1 to 2 pills.

PIL. QUININE IRON AND ZINC VALERIANATES.

Formula—Each pill contains: Quinine valerianate, Iron valerianate, Zinc valerianate, of each, 1 gr.

Action and uses—Tonic and nervine. Useful in nervous debility and hysteria.

Dose, 1 to 2 pills.

PIL. QUININE, IRON AND ZINC VALERIANATES AND CANNABIS INDICA.

Formula—Each pill contains: Quinine valerianate, Iron valerianate, Zinc valerianate, of each, 1 gr.; Ext. Cannabis indica, ¼ gr.

Action and uses—Tonic and nervine.

Dose, 1 to 2 pills.

PIL. QUININE NUX VOMICA AND ARSENIC.

Formula—Each pill contains: Quinine sulphate, 1 gr.; Ext. Nux vomica, ¼ gr.; Arsenous acid, 1-60 gr.

Action and uses—Tonic and alterative.

Dose, 1 to 2 pills.

PIL. QUININE AND STRYCHNINE, NO. 1.

Formula—Each pill contains: Quinine sulphate, 1 gr.; Strychnine, 1-60 gr.

Action and uses—Tonic, nerve stimulant.

Dose, 1 to 2 pills.

PIL. RHEUMATIC.

Formula—Each pill contains: Ext. Colocynth comp., 1½ grs.; Ext. Colchicum, acetic, 1 gr.; Ext. Hyoscyamus, Calomel, of each, ½ gr.

Action and uses—Antirheumatic and purgative.

Dose, 1 to 3 pills.

PIL. RHEUMATIC, WITHOUT MERCURY.

Formula—Each pill contains: Ext. Colocynth, 1½ grs.; Ext. Colchicum, acetic, ½ gr.; Podophyllin, Capsicum, of each, ¼ gr.; Ext. Belladonna, Ext. Nux vomica, of each, 1-10 gr.

Action and uses—Antirheumatic and purgative.

Dose, 1 to 3 pills.

PIL. RHUBARB, U. S.

Formula—Each pill contains: Rhubarb, 3 grs.; Soap, 1 gr.

Action and uses—Rhubarb is tonic, cathartic, stomachic and astringent. Valuable in dyspepsia attended with constipation; in diarrhea, when purging is indicated; in secondary stages of cholera infantum; in chronic dysentery and in almost all typhus diseases when fecal matter has accumulated in the intestines. See Fl. Ext. Rhubarb, page 99.

Dose, 1 to 3 pills.

PIL. RHUBARB COMP., U. S.

Formula—Each pill contains: Rhubarb, 2 grs.; Purified aloes, 1½ grs.; Myrrh, 1 gr.; Oil Peppermint, 1-10 gr.

Action and uses—Tonic and laxative. Useful in costiveness with debility of the stomach.

Dose, 1 to 2 pills.

PIL. SALICIN, 2 1-2 grs., 5 grs.

Action and uses—Tonic, antiperiodic and reputed antiseptic. It has been found efficacious in acute rheumatism, and by some authorities considered not less certain than quinine for intermittent fevers.

Dose, 2 1-2 to 15 grs.

PIL. SALICYLIC ACID, 2 1-2 grs., 3 grs., 5 grs.

Action and uses—A most efficient remedy in acute rheumatism, rapidly reducing temperature, relieving pain, in fact cutting short the disease. In an ordinary case of acute articular rheumatism we count upon relieving the patient in two or three days, the pain going first and then the fever. It is well to continue the drug ten to fifteen days after the apparent cure, to prevent relapse.

Dose, 2 1-2 to 15 grs.

PIL. SALINE CHALYBEATE TONIC, FLINT.

Formula—Each pill contains: Sodium chloride, 3 grs.; Potassium chloride, 1-20 gr.; Potassium sulphate, 1-10 gr.; Potassium carbonate, 1-20 gr.; Sodium carbonate, 3-5 gr.; Magnesium carbonate, 1-20 gr.; Calcium phosphate, precip., 1⁄2 gr.; Calcium carbonate, 1-20 gr.; Iron, reduced, 9-20 gr.; Iron carbonate, 1-20 gr.

Dose, 1 to 2 pills.

PIL. SALOL, 2 1-2 grs., 5 grs.

Action and uses—Febrifuge and antirheumatic.

Dose, 2 1-2 to 20 grs.

PIL. SANDALWOOD COMP.

Formula—Each pill contains: Oil Sandalwood, Ext. Cubeb, Balsam Copaiba, of each, 1 gr.

Action and uses—Valuable in obstinate cases of gonorrhea and gleet.

Dose, 1 to 3 pills.

PIL. SEAWRACK EXT., 3 grs.; See Pil. Bladderwrack Ext.

PIL. SILVER NITRATE, 1-8 gr., 1-4 gr.

Action and uses—In that form of dyspepsia characterized by the vomiting of large quantities of yeasty fluid it has yielded better results than any other remedy, and the same may be said of chronic gastritis or gastric ulcer. Nitrate of silver should be administered in pill form 1⁄8 to 1⁄3 grain three or four times a day when the stomach is empty. In chronic enteritis or colitis, nitrate of silver is sometimes of great service, especially if there be ulceration.

Dose, 1-8 to 1-2 grs.

PIL. SODIUM SALICYLATE, 5 grs.

Action and uses—Useful in affections dependent upon the rheumatic diathesis, in the various forms of neuralgia, especially migraine, trifacial neuralgia and sciatica, chorea, tonsilitis and urticaria.

Dose, 5 to 20 grs.

PIL. STROPHANTHUS, 1-20 gr., 1-4 gr.

Action and uses—A cardiac stimulant. Especially useful in progressive heart failure of elderly patients with attacks of dyspnea, simulating angina. Cardiac dropsy is relieved by it.

Dose, 1-20 to 1-4 grs.

PIL. STROPHANTHUS COMP.

Formula—Each pill contains: Tr. Strophanthus, 2 m.; Tr. Digitalis, 3 m.

Action and uses—See Pil. Strophanthus.

Dose, 1 to 2 pills.

PIL. STROPHANTHUS AND IRON.

Formula—Each pill contains: Strophanthus, 1⁄4 gr.; Iron sulphate, Potassium carbonate, of each, 1 1⁄2 grs.

Action and uses—See Pil. Strophanthus.

Dose, 1 to 2 pills.

PIL. STRYCHNINE, 1-200 gr., 1-100 **gr.**, **1-60 gr.**, 1-50 gr., 1-40 gr., 1-32 gr., 1-30 gr., 1-20 gr., 1-**16 gr.**

Action and uses—Nerve tonic, acting well in simple debility, nervous exhaustion and incontinence of urine. It is a valuable remedy in paraplegia, hemiplegia, diphtheritic paralysis and wrist drop. Strychnine is an excellent tonic, improving the appetite in a marked degree. In chorea it has been highly praised. One-half grain by the mouth has killed an adult. See Fl. Ext. Nux vomica, U. S., page 87.

Dose, 1-200 to 1-16 gr.

PIL. STRYCHNINE ARSENATE, 1-200 **gr.**

Action and uses—Nerve tonic and alterative.

Dose, 1-200 to 1-20 gr.

PIL. STRYCHNINE NITRATE, **Pil. Dipsomania**, 1-60 **gr.**, 1-50 **gr.**, 1-40 gr., 1-30 **gr.**

Action and uses—See Pil. Strychnine. Especially valuable in the treatment of alcoholism. Send for pamphlet.

Dose, 1-60 to 1-20 gr.

PIL. STRYCHNINE SULPHATE, 1-200 **gr.**, 1-100 gr., 1-60 **gr.**, 1-50 gr., 1-40 gr., 1-32 gr., 1-30 gr., 1-20 gr., 1-16 gr.

Action and uses—See Pil. Strychnine.

Dose, 1-200 to 1-16 gr.

PIL. STRYCHNINE COMP.

Formula—Each pill contains: Strychnine, Phosphorus, of each, 1-100 gr.; Ext. Cannabis indica, 1-16 gr.; Ginseng, Iron carbonate, of each, 1 gr.

Action and uses—Nerve tonic and stimulant. A good general tonic increasing the appetite and aiding digestion.

Dose, 1 to 2 pills.

PIL. SUMBUL COMP.

Formula—Each pill contains: Ext. Sumbul, Iron sulph. exsic., of each, 1 gr.; Asafetida, 2 gr.; Arsenous acid, 1-10 gr.

Action and uses—See Fl. Ext. Musk root, page 86.

Dose, 1 to 3 pills.

PIL. SUMBUL COMP., BOSWELL.

Formula—Each pill contains: Ext. Sumbul, 1 gr.; Aloes, purified, 1-6 gr.; Arsenous acid, Strychnine sulphate, of each, 1-50 gr.; Asafetida, 2 grs.; Iron sulph. exsic., 1 gr.

Action and uses—Nerve stimulant, tonic, antispasmodic and alterative.

Dose, 1 to 2 pills.

PIL. SYPHILITIC.

Formula—Each pill contains: Potassium iodide, 2½ grs.; Corrosive sublimate, 1-40 gr.

Action and uses—Alterative.

Dose, 1 to 2 pills.

PIL. SYPHILITIC, RICORD, MODIFIED.

Formula—Each pill contains: Mercury protiodide, Lactucarium, of each, ½ gr.; Ext. Opium, 1-10 gr.; Ext. Conium seed, 1½ grs.

Action and uses—Alterative.

Dose, 1 to 2 pills.

PIL. TERPIN HYDRATE, 2 grs., 5 grs.
Action and uses—Used in treatment of bronchial affections, coughs, colds and catarrhs.
Dose, 2 to 10 grs.

PIL. THREE VALERIANATES AND GOLD.
Formula—Each pill contains: Quinine valerianate, Iron valerianate, of each, ½ gr.; Zinc valerianate, 1 gr.; Gold and Sodium chloride, 1-20 gr.
Action and uses—Tonic and stimulant to the nerves.
Dose, 1 to 2 pills.

PIL. TONIC, AIKEN.
Formula—Each pill contains: Quinine sulphate, 1 gr.; Iron by hydrogen, ⅔ gr.; Arsenous acid, Strychnine, of each, 1-50 gr.
Action and uses—Tonic and antiperiodic.
Dose, 1 pill three times a day in chronic ague.

PIL. TONIC, HEMATIC, WITH CINCHONIDINE.
Formula—Each pill contains: Cinchonidine sulphate, 1 gr.; Iron by hydrogen, 1½ grs.; Ipecac, ⅛ gr.; Arsenous acid, Strychnine sulphate, of each, 1-40 gr.
Action and uses—Tonic and antiperiodic.
Dose, 1 to 2 pills.

PIL. TONIC, MADDIN.
Formula—Each pill contains: Zinc valerianate, Quinine valerianate; Iron, carbonate, Vallet, of each, 1 gr., Ext. Nux vomica, ½ gr.; Ext Aloes, ¼ gr.
Action and uses—Nerve tonic.
Dose, 1 to 2 pills.

PIL. TONIC, WALKER.
Formula—Each pill contains: Quinine sulphate, Iron carbonate, Vallet, of each, 2 grs.; Arsenous acid, 1-40 gr.; Strychnine, 1-60 gr.
Action and uses—Especially valuable in chronic ague.
Dose, 1 to 2 pills.

PIL. TRIPLE VALERIANATES; See Pil. Quinine, Iron and Zinc Valerianates.

PIL. TRIPLEX.
Formula—Each pill contains: Purified aloes, 2 grs.; Blue mass, 1 gr. Podophyllin, ¼ gr.
Action and uses—Cathartic with special action on the liver.
Dose, 1 to 3 pills.

PIL. TRIPLEX, FRANCIS.
Formula—Each pill contains: Purified aloes, Scammony, Blue mass, of each, 1 1-5 grs.; Myrrh, ¼ gr.; Oil Caraway, 1-5 gr.; Oil Croton, 1-20 gr.
Action and uses—As an aperient or laxative, one pill may be given every night upon retiring.
Dose, 1 to 2 pills.

PIL. VALERIAN EXT., 3 grs.
Action and uses—See Fl. Ext. Valerian, U. S., page 126.
Dose, 3 to 12 grs.

PIL. WARBURG'S TINCTURE, 1-2 dram, 1 dram.

Action and uses—A palatable and effective method of administering this invaluable remedy.

The original formula for Warburg's Tincture is as follows:

Socotrine Aloes	1 lb.	Gentian root	1 oz.
East India Rhubarb	4 ozs.	Zedoary root	1 oz.
Angelica seed	4 ozs.	Cubeb	1 oz.
Confection of Damocrates	4 ozs.	Electuary of Myrrh	1 oz.
Elecampane root	2 ozs.	Camphor	1 oz.
Spanish Saffron	2 ozs.	Purging Agaric	1 oz.
Fennel seed	2 ozs.	Sulphate of Quinine	10 ozs.
Prepared Chalk	2 ozs.	Diluted Alcohol	500 ozs.

DR. McLEAN states: "I have treated remittent fevers of every degree of severity, contracted in the jungles of the Deccan and Mypore and at the base of mountainous ranges in India, on the Coromandel coast, in the pestilential highlands of the northern division of the Madras Presidency, on the malarial rivers of China, and in men brought to Nettley Hospital from the swamps of the Gold Coast, and I affirm that I have never seen quinine, when given alone, act in the manner characteristic of this tincture; and, although I yield to no one my high opinion of the estimable value of quinine, I have never seen a single dose of it, given alone to the extent of 9½ grains, suffice to arrest an exacerbation of remittent fever, much less prevent its recurrence, while nothing is more common than to see the same quantity of the alkaloid in Warburg's Tincture bring about such results."—*Medical Times and Gazette.*

We confidently recommend to physicians the Pil. Warburg's Tincture, Lilly, as containing all the medicinal virtues of the tincture, in a form not obnoxious to patients.

We also prepare Pil. Warburg's Tincture, **without Aloes**, for the use of physicians desiring such a combination.

Dose, 1 to 3 pills.

PIL. WARBURG'S TINCTURE, WITHOUT ALOES, 1-2 dram, 1 dram.

Action and uses—See Pil. Warburg's Tincture.

Dose, 1 to 3 pills.

PIL. ZINC PHOSPHIDE, 1-10 gr., 1-8 gr., 1-6 gr., 1-4 gr., 1-2 gr.

Action and uses—Zinc phosphide has been largely used in the same class of cases as phosphorus, and by some physicians considered preferable. It has been used with good effect in treatment of brain diseases, and with excellent results in severe cases of neuralgia, palsy, etc.

Dose, 1-10 to 1 gr.

PIL. ZINC PHOSPHIDE COMP.

Formula—Each pill contains: Zinc phosphide, Ext. Nux vomica, Ext. Cannabis indica, of each, ⅛ gr.

Action and uses—Nerve tonic, stimulant and aphrodisiac.

Dose, 1 to 3 pills.

PIL. ZINC PHOSPHIDE AND NUX VOMICA.

Formula—Each pill contains: Zinc phosphide, 1-10 gr.; Ext. Nux vomica, ¼ gr.

Action and uses—See Pil. Zinc phosphide.

Dose, 1 to 3 pills.

PIL. ZINC SULPHOCARBOLATE, 1-4 gr., 1-2 gr., 1 gr., 2 1-2 grs., 5 grs.

Action and uses—Useful as an intestinal antiseptic in typhoid fever, infantile diarrhea and cholera infantum.

Dose, 1-4 to 5 grs.

PIL. ZINC VALERIANATE, 1-2 gr., 1 gr., 2 grs.

Action and uses—Antispasmodic. Valuable in neuralgic affections and in nervous diseases attended with palpitation of the heart, constriction of the throat and pain in the head. Useful in epilepsy and in the nervous affections which accompany chlorosis.

Dose, 1-2 to 4 grs.

ELI LILLY & COMPANY'S.

ENTERIC PILLS.

The coating of these pills allow their passage through the stomach before solution, that operation being performed in the duodenum or intestines. They are very vaulable in cases of gastric irritation or where the action of the prescribed remedy is likely to be affected by the action of the gastric secretion.

PIL. ENT. ANTISEPTIC, INTESTINAL.
Formula—Each pill contains: Mercury protiodide, ¼ gr.; Ext. Hyoscyamus, Aloin, Podophyllin, Ext. Nux vomica, of each, 1-16 gr. See Pil. Antiseptic, Intestinal, page 77.

PIL. ENT. CALCIUM SULPHIDE, 1-4 gr.; See Pil. Calcium sulphide, page 141.

PIL. ENT. CALOMEL, 1-2 gr., 1 gr., 2 grs.; See Pil. Calomel, page 141.

PIL. ENT. CATHARTIC IMPROVED.
Formula—Each pill contains: Ext. Colocynth comp., 1 gr.; Ext Jalap, Ext. Gentian, of each, ½ gr.; Leptandrin, Podophyllin, Ext. Hyoscyamus, of each, ¼ gr., Oil Peppermint, q. s.
Action and uses—See Pil. Cathartic improved, page 143.

PIL. ENT. CORROSIVE SUBLIMATE, 1-100 gr., 1-50 gr.; See Pil. Corrosive sublimate, page 146.

PIL. ENT. CREASOTE, BEECHWOOD, 1-2 gr., 1 gr.; See Pil. Creasote, Beechwood, page 147.

PIL. ENT. MERCURY BINIODIDE, 1-4 gr.; See Pil. Mercury biniodide, page 155.

PIL. ENT. MERCURY PROTIODIDE, 1-4 gr.; See Pil. Mercury protiodide, page 155.

PIL. ENT. PODOPHYLLIN, 1-4 gr.; 1-2 gr.; See Pil. Podophyllin, page 161.

PRIVATE FORMULAS.

We make a specialty of the MANUFACTURE of PILLS from private formulas.

So small a number as one thousand can be made in Gelatin coating or three thousand in Sugar coating. We are prepared to execute, however, the largest orders with great promptness. Contracts taken for regular supplies.

BOOKLETS

Containing valuable information in reference to any of the following subjects will be sent by mail, postage paid, on request.

STRYCHNINE NITRATE in the treatment of Alcoholism.

PALMETTO CORDIAL; LILLY, in presenility, prostatic troubles, irritation of the bladder and urethral inflammation.

"YOUR SPECIAL FORMULA," What do you have made?

PIL. PALMETOL; LILLY, in prostatitis.

ESSENCE OF PEPSIN; LILLY.

HORSE NETTLE in the treatment of epilepsy, illustrated.

QUICKLY SOLUBLE HYPODERMIC TABLETS.

FORMASEPTOL; LILLY. The new and incomparable liquid antiseptic.

PRUNICODEINE, safe and reliable in acute and chronic bronchial affections.

FLUID EXTRACT OF ERGOT AND ERGOTIN.

PIL. A. S. B. AND I.; LILLY. Tonic laxative in chronic constipation.

GLYCONES; LILLY, "Painless peristaltic persuaders."

YERBAZIN; LILLY, A perfect mask for quinine.

PIL. APHRODISIACA; LILLY, A food and tonic to the nervous system.

SUCCUS ALTERANS; LILLY, in syphilis.

Address

ELI LILLY & COMPANY,
    MANUFACTURING CHEMISTS,
       INDIANAPOLIS, IND.

ELI LILLY & COMPANY'S

MEDICINAL ELIXIRS,

Syrups, Wines and Cordials.

Our products in these important lines, representing the most advanced methods of elegant pharmacy as applied to liquid medicines, are unexcelled.

No valuable quality is in any case sacrificed for the sake of producing a satisfactory flavor, but in every instance the flavors are so selected and combined as to effect the best result in concealing any nauseous taste in the medicament.

Also, these preparations will be found particularly free from any tendency to precipitation or other change.

ELI LILLY & COMPANY'S

MEDICINAL ELIXIRS.

ELIX. ADJUVANS, N. F.*
Action and uses—Exclusively used as an adjuvant, especially for acrid or saline remedies.

ELIX. ALETRIS COMP.
Formula—Each fluid ounce represents: Unicorn root, Squaw vine, of each, 30 grs.; Cramp bark, 15 grs.; Blue cohosh, 7½ grs.
Action and uses—Uterine tonic and antispasmodic. Useful in all cases where the functions of the internal reproductive organs are deranged, as in amenorrhœa, dysmenorrhœa, menorrhagia, leucorrhœa, and to overcome the tendency to habitual abortion. Especially valuable to pregnant women of delicate or nervous habit. One or two doses daily for several weeks before parturition imparts tone to the uterus, facilitates labor and removes the cramps to which some are liable during the latter weeks of uterogestation.
Dose 1 to 2 fluid ounces, as the occasion requires.

ELIX. AMMONIUM BROMIDE.
Formula—Each fluid dram contains: Ammonium bromide, 5 grs.
Action and uses—Considered by some practitioners preferable to potassium bromide. Peculiarly applicable to functional nervous diseases. Useful in epilepsy and in the milder forms of ovaritis, and in strumous opthalmia. Said to promote the absorption of fat.

* National Formulary.

ELIX. AMMONIUM VALERIANATE.
Formula—Each fluid dram contains: Ammonium valerianate, 2 grs.

Action and uses—Nerve tonic. A very efficacious remedy in nervous headache, insomnia, hysteria and kindred complaints.

Dose 1 to 4 fluid drams, as required.

ELIX. AMMONIUM VALERIANATE AND MORPHINE.
Formula—Each fluid dram contains: Ammonium valerianate, 2 grs.; Morphine valerianate, 1-16 gr.

Action and uses—Nerve tonic and sedative. Valuable in nervous headache, insomnia, hysteria, high nervous excitement, delirium tremens, etc.

Dose 1 to 2 fluid drams.

ELIX. AROMATIC, U. S.
Action and uses—Used entirely as a vehicle replacing the former official Elixir Orange.

ELIX. BARK AND IRON, Iron protoxide and Peruvian bark.
Formula—Each fluid ounce represents: Calisaya bark, 8 grs.; Iron protoxide, 2 grs.

Action and uses—This preparation combines a protosalt of iron, with the medicinal elements of true calisaya bark, without the inky flavor common to many such compounds. It is valuable in debilitated conditions of the system, in dyspepsia and nervous prostration, loss of appetite, in anemia, and wherever a gentle tonic is needed.

Dose 1 to 4 fluid drams.

ELIX. BERBERINE AND IRON.
Formula—Each fluid dram contains: Berberine phosphate, ¼ gr.; Iron pyrophosphate, 1 gr.

Action and uses—Antiperiodic, stomachic and tonic. Useful in malarial affections, amenorrhea, enlargement of spleen, anorexia, chronic intestinal catarrh, etc.

Dose 1 to 2 fluid drams.

ELIX. BISMUTH.
Formula—Each fluid dram contains: Bismuth and Ammonium citrate, 2 grs.

Action and uses—Stomachic and astringent. Useful in pyrosis, irritable stomach, gastrodynia and in dysentry and diarrhea.

Dose 1 fluid dram,

ELIX. BISMUTH AND PANCREATIN.
Formula—Each fluid dram contains: Bismuth and Ammonium citrate, Pancreatin, of each, 1 grain.

Action and uses—Stomachic, astringent and aid to duodenal digestion. Valuable in dyspepsia, irritable stomach, dysentry and diarrhea.

Dose 1 to 2 fluid drams.

ELIX. BISMUTH AND STRYCHNINE.
Formula—Each fluid dram contains: Bismuth and Ammonium citrate, 2 grs.; strychnine, 1-60 gr.

Action and uses—Valuable in dyspepsia and in debilitated conditions of the stomach. The strychnine, by its tonic influence, improves the digestion, and in its combination with bismuth is beneficial in flatulent dyspepsia.

Dose 1 fluid dram.

ELIX. BISMUTH QUININE AND STRYCHNINE.
Formula—Each fluid dram contains: Bismuth and Ammonium citrate, 2 grs.; Quinine sulphate, ¼ gr.; Strychnine, 1-60 gr.

Action and uses—Stomachic, astringent and tonic.

Dose 1 fluid dram.

ELIX. BROMOCHLORAL COMP.

Formula—Each fluid ounce represents: Potassium bromide, Chloral hydrate, of each, 120 grs.; Ext. Hyoscyamus, Ext. Cannabis Indica, of each, 1 gr.

Action and uses—Anti-epileptic, hypnotic, sedative, antispasmodic. Induces sleep. Used in epilepsy, neurasthenia, mania, delirium tremens, tetanus, etc. Contra-indicated in inflamed stomach. Large doses must not be given in heart disease; children and the aged with caution.

Dose 1-2 to 2 fluid drams. In delirium tremens, acute mania and tetanus the dose may with caution be largely increased.

ELIX. BUCHU.

Formula—Each fluid dram represents: Buchu, 15 grs.

Action and uses—Of especial value in chronic affection of the genito-urinary mucous membrane, acting topically. A very useful remedy in cystitis and urethritis, also in lithiasis, chronic bronchitis and affections of the prostate gland.

Dose 1 to 4 fluid drams.

ELIX. BUCHU COMP.

Formula—Each fluid ounce represents: Buchu, Pareira Brava, of each, 16 grs.; Juniper berries, 20 grs.; Cubebs, 6½ grs.

Action and uses—An elegant and efficient preparation. Valuable in chronic bladder affections, and the various mucous discharges from the genito-urinary organs, depending upon a relaxed condition of the affected parts. Largely used in subacute and chronic gonorrhea, chronic cystitis, and irritation of the bladder. It also stimulates the kidneys.

Dose 1 to 4 fluid drams.

ELIX. BUCHU AND JUNIPER COMP.

Formula—Each fluid dram represents: Buchu, 3 grs.; Barberry bark, Juniper berries, of each, 1½ grs.; Sodium salicylate, 1¼ grs.

Action and uses—An active diuretic and antirheumatic.

Dose 1 to 4 fluid drams.

ELIX. BUCHU, JUNIPER AND POTASSIUM ACETATE.

Formula—Each fluid ounce represents: Buchu, 45 grs.; Juniper berries, 12 grs.; Potassium acetate, 16 grs.

Action and uses—Valuable in the treatment of diseases of the bladder, affections of the genito-urinary mucous membrane, inflammation of the kidneys, etc.

Dose 1 to 4 fluid drams.

ELIX. BUCHU AND PAREIRA BRAVA.

Formula—Each fluid dram represents: Buchu, Pareira Brava, of each, 15 grs.

Action and uses—A very useful remedy in chronic diseases of the urinary passages, kidneys and bladder.

Dose 1 to 4 fluid drams.

ELIX. BUCHU AND POTASSIUM ACETATE.

Formula—Each fluid dram represents: Buchu, 7 grs.; Potassium acetate, 5 grs.

Action and uses—Diuretic and aperient. Valuable in the treatment of diseases of the bladder, affections of the genito-urinary mucous membrane, inflammation of the kidneys, etc.

Dose 1 to 4 fluid drams.

ELIX. CAFFEINE BROMIDE, Caffeine hydrobromate.

Formula—Each fluid dram contains: Caffeine bromide, ½ gr.

Action and uses—Principally used as a diuretic and cardiac stimulant in renal and cardiac dropsy; also in nervous headache, neuralgia, etc.

Dose 1 to 4 fluid drams.

ELIX. CAFFEINE AND POTASSIUM BROMIDE; See Elix. Potassium bromide and Caffeine.

ELIX. CALCIUM LACTOPHOSPHATE.

Formula—Each fluid dram contains: Calcium lactophosphate, 2 grs.

Action and uses—Stimulant and nutrient. Used with benefit in all diseases of malnutrition and where the repair or development of the bones is required.

Dose 1 to 4 fluid drams.

ELIX. CALISAYA BARK.

Formula—Each fluid dram represents: Calisaya bark, 5 grs.

Action and uses—Tonic, febrifuge and antiperiodic. Represents the combined alkaloidal strength of the highest grade of calisaya bark. An excellent stomachic cordial, especially valuable in convalescence from malarial disease.

Dose 1 to 4 fluid drams.

ELIX. CALISAYA BARK AND BISMUTH.

Formula—Each fluid dram represents: Calisaya bark, 5 grs.; Bismuth and Ammonium citrate, 2 grs.

Action and uses—Used as a tonic, stomachic and astringent in dyspepsia, irritable stomach, etc.

Dose 1 fluid dram.

ELIX. CALISAYA BARK, BISMUTH AND STRYCHNINE.

Formula—Each fluid dram represents: Calisaya bark, 5 grs.; Bismuth and Ammonium citrate, 2 grs.; strychnine, 1-60 gr.

Action and uses—A pronounced tonic, to which is added the stomachic and astringent qualities of the bismuth. An excellent remedy in some forms of dyspepsia where there is general lack of tone in the system.

Dose 1 fluid dram.

ELIX. CALISAYA BARK; Detannated.

Formula—Each fluid dram represents: Calisaya bark, 5 grs.

Action and uses—Tonic, febrifuge and antiperiodic. This elegant preparation is used principally for making solutions of iron salts, which it is often desirable to combine with cinchona, as in such cases it does not form an inky precipitate.

Dose 1 to 4 fluid drams.

ELIX. CALISAYA BARK AND IRON.

Formula—Each fluid dram represents: Calisaya bark, 5 grs.; Iron pyrophosphate, 2 grs.

Action and uses—One of our most valuable nutritive tonics. Indicated in debilitated conditions of the system, in recovering from febrile diseases, in anemia, chlorosis, amenorrhea, and whenever a chalybeate tonic is desired. It is free from any nauseous or inky taste.

Dose 1 to 4 fluid drams.

ELIX. CALISAYA BARK, IRON AND BISMUTH.

Formula—Each fluid dram represents: Calisaya bark, 5 grs.; Iron pyrophosphate, 2 grs.; Bismuth and Ammonium citrate, 1 gr.

Action and uses—An efficient tonic, nutritive and stomachic in cases of debility associated with gastritis or enfeebled digestion.

Dose 1 to 2 fluid drams.

ELIX. CALISAYA BARK, IRON, BISMUTH, PEPSIN AND STRYCHNINE.

Formula—Each fluid dram represents: Calisaya bark, Pepsin, saccharated, U. S., of each, 5 grs.; Iron pyrophosphate, 2 grs.; Bismuth and Ammonium citrate, 1 gr.; Strychnine, 1-60 gr.

Action and uses—Stimulant, tonic, digestive and astringent. Where there is great debility with loss of digestive power and irritability of the stomach it is a very valuable combination.

Dose 1 fluid dram.

ELIX. CALISAYA BARK, IRON, BISMUTH AND STRYCHNINE.

Formula—Each fluid dram represents: Calisaya bark, 5 grs.; Iron pyrophosphate, 2 grs.; Bismuth and Ammonium citrate, 1 gr.; Strychnine, 1-60 gr.

Action and uses—A valuable tonic; increasing the appetite, giving tone to the stomach, and relieving nervous prostration.

Dose 1 fluid dram.

ELIX. CALISAYA BARK, IRON AND PEPSIN.

Formula—Each fluid dram represents: Calisaya bark, Pepsin, saccharated, U. S., of each, 5 grs.; Iron pyrophosphate, 2 grs.

Action and uses—Nutritive tonic and digestive.

Dose 1 to 4 fluid drams.

ELIX. CALISAYA BARK, IRON AND PHOSPHORUS.

Formula—Each fluid dram represents: Calisaya bark, 5 grs.; Iron pyrophosphate, 1 gr.; Phosphorus, 1-50 gr.

Action and uses—Nutritive tonic, especially valuable in nervous disorders.

Dose 1 to 2 fluid drams.

ELIX. CALISAYA BARK, IRON, PHOSPHORUS AND STRYCHNINE.

Formula—Each fluid dram represents: Calisaya bark, 5 grs.; Iron pyrophosphate, 1 gr.; Phosphorus, 1-50 gr.; Strychnine, 1-60 gr.

Action and uses—Nutritive tonic and stimulant. Useful in nervous disorders associated with general debility.

Dose 1 to 2 fluid drams.

ELIX. CALISAYA BARK, IRON AND QUININE.

Formula—Each fluid dram represents: Calisaya bark, 5 grs.; Iron pyrophosphate, 2 grs.; Quinine sulphate, 1 gr.

Action and uses—A valuable remedy in cases where calisaya bark and iron is indicated but a more decided tonic effect is required.

Dose 1 to 2 fluid drams.

ELIX. CALISAYA BARK, IRON, QUININE AND STRYCHNINE.

Formula—Each fluid dram represents: Calisaya bark, 5 grs.; Iron pyrophosphate, 2 grs.; Quinine sulphate, ½ gr.; Strychnine, 1-60 gr.

Action and uses—A decided nutritive tonic and stimulant.

Dose 1 fluid dram.

ELIX. CALISAYA BARK, IRON AND STRYCHNINE.

Formula—Each fluid dram represents: Calisaya bark, 5 grs.; Iron pyrophosphate, 2 grs.; Strychnine, 1-60 gr.

Action and uses—An excellent tonic in nervous and general debility, giving tone to the digestive apparatus.

Dose 1 fluid dram.

ELIX. CALISAYA BARK, IRON, STRYCHNINE AND PEPSIN.

Formula—Each fluid dram represents: Calisaya bark, Pepsin, saccharated, U. S., of each, 5 grs.; Iron pyrophosphate, 2 grs.; Strychnine, 1-60 gr.

Action and uses—An excellent digestive tonic and stimulant, valuable in nervous and general debility from impaired digestion.

Dose 1 fluid dram.

ELIX. CALISAYA BARK AND PEPSIN.

Formula—Each fluid dram represents: Calisaya bark, Pepsin, saccharated, U. S., of each, 5 grs.

Action and uses—An excellent digestive tonic of wide application in cases where there is simple lack of tone caused by indigestion.

Dose 1 to 4 fluid drams, after each meal.

WHEN ORDERING OR PRESCRIBING.

ELIX. CALISAYA BARK, PEPSIN AND BISMUTH.

Formula—Each fluid dram represents: Calisaya bark, Pepsin, saccharated, U. S., of each, 5 grs.; Bismuth and Ammonium citrate, 1 gr.

Action and uses—Indicated in dyspepsia, and when there are evidences of gastric irritability.

Dose 1 to 4 fluid drams.

ELIX. CALISAYA BARK, PEPSIN, BISMUTH AND STRYCHNINE.

Formula—Each fluid dram represents: Calisaya bark, Pepsin, saccharated, U. S., of each, 5 grs.; Bismuth and Ammonium citrate, 1 gr.; Strychnine, 1-60 gr.

Action and uses—Nutritive tonic, astringent and stimulant. Useful where there is want of tone of the digestive organs accompanied with general debility.

Dose 1 fluid dram.

ELIX. CALISAYA BARK, PEPSIN AND STRYCHNINE.

Formula—Each fluid dram represents: Calisaya bark, Pepsin, saccharated, U. S., of each, 5 grs.; Strychnine, 1-60 gr.

Action and uses—Digestive, tonic and stimulant. Valuable in dyspepsia with debility.

Dose 1 fluid dram.

ELIX. CALISAYA BARK, QUININE AND STRYCHNINE.

Formula—Each fluid dram represents: Calisaya bark, 5 grs.; Quinine sulphate, ½ gr.; strychnine, 1-60 gr.

Action and uses—Tonic, antiperiodic and stimulant.

Dose 1 fluid dram.

ELIX. CALISAYA BARK AND STRYCHNINE.

Formula—Each fluid dram represents: Calisaya bark, 5 grs.; Strychnine, 1-60 gr.

Action and uses—Tonic, antiperiodic and stimulant.

Dose 1 fluid dram.

ELIX. CASCARA SAGRADA AROMATIC.

Formula—Each fluid dram represents: Cascara sagrada, 15 grs.

Action and uses—Tonic, febrifuge and cathartic. Recommended in the treatment of habitual constipation, especially in those cases in which atony of the stomach and bowels is a feature.

Dose 1 to 4 fluid drams.

ELIX. CASCARA SAGRADA COMP.

Formula—Each fluid dram represents: Cascara sagrada, Senna, Rhubarb, of each, 5 grs.

Action and uses—Cathartic and laxative.

Dose 1 to 4 fluid drams.

ELIX. CELERY COMP.

Formula—Each fluid dram represents: Celery seed, Coca leaves, Black haw bark, of each, 3 grs.

Action and uses—Anodyne, antispasmodic and nervine. Recommended in nervous disorders.

Dose 2 to 4 fluid drams.

ELIX. CELERY AND GUARANA.

Formula—Each fluid dram represents: Celery seed, 5 grs.; Guarana, 10 grs.

Action and uses—Stimulant, stomachic and nervine. Valuable in nervous prostration, sick headache and the cephalalgia sometimes following menstruation and that following dissipation.

Dose 1 to 4 fluid drams.

ELIX. CELERY, KOLA AND COCA COMP.

Formula—Each fluid ounce represents: Celery seed, Kola nuts, Coca leaves, Black haw bark, of each, 40 grs.

Action and uses—Valuable in nervous prostration, as a stimulant in extreme fatigue and for neutralizing the intoxicating effects of alcohol.

Dose 1 to 4 fluid drams.

ELIX. CHLORAL HYDRATE.

Formula—Each fluid dram contains: Chloral hydrate, 5 grs.

Action and uses—Hypnotic, antispasmodic, analgesic. Produces sleep. Used in puerperal eclampsia, mania, delirium tremens, convulsions, chorea, tetanus, hysteria, epilepsy, local spasms, asthma, strangulated hernia, incontinence of urine, spasmodic croup, spasm of glottis, etc. Contra-indicated in inflamed stomach. Large doses must not be given in heart disease, caution must be used with children and the aged.

Antidote—See "Poisons and Antidotes," Index.

Dose 1 to 6 fluid drams.

ELIX. COCA.

Formula—Each fluid dram represents: Coca leaves, 15 grs.

Action and uses—Anodyne and antispasmodic. A powerful nerve stimulant. Increases the muscular power to sustain fatigue.

Dose 1 to 4 fluid drams.

ELIX. CODEINE SULPHATE.

Formula—Each fluid dram contains: Codeine sulphate, ¼ gr.

Action and uses—Very valuable in place of morphine when pain is not severe, as a habit is not established. Used in bronchitis, irritating cough, ovarian pains, pains from tumors, insomnia, when not due to violent pains, to abate desire in morphine habit, diabetes mellitus, diseases of the respiratory organs, etc. Less poisonous than morphine.

Antidotes—See "Poisons and Antidotes," Index.

Dose 1 to 4 fluid drams.

ELIX. CORYDALIS COMP.

Formula—Each fluid dram represents: Turkey corn, 4 grs.; Stillingia, Prickly ash bark, Twin leaf, of each, 2 grs.; Blue flag, Sheep laurel, Potassium iodide, of each, 1 gr.

Action and uses—A valuable alterative elixir, used in blood diseases generally, liver affections and rheumatism.

Dose 1 fluid dram, three or four times a day.

ELIX. CRAMP BARK COMP.; See Elixir Viburnum comp.

ELIX. DANDELION COMP.

Formula—Prepared from Dandelion, Wild cherry and Gentian, with aromatics, after the formula published by the American Pharmaceutical Association.

Action and uses—Intended chiefly as a vehicle or corrigent to cover the bitter taste of quinine and similar substances. For this purpose however, it is quite inferior to XERMAZIN, Lilly, see page 327

ELIX. DIURETIC.

Formula—Each fluid dram represents: Buchu, 15 grs.; Uva Ursi, Cleavers, of each, 8 grs.; Juniper berries, 5 grs.

Action and uses—Valuable in suppression of urine and in inflammation of the kidneys and bladder.

Dose 1 to 4 fluid drams.

ELIX. EMMENAGOGUE.

Formula—Each fluid dram represents: Aloes, purified, 1½ grs.; Rue, Saffron, Savin, of each, ¾ gr.

Action and uses—Stimulant, emmenagogue and diaphoretic. Restores the menstrual discharge when suppressed by cold.

Dose 1 to 4 fluid drams in hot water.

WHEN ORDERING OR PRESCRIBING.

ELIX. EUCALYPTUS.

Formula—Each fluid dram represents: Eucalyptus, 10 grs.

Action and uses—Considered valuable in malarial fevers, and has been used as a substitute for quinine, although authorities differ as to its antiperiodic properties. It has been successfully employed in bronchial affections with fetid expectoration, in ozena and in fetid or profuse mucous discharge.

Dose 1 to 2 fluid drams.

ELIX. EUCALYPTUS COMP.

Formula—Each fluid dram represents: Eucalyptus, 10 grs.; Prickly ash berries, Grindelia, of each, 5 grs.; Golden seal, 2½ grs.

Action and uses—A valuable stimulant tonic, an efficient remedy in intermittent fever and other malarial affections; also to remove splenic enlargement so frequently following these disorders.

Dose 1 to 2 fluid drams.

ELIX. GENTIAN.

Formula—Each fluid dram represents: Gentian, 4 grs.

Action and uses—A very agreeable pure bitter tonic. Useful in dyspepsia and in debility with loss of appetite.

Dose 1 to 4 fluid drams.

ELIX. GENTIAN COMP.

Formula—Each fluid dram represents the same amount of Infusion Gentian comp., U. S., 1870.

Action and uses—Aromatic tonic and stomachic.

Dose 1 to 4 fluid drams.

ELIX. GENTIAN FERRATED.

Action and uses—An elegant ferruginous tonic.

Dose 1 to 2 fluid drams.

ELIX. GENTIAN AND IRON CHLORIDE.

Formula—Each fluid dram represents: Gentian, 4 grs.; Tinct. Iron chloride, 5 m.

Action and uses—Ferruginous tonic. So combined as to be free from astringency and inky flavor. It may be given to delicate women and children without disagreeing with the most sensitive stomach.

Dose 1 to 2 fluid drams.

ELIX. GENTIAN AND IRON CHLORIDE WITH LACTATED PEPSIN.

Formula—Each fluid dram represents: Gentian, 2 grs.; Tinct. Iron chloride, 2 m., Lactated pepsin, 2½ grs.

Action and uses—An excellent digestive and tonic in dyspepsia.

Dose 1 to 2 fluid drams.

ELIX. GENTIAN, IRON CHLORIDE AND PEPSIN.

Formula—Each fluid dram represents: Gentian, 4 grs.; Tinct. Iron chloride, 5 m., Pepsin, saccharated, 2 grs.

Action and uses—Valuable in indigestion.

Dose 1 to 2 fluid drams.

ELIX. GENTIAN, IRON AND STRYCHNINE.

Formula—Each fluid dram represents: Gentian, 4 grs.; Iron pyrophosphate, 2 grs.; Strychnine, 1-60 gr.

Action and uses—Nutritive tonic and stimulant. Valuable where strychnine is indicated.

Dose 1 fluid dram.

ELIX. GRINDELIA.

Formula—Each fluid dram represents: Grindelia robusta, 15 grs.

Action and uses—Highly recommended in asthma and chronic bronchitis.

Dose 1 to 2 fluid drams.

ELIX. GUARANA.

Formula—Each fluid dram represents: Guarana, 15 grs.

Action and uses—Serviceable in cases where the brain becomes depressed by over mental exertion or where there is a sensation of exhaustion or fatigue. It is especially valuable in nervous headache, and cephalalgia sometimes accompanying menstruation and that following a course of dissipation.

Dose 1 to 2 fluid drams.

ELIX. GUARANA AND CELERY; See Elix. Celery and Guarana.

ELIX. HELONIAS.

Formula—Each fluid dram represents: Helonias root, 10 grs.

Action and uses—Tonic and diuretic. Beneficial in nocturnal emissions and as a uterine tonic, removing abnormal conditions and imparting vigor.

Dose 1 to 4 fluid drams.

ELIX. HELONIAS COMP.

Formula—Each fluid ounce represents: Partridgeberry, 110 grs. Helonias root, High Cranberry, Blue cohosh, of each, 28 grs.

Action and uses—Valuable uterine tonic and antispasmodic. It may be used in all cases where the functions of the internal reproductive organs are deranged, as in amenorrhea, dysmenorrhea, menorrhagia, leucorrhea, and to overcome tendency to habitual abortion. Pregnant women of a delicate or nervous temperament will find it beneficial to take one or two doses daily for several weeks previous to prostration, as it facilitates labor and removes cramps to which they are sometimes liable. It appears to exert a specific influence on the uterus

Dose 1 to 2 fluid ounces three times a day.

ELIX. HYPNOTIC.

Formula—Each fluid ounce represents: Chloral hydrate, 60 grs.; Potassium bromide, 60 grs.; Ext. Cannabis Indica, Ext. Hyoscyamus, of each, 1 gr.

Action and uses—Antiepileptic, hypnotic, sedative, antispasmodic. Used in epilepsy, neurasthenia, mania, delirium tremens, tetanus, etc. Contra-indicated where there is inflammation of the stomach. Large doses must not be given in heart disease; children and the aged with caution.

Dose 1 to 4 fluid drams. In delirium tremens, acute mania and tetanus the dose may, with caution, be largely increased.

ELIX. IRON PYROPHOSPHATE AND QUININE.

Formula—Each fluid dram contains: Iron pyrophosphate, 2 grs.; Quinine sulphate, 1 gr.

Action and uses—A reliable tonic elixir, especially where nutrition is poor.

Dose 1 to 2 fluid drams.

ELIX. IRON PYROPHOSPHATE, QUININE AND STRYCHNINE.

Formula—Each fluid dram contains: Iron pyrophosphate, 2 grs.; Quinine sulphate, 1 gr.; Strychnine, 1-60 gr.

Action and uses—Nutritive tonic, antiperiodic and stimulant. Preferred by some to Elixir Iron, Quinine and Strychnine phosphates in the treatment of chronic ague, in convalescence from malarial fevers and whenever a general tonic is needed.

Dose 1 fluid dram three times a day, just before or after meals.

ELIX. IRON PYROPHOSPHATE AND STRYCHNINE.
Formula—Each fluid dram contains: Iron pyrophosphate, 2 grs.; Strychnine, 1-60 gr.
Action and uses—Nutritive tonic and stimulant.
Dose 1 fluid dram.

ELIX. IRON, QUININE AND STRYCHNINE CITRATE.
Formula—Each fluid dram contains: Iron, Quinine and Strychnine citrate, 4 grs.
Action and uses—An efficient antiperiodic in chronic ague, also valuable in convalescence from malarial attacks and as a general tonic.
Dose 1 fluid dram three times a day, before or after meals.

ELIX. IRON, QUININE AND STRYCHNINE PHOSPHATES.
Formula—Each fluid dram contains: Iron phosphate, 2 grs.; Quinine phosphate, 1 gr.; Strychnine phosphate, 1-60 gr.
Action and uses—This prescription has been long and favorably known to the profession and successfully used in the treatment of chronic ague, in convalescence from malarial fevers, and whenever a general tonic is needed.
Dose for adult, 1 fluid dram three times a day, just before or after meals.

ELIX. IRON, QUININE AND STRYCHNINE PHOSPHATES WITH LACTATED PEPSIN.
Formula—Each fluid dram represents: Iron phosphate, 2 grs.; Quinine phosphate, ½ gr.; Strychnine, 1-60 gr.; Lactated pepsin, 2½ grs.
Action and uses—An excellent remedy in all cases where a tonic is needed in combination with a digestive.
Dose 1 fluid dram three times daily, before or after meals.

ELIX. IRON AND STRYCHNINE PHOSPHATES.
Formula—Each fluid dram contains: Iron phosphate, 2 grs.; Strychnine phosphate, 1-60 gr.
Action and uses—Nutritive tonic and stimulant.
Dose 1 fluid dram.

ELIX. JABORANDI.
Formula—Each fluid dram represents: Jaborandi, 10 grs.
Action and uses—Valuable for the removal of serous effusions, as in hydrothorax, anasarca, ascites, chronic pleurisy, etc.
Dose 1 to 4 fluid drams.

ELIX. KOLA COMP.
Formula—Each fluid dram represents: Kola, Celery seed, Coca leaves, of each, 5 grs.
Action and uses—Valuable in nervous prostration, as a stimulant in extreme fatigue and for neutralizing the intoxicating effects of alcohol.
Dose 1 to 4 fluid drams.

ELIX. LACTATED PEPSIN.
Formula—Each fluid dram represents: Lactated Pepsin, 5 grs., containing Pepsin 1:3000, Pancreatin, of each, ½ gr., with Lactic acid, Hydrochloric acid, Maltose and Diastase.
Action and uses—Lactated pepsin, combining as it does the several digestive ferments, has a wider range of application than simple pepsin. It is therefore preferable in cases where there is not only lack of digestion of the albuminoids, but where starchy and fatty foods are not assimilated.
Dose 1 to 2 fluid drams.

ELIX. LACTATED PEPSIN AND BISMUTH.

Formula—Each fluid dram represents: Lactated Pepsin, 5 grs.; Bismuth and Ammonium citrate, 1 gr.

Action and uses—Useful in many cases of dyspepsia, gastralgia, etc.

Dose 1 to 2 fluid drams.

ELIX. LACTATED PEPSIN, BISMUTH AND STRYCHNINE.

Formula—Each fluid dram represents: Lactated pepsin, 5 grs.; Bismuth and Ammonium citrate, 1 gr.; Strychnine, 1-128 gr.

Action and uses—A very valuable remedy in the treatment of gastralgia, dyspepsia and disorders dependent on lack of tone of the digestive apparatus.

Dose 1 to 2 fluid drams.

ELIX. LAXATIVE COMP.

Formula—Each fluid dram represents: Cascara sagrada, 8 grs.; Senna, 5 grs.; Butternut bark, 4 grs.; Licorice, Cardamom, of each, 1 gr.

Action and uses—Laxative and cathartic.

Dose 1 to 4 fluid drams.

ELIX. LICORICE AROMATIC; QUININE ELIXIR.

Action and uses—A vehicle for Quinine and other bitter or nauseous medicines.   Mix the quinine with the elixir at the time it is to be taken.   It is inferior for this purpose to YERBAZIN, Lilly, see page 327

ELIX. MANACA WITH SALICYLATES.

Formula—Each fluid ounce represents: Manaca, 80 grs.; Sodium salicylate, 64 grs.; Lithium salicylate, 32 grs.; Potassium salicylate, 8 grs.

Action and uses—Valuable in acute and subacute rheumatism, lithiasis, arthritis, etc.

Dose 1 to 2 fluid drams.

ELIX. MORPHINE VALERIANATE.

Formula—Each fluid dram contains: Morphine valerianate, ½ gr.

Action and uses—Used in hysteria, nervousness, delirium tremens, etc.

Dose 1 to 2 fluid drams. In extreme cases 4 fluid drams may be given repeated not more than four times per day.

ELIX. ORANGE.

Action and uses—This preparation is merely a base or vehicle for use in the extemporaneous preparation of compound elixirs and in most cases the medicinal substance may be simply dissolved in the elixir.

ELIX. PANCREATIN.

Formula—Each fluid dram contains: Pancreatin, 1 gr.

Action and uses—An elegant form for the administration of pancreatin.   Used as an aid to duodenal digestion.

Dose 2 to 4 fluid drams.

ELIX. PEPSIN.

Formula—Each fluid dram contains: Pepsin, saccharated, U. S., 5 grs.

Action and uses—An elegant and effective preparation of pepsin, applicable in cases where the albuminoids are badly digested.

Dose 1 to 4 fluid drams after meals.

ELIX. PEPSIN LACTATED; See Elix. Lactated Pepsin.

ELIX. PEPSIN AND BISMUTH.

Formula—Each fluid dram represents: Pepsin, saccharated, U. S., 5 grs.; Bismuth and Ammonium citrate, 1 gr.

Action and uses—Used in many cases of dyspepsia, gastralgia, etc.

Dose 1 to 2 fluid drams.

ELIX. PEPSIN, BISMUTH AND IRON.

Formula—Each fluid dram contains: Pepsin, saccharated, U. S., 5 grs.; Bismuth and Ammonium citrate, 1 gr.; Iron pyrophosphate, 2 grs.

Action and uses—Employed in dyspepsia and to give tone to the digestive apparatus, especially where anemic conditions are a feature.

Dose 1 to 2 fluid drams.

ELIX. PEPSIN, BISMUTH, IRON AND QUININE.

Formula—Each fluid dram contains: Pepsin, saccharated, U. S., 5 grs.; Bismuth and Ammonium citrate, 1 gr.; Iron pyrophosphate, 2 grs., Quinine sulphate, ¼ gr.

Action and uses—Valuable in indigestion when accompanied by stomachic and intestinal irritation and anemia with general debility.

ELIX. PEPSIN, BISMUTH, IRON, QUININE AND STRYCHNINE.

Formula—Each fluid dram contains: Pepsin, saccharated, U. S., 5 grs.; Bismuth and Ammonium citrate, 1 gr.; Iron pyrophosphate, 2 grs.; Quinine sulphate, ¼ gr.; Strychnine, 1-60 gr.

Action and uses—A decided tonic in dyspepsia accompanied by gastralgia and general debility.

Dose 1 fluid dram.

ELIX. PEPSIN, BISMUTH AND STRYCHNINE.

Formula—Each fluid dram contains: Pepsin, saccharated, U. S., 5 grs.; Bismuth and Ammonium citrate, 1 gr.; Strychnine, 1-60 gr.

Action and uses—This valuable and popular preparation has been largely used by the profession in the treatment of gastralgia, dyspepsia, and disorders dependent upon a lack of tone of the digestive apparatus.

Dose 1 to 2 fluid drams.

ELIX. PEPSIN, BISMUTH AND WAFER ASH.

Formula—Each fluid dram represents: Pepsin, saccharated, U. S., 5 grs.; Bismuth and Ammonium citrate, 1 gr.; Wafer ash, 10 grs.

Action and uses—Useful in dyspepsia and debility consequent on gastro-enteric irritation.

Dose 1 to 2 fluid drams.

ELIX. PEPSIN, IRON, QUININE AND STRYCHNINE.

Formula—Each fluid dram represents: Pepsin, saccharated, U. S., 5 grs.; Iron pyrophosphate, 2 grs.; Quinine sulphate, ¼ gr.; Strychnine, 1-60 gr.

Action and uses—Tonic, digestive and stimulant.

Dose 1 fluid dram.

ELIX. PEPSIN, IRON AND STRYCHNINE.

Formula—Each fluid dram contains: Pepsin, saccharated, U. S., 5 grs.; Iron pyrophosphate, 2 grs.; Strychnine, 1-60 gr.

Action and uses—Tonic, digestive and stimulant.

Dose 1 fluid dram.

ELIX. PEPSIN AND PANCREATIN.

Formula—Each fluid dram contains: Pepsin 1:3000, Pancreatin, of each, 1 gr.

Action and uses—An excellent combination in cases where in addition to lack of digestion of starchy food, fatty matter is not assimilated.

Dose 1 to 4 fluid drams.

ELIX. PEPSIN, PANCREATIN AND BISMUTH.

Formula—Each fluid dram contains: Pepsin 1:3000, Pancreatin, Bismuth and Ammonium citrate, of each, 1 gr.

Action and uses—In dyspepsia with gastro-enteritis.

Dose 1 to 4 fluid drams.

ELIX. PEPSIN, PANCREATIN, BISMUTH AND STRYCHNINE.

Formula—Each fluid dram contains: Pepsin 1:3000, Pancreatin, Bismuth and Ammonium citrate, of each, 1 gr.; Strychnine, 1-60 gr.

Action and uses—Valuable in many forms of dyspepsia accompanied with gastro-enteritis and general debility.

Dose 1 fluid dram.

ELIX. PEPSIN POWDER COMP.; See Elix. Lactated Pepsin.

ELIX. PEPSIN AND STRYCHNINE.

Formula—Each fluid dram contains: Pepsin, saccharated, U. S., 5 grs.; Strychnine, 1-60 gr.

Action and uses—Digestive and tonic. Used in dyspepsia with general debility.

Dose 1 fluid dram.

ELIX. PHOSPHORUS.

Formula—Each fluid dram contains: Phosphorus, 1-50 gr.

Action and uses—Stimulant and nutritive to the osseous and nervous tissue. Useful in chronic nervous exhaustion when the nerve centers are implicated, in osteomalacia, rachitis, progressive locomotor ataxia, threatened cerebral softening, paraplegia and functional impotence.

Dose 1 to 2 fluid drams.

ELIX. PHOSPHORUS AND NUX VOMICA.

Formula—Each fluid dram contains: Phosphorus, 1-50 gr.; Ext. Nux vomica, ¼ gr.

Action and uses—Tonic, stimulant and nutritive. Valuable in atonic dyspepsia, mental overwork and depression, and generally in cases where the tonic effect of nux vomica is indicated in connection with phosphorus.

Dose 1 fluid dram.

ELIX. PHOSPHORUS, NUX. VOMICA AND DAMIANA.

Formula—Each fluid dram represents: Phosphorus, 1-100 gr.; Nux vomica, 1 gr.; Damiana, 8 grs.

Action and uses—Nutritive tonic, stimulant and aphrodisiac. Less convenient than Pil. Aphrodisiaca, see page 324

Dose 1 to 2 fluid drams.

ELIX. PHOSPHORUS, NUX VOMICA, DAMIANA AND IRON.

Formula—Each fluid dram represents: Phosphorus, 1-200 gr.; Nux vomica, 1 gr.; Damiana, 8 grs.; Iron pyrophosphate, 1 gr.

Action and uses—Applicable in cases of cerebral or sexual exhaustion, etc., where anemia is a factor.

Dose 1 to 2 fluid drams.

ELIX. POTASSIUM BROMIDE.

Formula—Each fluid dram contains: Potassium bromide, 10 grs.

Action and uses—Used extensively in the treatment of convulsive and spasmodic affections, more especially in epilepsy. It is also of great benefit in convulsive seizures of children, in laryngismus stridulus, night terrors etc. It is of service in incontinence of urine, pertussis, cramp of lower limbs, chorea, delirium tremens, mental depression, nervous headache. It is an excellent hypnotic, and causes refreshing sleep, more especially in cases of worry, mental anxiety, a full dose being given at bed time. It has been used in diabetes, and in those forms of menorrhagia dependent on ovarian irritability.

Dose in epilepsy, 10 to 60 grs. of the salt, gradually increased and **continued** for long periods. As a hypnotic, 20 to 30 grs.; **to a child, 2 to 3** grs.

ELIX. POTASSIUM BROMIDE AND CAFFEINE.

Formula—Each fluid dram contains: Potassium bromide, 10 grs.; Caffeine bromide, ½ gr.

Action and uses—Largely used in nervous headache, neuralgia, mental anxiety and worry, producing quiet sleep.

Dose 1 to 4 fluid drams.

ELIX. POTASSIUM BROMIDE AND CHLORALHYDRATE.

Formula—Each fluid dram contains: Potassium bromide, 10 grs.; Chloral hydrate, 5 grs.

Action and uses—Anti-epileptic, hypnotic, sedative, antispasmodic. Used in epilepsy, neurasthenia, mania, delirium tremens, tetanus, etc.; should not be used where there is gastric inflammation nor in large doses where there is heart disease. To the aged and children with caution.

Dose 1 to 4 fluid drams. In delirium tremens, acute mania and tetanus the dose may be largely but cautiously increased.

ELIX. PURGANS, LILLY.

Constituents—Rhamnus Purshiana, Euonymus atropurpureus, Cassia acutifolia, purif., Iris versicolor, Hyoscyamus niger and aromatics.

"A perfect liquid cathartic."

ELIXIR PURGANS, LILLY, reliably stimulates the dormant liver without undue irritation, and, by its gentle yet positive effect upon the alimentary tract, calls into useful action those rebellious physiological functions which act as the most potent causes in producing a condition of chronic or obstinate constipation. This is ESPECIALLY TRUE IN HABITUAL CONSTIPATION so common in WOMEN and CHILDREN, and it will be found also particularly useful in that large class to whom pills and powders are so repugnant. Its endorsement at Bellvue and many other prominent hospitals east and west, as well as its employment in general practice by the most eminent medical men, confirms the experience of years in its use. Physicians in prescribing should be careful to write "ELIXIR PURGANS, LILLY, that other preparations may not be substituted.

Dose, as a Cathartic, 2 to 4 teaspoonfuls; **as a Laxative,** 1 to 2 teaspoonfuls; **as an Aperient,** ½ to 1 teaspoonful.

ELIX. QUININE AND STRYCHNINE.

Formula—Each fluid dram contains: Quinine sulphate, 1 gr.; Strychnine, 1-60 gr.

Action and uses—Tonic and antiperiodic.

Dose 1 fluid dram.

ELIX. RHEUMATIC; See Elix. Buchu and Juniper comp.

ELIX. RHUBARB, ALKALINE WITH PANCREATIN.

Formula—Rhubarb, Golden seal, Cinnamon, Potassium bicarbonate, Pancreatin.

Action and uses—An agreeable laxative, antacid, tonic and digestive. Valuable in obstinate constipation, acidity of the stomach, dyspepsia and in diarrhea, dysentery, cholera morbus and cholera infantum. All derangements of the stomach are corrected without unpleasant after effects.

Dose 1 to 2 fluid drams.

ELIX. SALICYLIC ACID.

Formula—Each fluid dram contains: Salicylic acid, 2½ grs.

Action and uses—Antipyretic and antiseptic. An efficient remedy in acute rheumatism, rapidly reducing temperature, relieving pain and cutting short the attack. In ordinary cases of acute articular rheumatism we count upon relieving the patient in two or three days, the pain going first then the fever. The use of the drug in such cases should be continued for ten to fifteen days after apparent cure, to prevent relapse.

Dose 1 to 6 fluid drams.

ELIX. SALICYLIC ACID COMP.

Formula—Each fluid dram represents: Salicylic acid, Black cohosh, of each, 5 grs.; Gelsemium, Potassium iodide, of each, 1 gr.; Sodium bicarbonate, q. s.

Action and uses—An excellent combination in acute rheumatism, cutting short the attack usually in from two to three days. The use of the remedy should be continued ten or fifteen days after the abatement of the disease.

Dose 1-2 to 3 fluid drams.

ELIX. SAW PALMETTO COMP.

Formula—Saw palmetto berries, Sandalwood, Damiana, Coca leaves, Nux vomica, Kola nut, Potassium acetate.

Action and uses—Tonic, stimulant and diuretic.

Dose 1 to 2 fluid drams.

ELIX. SIMPLE WHITE, LILLY'S FORMULA.

Also supplied colored red when desired.

Action and uses—An excellent vehicle for administration of nauseous remedies. A combination of aromatics of fine flavor. It is convenient as a solvent for many salts, as the bromides of potassium, sodium and ammonium; chloral hydrate, and many others that will readily occur to the prescriber.

ELIX. SODIUM BROMIDE.

Formula—Each fluid dram contains: Sodium bromide, 10 grs.

Action and uses—It is considered by some more eligible than potassium bromide, as its administration produces no eruption of acne. The dose is the same as potassium bromide. See Elixir Potassium bromide.

Dose 1 to 6 fluid drams.

ELIX. SODIUM SALICYLATE.

Formula—Each fluid dram contains: Sodium salicylate, 5 grs.

Action and uses—Useful in affections dependent upon the rheumatic diathesis, in the various forms of neuralgia, especially migraine, trifacial neuralgia and sciatica, chorea, tonsillitis and urticaria.

Dose 1 to 4 fluid drams.

ELIX. STRONTIUM IODIDE.

Formula—Each fluid dram contains: Strontium iodide, 2 grs., sweetened with saccharine.

Action and uses—Preferred by some practitioners to potassium iodide as an alterative and especially as a uric acid solvent for which purpose saccharine is used in sweetening this elixir instead of cane sugar.

ELIX. SUMBUL COMP.

Formula—Each fluid dram represents: Musk root, 10 grs.; Scullcap, 2 grs.; Valerian, ½ gr.

Action and uses—A valuable combination applicable in a wide range of nervous disorders which are relieved without the distressing effects following the use of narcotics. It is especially useful in hysteria, though very effectual in chorea, convulsions, delirium tremens, etc.

Dose 1-2 to 2 fluid drams.

ELIX. TERPIN HYDRATE.

Formula—Each fluid dram contains: Terpin hydrate, 1 gr.

Action and uses—Used in treatment of bronchial affections, coughs, colds and catarrhs. See PRUNICODEINE, LILLY, page 221.

ELIX. TERPIN HYDRATE AND CODEINE.

Formula—Each fluid dram contains: Terpin hydrate, 1 gr.; Codeine sulphate, ⅛ gr.

Action and uses—Used in the treatment of bronchial affections coughs, colds and catarrh. See PRUNICODEINE, LILLY, page 221.

ELIX. VIBURNUM COMP.

Formula—Each fluid dram represents: Viburnum opulus, Aletris, of each, 5 grs.; Trillium, 10 grs.

Action and uses—Uterine tonic and antispasmodic. Especially valuable in its tonic influence upon the female generative organs, overcoming the tendency to repeated miscarriages. It relieves the cramps of pregnant women and hastens parturition.

Dose 1 to 6 fluid drams.

ELIX. WAFER ASH.

Formula—Each fluid dram represents: Wafer ash, 10 grs.

Action and uses—A pure tonic, acting without irritation. Advantageously used in convalescence from fevers and in debility from gastro-enteritis. It promotes the appetite, gives tone to the stomach and is tolerated when other tonics are rejected.

Dose 1 to 3 fluid drams.

ELIX. WAHOO.

Formula—Each fluid dram represents: Wahoo root bark, 10 grs.

Action and uses—Highly recommended as a hepatic stimulant and in hepatic dyspepsia or biliousness. Its effects are felt most about forty-eight hours after taking.

Dose 2 to 4 fluid drams.

ELIX. ZINC VALERIANATE.

Formula—Each fluid dram contains: Zinc valerianate, 1 gr.

Action and uses—Antispasmodic. Valuable in neuralgic affections and in nervous diseases attended with palpitation of the heart, constriction of the throat and pain in the head. Useful in epilepsy and the nervous affections which accompany chlorosis.

Dose 1-2 to 2 fluid drams.

ELI LILLY & COMPANY'S

MEDICINAL SYRUPS.

SYR. ANODYNE PINE EXPECTORANT; See Syr. White pine comp.

SYR. CALCIUM HYPOPHOSPHITE.

Formula—Each fluid dram contains: Calcium hypophosphite, 2 grs.

Action and uses—Used in phthisis, rachitis, chlorosis, defective nutrition of nervous and bony tissue. Contra-indicated in fever.

Dose 1 to 4 fluid drams.

SYR. CALCIUM IODIDE.

Formula—Each fluid dram contains: Calcium iodide, 1 gr.

Action and uses—Used in syphilis, hepatitis, asthma, struma, etc., instead of potassium iodide and is said to act better than the potassium salt.

Dose 2 to 4 fluid drams.

SYR. CALCIUM LACTOPHOSPHATE.

Formula—Each fluid dram contains: Calcium lactophosphate, 2 grs.

Action and uses—Stimulant and nutrient. Beneficial in all diseases of malnutrition and where the repair or development of the bones is required.

Dose 1 to 4 fluid drams.

SYR. CALCIUM AND SODIUM HYPOPHOSPHITES.

Formula—Each fluid dram contains: Calcium hypophosphite, Sodium hypophosphite, of each, 2 grs.

Action and uses—Used in phthisis, rachitis, chlorosis, defective nutrition of nervous and bony tissue. Contra-indicated in fever.

Dose 1 to 2 fluid drams.

SYR. CALCIUM AND SODIUM LACTOPHOSPHATES.

Formula—Each fluid dram contains: Calcium lactophosphate, 2 grs., Sodium lactophosphate, 1 gr.

Action and uses—Stimulant and nutrient. Beneficial in all diseases of malnutrition and where the repair or development of the bones is required.

Dose 1 to 2 fluid drams.

SYR. CALCIUM, SODIUM AND IRON HYPOPHOSPHITES.

Formula—Each fluid dram contains: Calcium hypophosphite, Sodium hypophosphite, of each, 2 grs.; Iron hypophosphite, ½ gr.

Action and uses—Tonic, stimulant and nutrient. Used in phthisis, rachitis, chlorosis, defective nutrition of nervous and bony tissue, especially where anæmia is present.

Dose 1 to 2 fluid drams.

SYR. CALCIUM, SODIUM AND POTASSIUM HYPOPHOSPHITES; See Syr. hypophosphites comp., Churchill's formula.

SYR. DOVER'S POWDER.

Formula—Each fluid ounce represents: Dover's powder, 40 grs.

Action and uses—Anodyne and soporific. A convenient and pleasant form in which to administer Dover's powder as a liquid.

SYR. HEMATIC HYPOPHOSPHITES; See Syr. Hypophosphites comp., hematic.

SYR. HOREHOUND COMP.

Formula—Each fluid ounce represents: Horehound, Jersey tea, Elecampane, Spikenard, Comfrey, Wild cherry, of each, 15 grs.; Blood root, 7½ grs.

Action and uses—Often employed in obstinate cough and in pulmonary and bronchial affections generally.

SYR. HYDRIODIC ACID, U. S., 1 per cent.

NOTE—We also prepare a Syrup Hydriodic acid, 2%, which is sometimes demanded. The following statements refer only to the official 1% preparation.

Action and uses—LILLY'S SYRUP HYDRIODIC ACID is a handsome, permanently colorless syrup of grateful acid taste. Dose, 15 minims to half a fluid ounce, diluted with water. Fifteen minims frequently repeated gives prompt relief in bronchial and asthmatic difficulties. In psoriasis, enlargements of the thyroid gland and other glandular enlargements the dose should be from one to two teaspoonfuls three times daily with meals. It is a valuable means of introducing iodine to the system, is readily absorbed and assimilated and its use may be continued for a longer time without objection by the patient than other iodides. It does not produce irritation of the stomach, as frequently occurs when using iodide potassium. It is incompatible with some metallic salts, though combinations may be made with vegetable tinctures and fluid extracts, bichloride of mercury and Fowler's solution. One teaspoonful of the syrup is equal in therapeutic strength to about five grains iodide potassium. Specify LILLY'S SYRUP HYDRIODIC ACID in ordering or prescribing.

SYR. HYPOPHOSPHITES, U. S.

Action and uses—Same as Syr. Hypophosphites comp., calcium, sodium, potassium and iron, except that the iron salt is omitted.

SYR. HYPOPHOSPHITES COMP., CALCIUM, SODIUM, POTASSIUM AND IRON.

Formula—Each fluid dram contains: Calcium hypophosphite, Sodium hypophosphite, of each, 2 grs.; Potassium hypophosphite, 1 gr.; Iron hypophosphite ½ gr.

Action and uses—Used with benefit in all diseases of malnutrition and when the repair or development of the bones is required. Particularly useful in protracted suppuration, osteomalacia, rachitis, caries, scrofulosis, chronic phthisis and in the anemia and bone softening of lactation. Much employed in nervous and general debility and in chronic lung diseases.

SYR. HYPOPHOSPHITES COMP., CHURCHILL'S FORMULA.

Formula—Each fluid dram contains: Calcium hypophosphite, Sodium hypophosphite, of each, 2 grs.; Potassium hypophosphite, 1 gr.

Action and uses—Same as Syr. Hypophosphites comp., Calcium, sodium, potassium and iron, except that the iron salt is omitted.

SYR. HYPOPHOSPHITES COMP., HEMATIC.

Formula—Each fluid ounce contains: Potassium hypophosphite, **Iron** hypophosphite, of each, 1½ grs.; Calcium hypophosphite, Manganese hypophosphite, of each, 1 gr.; Quinine hypophosphite, 7-16 gr.; Strychnine hypophosphite, 1-16 gr.

Action and uses—This is an excellent tonic and alterative to the nerve and brain tissue, and may be used in phthisis, scrofula, cachexy, excessive debility from over mental exertion, sexual excesses; in convalescence from exhausting diseases; in remittent fever attacking enfeebled subjects. It has been used successfully in chronic bronchitis, asthma, dyspepsia, neuralgia, paralysis agitans, night sweats, etc.

Dose 1 to 2 fluid drams in water three times a day at meals.

SYR. HYPOPHOSPHITES COMP. AND MANGANESE.

Formula—Each fluid dram contains: Calcium hypophosphite, Sodium hypophosphite, of each, 2 grs.; Potassium hypophosphite, 1 gr.; Iron hypophosphite, Manganese hypophosphite, of each, ½ gr.

Action and uses—Similar to Syr. Hypophosphites comp., calcium, sodium, potassium and iron, the iron salt being replaced by manganese.

SYR. HYPOPHOSPHITES COMP. WITH MANGANESE AND QUININE.

Formula—Each fluid dram contains: Calcium hypophosphite, Sodium hypophosphite, of each, 2 grs.; Potassium hypophosphite, 1 gr.; Iron hypophosphite, Manganese hypophosphite, of each, ½ gr.; Quinine hypophosphite, ¼ gr.

Action and uses—Same as Syr. Hypophosphites comp. and Manganese, the tonic quality being increased by the addition of quinine.

SYR. HYPOPHOSPHITES COMP., N. F.

Action and uses—Similar to Syr. Hypophosphites comp. with Manganese and Quinine.

SYR. HYPOPHOSPHITES COMP. AND QUININE.

Formula—Each fluid dram contains: Calcium hypophosphite, Sodium hypophosphite, of each, 2 grs.; Potassium hypophosphite, 1 gr.; Iron hypophosphite, ½ gr.; Quinine hypophosphite, ¼ gr.

Action and uses—Similar to Syr. Hypophosphites comp., calcium, sodium, potassium and iron with the addition of quinine.

SYR. HYPOPHOSPHITES COMP. WITH QUININE AND STRYCHNINE.

Formula—Each fluid dram contains: Calcium hypophosphite, 1½ grs.; Potassium hypophosphite, 1 gr.; Manganese hypophosphite, ½ gr.; Iron hypophosphite, Quinine hypophosphite, of each, ¼ gr.; Strychnine hypophosphite, 1-60 gr.

Action and uses—Similar to Syr. Hypophosphites comp., hematic, not however, of such general application as a hematinic.

Dose 1 fluid dram.

SYR. IPECAC, U. S.

Action and uses—Emetic and expectorant.

Dose as an Emetic, 4 to 8 fluid drams; **as an Expectorant,** ½ to 1 fluid dram.

SYR. IRON CHLORIDE.

Formula—Each fluid ounce contains: 40 drops Tincture Iron chloride.

Action and uses—An elegant and palatable form in which to administer Tincture Iron chloride.

Dose 1 to 4 fluid drams.

SYR. IRON IODIDE, U. S.

Action and uses—Alterative and tonic.

Dose 15 to 30 minims diluted with water. The dilution should be made at the moment it is taken and the mouth should be carefully washed after each dose.

SYR. IRON PYROPHOSPHATE.

Formula—Each fluid dram contains: Iron pyrophosphate, 4 grs.

Action and uses—A mild and efficient chalybeate, employed with marked success in anemic diseases.

Dose 1 to 2 fluid drams.

SYR. IRON AND MANGANESE HYPOPHOSPHITES.

Formula—Each fluid dram contains: Iron hypophosphite, 1 gr.; Manganese hypophosphite, ½ gr.

Action and uses—M. Hannon considers that manganese is peculiarly suited to the treatment of anemic cases in which iron has failed or acts but slowly, but he prefers to give the manganese and iron combined. This syrup presents a very eligible form for its administration.

Dose 1 to 2 fluid drams.

SYR. IRON AND MANGANESE IODIDES.

Formula—Each fluid dram contains: Iron iodide, 2 grs.; Manganese iodide, ½ gr.

Action and uses—Alterative and tonic.

Dose 1 to 2 fluid drams diluted with water. The dilution should be made at the moment of taking, after which the mouth should be carefully washed.

SYR. IRON, QUININE AND STRYCHNINE PHOSPHATES.

Formula—Each fluid dram contains: Iron phosphate, 2 grs.; Quinine phosphate, 1 gr.; Strychnine phosphate, 1-60 gr.

Action and uses—A valuable tonic; useful in convalescence from malarial fevers, and enfeebled conditions of the system generally.

Dose 1 to 2 fluid drams.

SYR. LACTUCARIUM, U. S.

Action and uses—Hypnotic and anodyne.

Dose 1-2 to 2 fluid drams.

SYR. MANGANESE IODIDE.

Formula—Each fluid dram contains: Manganese iodide, ½ gr.

Action and uses—Alterative and tonic.

Dose 1 to 4 fluid drams.

SYR. PHOSPHATES COMP.; CHEMICAL FOOD.

Formula—Each fluid dram contains: Calcium phosphate, 2 grs.; Iron phosphate, Sodium phosphate, of each, 1 gr.; Potassium phosphate, ½ gr.

Action and uses—A valuable chalybeate tonic and reconstructive. Used principally in malnutrition.

Dose 1 to 2 fluid drams.

SYR. RHUBARB AROMATIC, U. S.

Action and uses—A warm stomachic laxative well calculated for the bowel complaints of children.

Dose for an infant with diarrhea, 1 fluid dram.

SYR. RHUBARB AND POTASSIUM COMP.; NEUTRALIZING CORDIAL.

Formula—Rhubarb, Goldenseal, Cassia, Oil Peppermint, Potassium bicarbonate.

Action and uses—An agreeable laxative, antacid and tonic. Valuable in obstinate constipation, acidity of the stomach, dyspepsia and in diarrhea, dysentry, cholera morbus and cholera infantum. All derangements of the stomach are corrected without unpleasant after effects.

Dose 1 to 2 fluid drams.

SYR. SARSAPARILLA.

Action and uses—Mildly alterative.   Used principally as a vehicle.
Dose 2 to 4 fluid drams.

SYR. SARSAPARILLA COMP., U. S.

Action and uses—Mildly alterative.   Used principally as a vehicle.
Dose 2 to 4 fluid drams.

SYR. SAW PALMETTO WITH HYPOPHOSPHITES.

Formula—Each fluid dram represents: Saw palmetto, 5 grs.; Calcium
hypophosphite, 2 grs.; Sodium hypophosphite, Potassium hypophosphite, of each, 1 gr.

Action and uses—On account of its tonic and expectorant properties
saw palmetto is of service in phthisis and it is for this reason that it is
here combined with the hypophosphites.

Dose 1 to 2 fluid drams.

SYR SODIUM HYPOPHOSPHITE.

Formula—Each fluid dram contains: Sodium hypophosphite, 2 grs.

Action and uses—Has the general properties of the alkaline hypophosphites.   See Syr. Hypophosphites comp.

Dose 1 to 4 fluid drams.

SYR. SQUAW VINE COMP.; MOTHER'S CORDIAL.

Formula—Each fluid ounce represents: Squaw vine, 45 grs.; Helonias
root, High cranberry bark, Blue cohosh root, of each, 15 grs.

Action and uses—Uterine tonic and antispasmodic.   One or two doses
daily to pregnant women for several weeks previous to parturition imparts energy to the uterine nervous system and relieves the cramps often
experienced during this period.

Dose 1-2 to 1 fluid ounce.

SYR. SQUILL, U. S.

Action and uses—Much employed as an expectorant.
Dose 1-2 to 1 fluid dram.

SYR. SQUILL COMP., U. S.

Action and uses—Emetic, diaphoretic and expectorant.

Dose for children from 10 drops to 1 fluid dram according
to age, and in croup it may be repeated every fifteen or twenty minutes
until it vomits.   Adult dose, as an expectorant, 20 to 50 drops.

SYR. STILLINGIA COMP.

Formula—Stillingia, Elder flowers, Turkey corn, Pipsissewa, Blue flag,
Coriander, Prickly ash berries.

Action and uses—Alterative.

Dose 1 to 4 fluid drams.

SYR. TAR, U. S.

Action and uses—An excellent method of administering tar.   Used
with advantage in chronic catarrh affections.

SYR. TOLU, U. S.

Action and uses—Used chiefly to impart its agreeable flavor to
mixtures.

SYR. TRIFOLIUM, COMP.

Formula—Each fluid ounce represents: Red clover, 32 grs.; Stillingia,
Burdock root, Poke root, Berberis aquifolium, Cascara amarga, of each,
16 grs.; Prickly ash bark, 4 grs.; Potassium iodide, 8 grs.

Action and uses—Alterative.
Dose 2 to 4 fluid drams.

SYR. WHITE PINE COMP.

Formula—Each fluid ounce represents: White pine bark, Cherry bark, of each, 30 grs.; Balm Gilead buds, Spikenard, of each, 4 grs.; Sanguinaria, 3½ grs.; Sassafras, 2 grs.; Morphine acetate, 3-16 gr.; Chloroform, 4 m.

Action and uses—A very popular and reliable remedy in bronchial and pulmonary diseases.

Dose 1 to 2 fluid drams.

SYR. WHITE PINE COMP. WITHOUT MORPHINE.

Formula—Same as Syr. White Pine comp., omitting Morphine acetate.

Dose 1 to 2 fluid drams.

SYR. WILD CHERRY, U. S.

Action and uses—Tonic and sedative. Largely used as a basis for cough mixtures.

Dose 2 to 4 fluid drams.

SYR. YELLOW DOCK COMP.; SCROFULOUS SYRUP.

Formula—Yellow dock, American ivy, False bittersweet, Figwort.

Action and uses—Alterative.

Dose 1 to 4 fluid drams.

SYR. YERBA SANTA AROMATIC; See Yerbazin, page 327

ELI LILLY & COMPANY'S.

MEDICINAL WINES.

WINE AMERICAN WHITE ASH.

Formula—Each fluid ounce represents: American White ash bark, 80 grs.

Action and uses—Tonic and cathartic. Used in constipation and in dropsical affections, also extensively in ague cake or enlarged spleen.

Dose 1 to 4 fluid drams.

WINE BEEF.

Formula—Each fluid ounce represents: Beef, 2 troy ozs.

Action and uses—Combines the nutritive effect of beef with the stimulating qualities of the best sherry wine.

Dose 2 to 4 fluid drams.

WINE BEEF AND IRON.

Formula—Each fluid ounce represents: Beef, 2 troy ozs.; Iron citrate, 4 grs.

Action and uses—Valuable in impaired nutrition, impoverishment of the blood, in convalescence from disease, and where there is enfeebled digestion, and in all cases where a nutritive tonic is indicated.

Dose 2 to 4 fluid drams.

WINE BEEF, IRON AND CINCHONA.

Formula—Each fluid ounce represents: Beef, 2 troy ozs.; Iron citrate, 4 grs.; Calisaya bark, 40 grs.

Action and uses—Similar to Wine Beef and Iron, the cinchona being added for its tonic effect.

Dose 2 to 4 fluid drams.

WINE BEEF, IRON AND PEPSIN.

Formula—Each fluid ounce represents: Beef, 2 troy ozs.; Iron citrate, 4 grs.; Pepsin, saccharated, U. S., 80 grs.

Action and uses—Similar to Wine Beef and Iron the pepsin being added to assist digestion in cases where necessary.

Dose 2 to 4 fluid drams.

WINE CINCHONA.

Action and uses—A mild tonic stimulant for invalids and convalescents.

Dose 2 to 4 fluid drams.

WINE COCA.

Formula—Each fluid ounce represents: Coca leaves, 80 grs.

Action and uses—Anodyne, antispasmodic, and nerve stimulant.

Dose 2 to 4 fluid drams.

WINE COCA AND BEEF.

Formula—Each fluid ounce represents: Coca leaves, 80 grs.; Beef, 2 troy ozs.

Action and uses—Anodyne, antispasmodic, nerve stimulant and nutritive.

Dose 2 to 4 fluid drams.

WINE COCA, BEEF AND IRON.

Formula—Each fluid ounce represents: Coca leaves, 80 grs.; Beef, 2 troy ozs.; Iron citrate, 4 grs.

Action and uses—Nerve stimulant and nutritive tonic.

Dose 2 to 4 fluid drams.

WINE COCA AND CELERY.

Formula—Each fluid ounce represents: Coca leaves, Celery seed, of each, 80 grs.

Action and uses—Anodyne, antispasmodic and nervine.

Dose 1 to 2 fluid drams.

WINE COCA WITH HYPOPHOSPHITES.

Formula—Each fluid ounce represents: Coca leaves, 80 grs., with Calcium, Sodium and Potassium hypophosphites.

Action and uses—This preparation is indicated in acute and chronic bronchitis, phthisis, and all wasting diseases, sleeplessness, loss of memory, lack of energy, nightsweats, dyspepsia, hysteria, mental overwork, etc.

Dose 1 to 4 fluid drams.

WINE COLCHICUM SEED, U. S.

Action and uses—Diaphoretic, diuretic, cathartic, anodyne and sedative. Valuable in rheumatism and gout. In the latter it should be given with an alkali and kept short of emetocatharsis.

Dose 10 to 30 minims.

WINE OF CONDURANGO.

Formula—Each fluid ounce represents: Condurango bark, 60 grs.

Action and uses—Aromatic tonic.

Dose 1 to 4 fluid drams.

WINE IPECAC, U. S.

Action and uses—Expectorant and diaphoretic.

Dose as an expectorant, 5 to 10 minims. Not eligible as an emetic as the contained alcohol counteracts the emetic action of the drug.

WINE IRON.
Formula—Each fluid ounce contains: Iron and Ammonium citrate, 8 grs.

Action and uses—A simple ferruginous tonic, slightly astringent. Used principally in anemic and chlorotic conditions.

Dose 1 to 4 fluid drams.

WINE IRON BITTER, U. S.
Action and uses—A mild ferruginous tonic, valuable in many cases of debility, loss of appetite and general prostration.

Dose 1 to 2 fluid drams.

WINE KOLA.
Formula—Each fluid ounce represents: Kola, 60 grs.

Action and uses—Astringent, stimulant and stomachic. Similar in action to guarana, tea, coffee, etc. See Fl. Ext. Kola nuts, page 72.

Dose 2 to 4 fluid drams.

WINE PEPSIN.
Formula—Each fluid ounce contains: Pepsin saccharated, U. S., 10 grs.

Action and uses—An excellent stomachic and digestive in doses of from 2 to 4 fluid drams after each meal.

WINE TAR.
Action and uses—Used in chronic catarrhal affections and in complaints of the urinary passages.

Dose 1 to 2 fluid drams.

WINE WILD CHERRY AND IRON.
Formula—Each fluid ounce represents: Wild cherry bark, 160 grs.; Iron pyrophosphate, 16 grs.

Action and uses—Tonic and sedative.

Dose 1 to 4 fluid drams.

ELI LILLY & COMPANY'S.

MEDICINAL CORDIALS.

ANTIRHEUMATIC CORDIAL.
Formula—Each fluid dram represents: Cascara sagrada, Sodium salicylate, of each, 2½ grs.

Action and uses—Useful in affections dependent upon the rheumatic diathesis, in various forms of neuralgia, especially migraine, sciatica, etc.

Dose 2 to 6 fluid drams.

BLACKBERRY CORDIAL.
Formula—The juice of the ripe berries with aromatics.

Action and uses—An elegant preparation of this old and favorite domestic remedy. Very useful in diarrhea of women and children, also as a stomachic.

Dose 2 to 8 fluid drams.

BUCKTHORN CORDIAL.
Formula—Each fluid dram represents: Buckthorn bark, 10 grs.

Action and uses—Useful in habitual constipation.

Dose 1 to 4 fluid drams.

WHEN ORDERING OR PRESCRIBING.

CALISAYA CORDIAL.

Formula - Each fluid dram represents: Calisaya bark, 5 grs.
Action and uses —An elegant simple tonic, especially adapted to delicate women and to convalescents.
Dose 1-2 to 1 fluid ounce.

CASCARA CORDIAL.

Formula— Each liter represents: Cascara sagrada, 125 gm.; Berberis aquifolium, 3.7 gm. and aromatics.
Action and uses- Laxative and stomachic.
Dose 2 to 4 fluid drams.

CURACAO CORDIAL, N. F.

Action and uses—A pleasant stimulating cordial, generally used as a vehicle.
Dose 1-2 to 1 fluid ounce.

COCA CORDIAL.

Formula—Each fluid ounce represents: Coca leaves, 60 grs.
Action and uses—See Fl. Ext. Coca, page 45.
Dose 1-2 to 1 fluid ounce.

HELONIAS CORDIAL.

Formula—Each fluid ounce represents: Unicorn root false, Blue cohosh, of each, 15 grs.; Squaw vine, Cramp bark, of each, 60 grs.; aromatics.
Action and uses—Uterine tonic and antispasmodic. Useful in amenorrhea, dysmenorrhea, menorrhagia, leucorrhea and to **overcome** tendency to habitual abortion. It facilitates labor **and removes cramps.**
Dose 2 to 4 fluid drams

KOLA CORDIAL.

Formula- Each fluid ounce represents: Kola, 120 grs.
Action and uses—See Fl. Ext. Kola, page 72.
Dose 2 to 4 fluid drams.

NEUTRALIZING CORDIAL.

Formula—Rhubarb, Golden seal, Cassia, Oil Peppermint and Potassium carbonate.
Action and uses—An agreeable laxative antacid and tonic. Used in obstinate constipation, acidity of the stomach and as a laxative in pregnancy and when piles are present. Valuable in diarrhea, dysentery, cholera morbus, cholera infantum.
Dose for an adult 1-2 to 1 fluid ounce repeated as often as required.

PEPSIN CORDIAL.

One fluid dram **(a teaspoonful) will curd two pints of milk at 100° F. in a** few minutes. **To prepare**
Junket—Take one-half pint of fresh milk heated lukewarm, add one teaspoonful of Pepsin Cordial, and stir just enough to mix. Let it stand till firmly curdled. It may be served plain or with sugar and grated nutmeg.
Whey—Curd warm **milk** with Pepsin Cordial as above directed; when firmly curdled beat up with a fork until the curd is finely divided; now strain and the whey is ready for use. Whey is highly nutritious food. It is always valuable as a means of variety in diet for the sick. It is frequently resorted to as a food for infants to tide over periods of indigestion, summer complaints, **etc.**

PALMETTO CORDIAL, LILLY; CORDIAL PALMETTO COMP.

Formula—Each fluid dram represents: Saw Palmetto, 20 grs.; Sandalwood, 10 grs., Aromatics.
Action and uses—For the treatment of diseases of the genito-urinary system. Specially indicated in presenility, prostatic troubles, irrita-

tion of bladder and urethral inflammation. Combines the virtues of the ripe berries of Serenœa serrulata and true Santalum album. Our investigation, both botanical and chemical, of the Saw Palmetto berry has demonstrated that the reconstructive and other therapeutically valuable principles reside in the fixed and volatile oils and in the resins; hence, our products of this valuable drug are offered with the assurance that the best possible results will be obtained by procuring Lilly's preparations of Saw Palmetto. The United States Dispensatory says, "Saw Palmetto berries are reported sedative, diuretic, tonic and expectorant, and are used in chronic bronchitis; also in sexual impotence." Shoemaker says, "On account of its tonic and expectorant properties, saw Palmetto berries are of service in phthisis pulmonalis. It is also valuable in atrophy of the mammæ, testes or uterus and exerts a beneficial influence upon the enlarged prostate." It has been used with success by many physicians in the treatment of enlargement of the prostate gland, and for dribbling urine when there seems to be want of power in the bladder. In cases of irritation of the bladder it has exerted its efficacy without the slightest inconvenience or impairment of any function. Santalum album is a valuable remedy in treatment of chronic and subacute inflammations of the mucous membrane, especially in bronchitis and gonorrhœa when the period of acute inflammation has passed, also recommended in gleet, cystitis and urethral hemorrhage. Palmetto Cordial, Lilly, is an elegant preparation uniting the therapeutic value of these two important remedies. The combination was suggested to us by a prominent physician for whom we prepared it in a different form. After thoroughly testing it he says "there is no doubt of its success in certain diseases of the genito-urinary system, especially as a remedy for irritable bladder, urethral inflammation and prostatic trouble. In presenility it would undoubtedly have a happy effect."

Dose 1 teaspoonful three times daily.

SEDATIVE CORDIAL.

Formula—Each fluid ounce represents: Black haw, Goldenseal, of each, 60 grs.; Jamaica dogwood, 30 grs.; Aromatics.

Action and uses—Uterine sedative and anodyne. Valuable in diseases of the female organs of generation, especially in nervous disorders of pregnancy, to prevent abortion and in spasmodic dysmenorrhea.

Dose 1 to 4 fluid drams.

ELI LILLY & COMPANY'S

GLYCEROLES.

GLYC. CALENDULA.

Formula—Each fluid ounce represents: Calendula flowers, 120 grs.

Action and uses—Exclusively used as a local application to promote the healing process in wounds, ulcers, burns and other breaches of tissue.

GLYC. HYDRASTIS; Glyceritum Hydrastis, U. S.

Formula—Each fluid ounce represents: Goldenseal, 480 grs.

Action and uses—See Fl. ext. Goldenseal, nonalcoholic, page 61.

GLYC. HYPOPHOSPHITES.

Formula—Each fluid ounce contains: Calcium hypophosphite, 6 grs.; Sodium hypophosphite, 5 grs.; Potassium hypophosphite, 5 grs.

Action and uses—See Syr. Hypophosphite comp., page 187.

Dose 1 to 2 fluid drams.

GLYC. PEPSIN; See Concentrated Solution Pepsin, page 232.

GLYC. TANNIC ACID; Glyceritum Acidi Tannici, U. S.

Action and uses—May be used internally or externally for nearly all purposes to which tannic acid is applied. Being a 20% solution it may be diluted by the addition of glycerin when a weaker preparation is desired.

GLYC. TAR.

Formula—Each fluid ounce represents: Tar, 30 grs.

Action and uses—A valuable remedy in chronic catarrhal affections

ELI LILLY & COMPANY'S

STANDARD TINCTURES.

The strength of these tinctures is based upon the official quantity of drug of a standard alkaloidal strength, when indicated as "standardized." In such cases the drugs are assayed and the quantity used is so calculated as to make the finished tinctures conform to the standards. The standards adopted, when not indicated below, are given upon the labels. The medicinal properties of the tinctures when not given here may be found under the appropriate head in the Fluid Extract list, pages 5 to 130.

TINCT. ACONITE ROOT, U. S., standardized.. ....Dose 1 to 5 m.

TINCT. BELLADONNA LEAVES, U. S., standardized. Dose 5 to 15 m.

TINCT. CANNABIS INDICA, U. S., standardized.... .....Dose 30 m., increased till its effects are experienced.

TINCT. COLCHICUM SEED, U. S., standardized...Dose 10 to 30 m.

TINCT. CINCHONA, U. S., standardized.........Dose 1 to 4 fl. drs.

TINCT. CINCHONA COMP., U. S., standardized.. Dose 1 to 4 fl. drs.

TINCT. CINCHONA COMP.; HUXHAM'S, standardized..............
                                                 Dose 1 to 4 fl. drs.

TINCT. CONIUM FRUIT... ....Dose 5 to 20 m.

TINCT. DIGITALIS, U. S., standardized ....Dose 5 to 10 m.

TINCT. GELSEMIUM, U. S., standardized.........Dose 10 to 20 m·

TINCT. GELSEMIUM, from green drug.........…Dose 10 to 20 m.

TINCT. HENBANE, U. S., standardized.......... .Dose 30 to 60 m.

TINCT. IPECAC AND OPIUM, U. S.; FL. DOVER... Dose 5 to 10 m.
     Standard of strength. One pint represents Ipecac and Opium, of each, 1¼ troy ounces or, each minim is equivalent to 1 grain Dover's powder. The morphine strength is 6 grains in each fluid ounce.

TINCT. LACTUCARIUM, U. S............ ....Dose 1 to 3 fl. drs.

TINCT. NUX VOMICA, U. S. ....   Dose 5 to 20 m.
     Standard of strength—100 c.c. yields 0.3 gm. total alkaloids when assayed by the method of the U. S. Pharmacopoeia, 1890.

TINCT. OPIUM, U. S............... ....Dose 5 to 15 m.
     Standard of strength—Each fluid ounce contains 6 grains of Morphine.

TINCT. OPIUM CAMPHORATED, U. S.......   Infant dose 5 to 10 m.;
                                              Adult dose 1 to 2 fl. drs.
     Standard of strength—Each fluid ounce contains 0.245 grain Morphine.

TINCT. OPIUM COMP.; SQUIBB'S DIARRHEA MIXTURE. ....
                                            Dose 10 to 30 m.
     Formula—Contains Tinct. Opium, Spirit Camphor, Tinct. Capsicum, Chloroform, Alcohol.

TINCT. OPIUM, DEODORIZED, U. S...............Dose 10 to 20 m.
     Standard of strength—Each fluid ounce contains 6 grains morphine.

TINCT. SOLANUM CAROLINENSE; from the berries...............
Dose 1 to 4 fl. drs.

TINCT. STRAMONIUM SEED U-S., standardized...Dose 5 to 20 m.

TINCT. STROPHANTHUS, U. S.......................Dose 4 to 8 m.,
gradually and very carefully increased.

Action and uses—In lethal doses, besides destroying the capacity of
the muscles to assume the normal state of partial flaccidity, strophanthus
causes the rigidity of contraction to become permanent and to pass into
the rigor of death. As a result of this action of the muscle, the heart is
early and powerfully affected. It receives a larger quantity in a given
time than any other muscle of the body, and therefore it is probable
that strophanthin, the active principle, affects the action of the heart
more distinctly and powerfully than that of the other striped muscles.
The various changes in the heart's action, found to result from the administration of strophanthus, are the ordinary changes found and described frequently in the case of digitalis and other members of this
group, and it has been administered in a large number of cases as a substitute for digitalis, with good results.

TINCT. VERATRUM VIRIDE, U.S., standardized...Dose 3 to 8 m.

TINCT. WARBURG'S ....Dose 1 2 to 3 fl. drs.

TINCT. WARBURG'S, MODIFIED...............Dose 1-2 to 3 fl. drs.

TINCT. WARBURG'S, WITHOUT ALOES......Dose 1-2 to 3 fl. drs.

SPECIAL PREPARATIONS.

We are constantly called upon to prepare special
Elixirs, Syrups, Wines, Cordials, Tinctures, Glyceroles,
etc., for those who furnish their own formulas. These
are made in almost any quantity desired and usually on
very short notice.

We especially call attention to our facilities for preparing cough syrups, etc., in lots of one barrel or more,
for druggists who bottle their own specialties.

Quotation will be cheerfully rendered on request.

ELI LILLY & COMPANY,
PHARMACEUTICAL CHEMISTS,
INDIANAPOLIS, IND.

ELI LILLY & COMPANY'S
COMPRESSED TABLETS,
SUGAR COATED
Compressed Tablets,
TABLET TRITURATES,
Hypodermic Tablets,
Veterinary Hypodermic Tablets
AND
Compressed Lozenges.

The departments devoted to the manufacture of these lines are fully equipped with the most modern apparatus for the production of goods of the most accurate and uniform character.

We are therefore prepared to manufacture, at very reasonable prices, compressions, either plain or sugar coated, triturates or hypodermic tablets from private formulas. The largest contracts promptly executed.

COMPRESSED TABLETS.

This department possesses every facility for making perfect goods in large quantities. We are therefore prepared to manufacture, at very reasonable charges, compressions from special formulas and will be pleased at all times to submit quotations on same in lots of not less than five pounds.

TAB. ACETANILID, 1 gr., 2 grs., 3 grs., 4 grs., 5 grs.
Action and uses—See Pil. Acetanilid, page 132.
Dose 2 to 10 grains.

TAB. ACETANILID COMP.; See Tab. Migraine.

TAB. ACETANILID COMP., SPECIAL.
Formula—Each tablet contains: Acetanilid, 3 grs.; Sodium bicarbonate, 1 gr.; Ammonium chloride, Caffeine citrate, of each, ½ gr.
Action and uses—Combines the effects of acetanilid and caffeine giving a wider range of application than either separately. Almost a specific in headache from any cause, especially in the sharp cutting pains of migraine and neuralgia.
Dose 1 to 2 tablets, repeated as required.

TAB. ACETANILID COMP., LILLY.

Formula—Each tablet contains: Acetanilid, 3 grs.; Sodium bicarbonate, ¼ gr.; Caffeine citrate, ½ gr.; Capsicum, 1-10 gr.

Action and uses—Similar to Tab. Acetanilid comp., with the added stimulating effect of capsicum.

Dose 1 to 2 tablets, repeated as required.

TAB. ALUM COMP., For injection.

Formula—Each tablet contains: Alum, 2½ grs.; Zinc sulphate, 2 grs.; Fl. ext. Golden seal, colorless, 1 min.; Morphine sulphate, 1-32 gr.

Action and uses—Used as a vaginal injection in leucorrhea, dissolved in varying proportions of water as required.

TAB. AMMONIUM CHLORIDE, 2 grs.

Action and uses—Efficient in bronchial catarrh when there is no fever and in chronic bronchitis when the secretion is scanty and tough. A tablet should be placed as far back in the mouth as possible and allowed to dissolve slowly, repeating the application every two or three hours in severe cases.

TAB. ANALGESIC.

Formula—Each tablet contains: Acetanilid, 3 grs.; Sodium bicarbonate, 1 gr.; Caffeine citrate, ½ gr.

Action and uses—Similar to Tab. Acetanilid comp., special.

Dose 1 to 2 tablets.

TAB. ANTICONSTIPATION.

Formula—Each tablet contains: Ext. Cascara sagrada, 1 gr.; Ext. Nux vomica, Podophyllin, Ipecac, Ext. Belladonna leaves, of each, ⅛ gr.

Dose 1 to 3 tablets.

TAB. ANTIDYSPEPSIA.

Formula—Each tablet contains: Pepsin, saccharated, U. S., 5 grs.; Bismuth subnitrate, Magnesium calcined, of each, 2 grs.; Ginger, 1 gr.; Ipecac, ½ gr.

Dose 1 to 2 tablets.

TAB. ANTISEPTIC, ALKALINE, SEILER.

Formula—Each tablet contains: Sodium bicarbonate, Sodium biborate, Sodium benzoate, sodium salicylate, Sodium chloride, Eucalyptol, Thymol, Menthol, Oil Wintergreen, in the proportions recommended by Dr. Carl Seiler.

Action and uses—The solution prepared from these tablets has been found exceedingly beneficial in nasal catarrh and as a very agreeable and efficient mouth wash in cases of stomatitis and retraction of the gums, etc., as well as a disinfecting and cleansing wash for all mucous surfaces. It is especially useful in cases of dry catarrh with ozena as it instantly destroys the odor. To prepare the solution dissolve one tablet in two fluid ounces of warm water to be used as a spray or wash. In catarrh, to be snuffed up the nose by the patient morning and night.

TAB. ANTISEPTIC, For external use only.

Formula—Each tablet contains: Corrosive sublimate, 7 3-10 grs.; Ammonium chloride, 7 7-10 grs.

Note—These tablets will be supplied either white or colored green, as desired.

Action and uses—Convenient for preparing antiseptic solutions. To prepare a 1 to 1000 solution, dissolve one tablet in one pint of water. The amount of water may be increased or diminished to secure any strength solution desired.

TAB. ANTISEPTIC, External, colored green.

Formula—See Tablet Antiseptic for external use.

TAB. BISMUTH SUBGALLATE, 2 grs., 5 grs.

Action and uses—Valuable in gastro-intestinal affections, diarrhea, dysentery, etc., and especially in fermentive dyspepsia.

Dose 2 to 10 grains.

TAB. BISMUTH AND CERIUM OXALATE.

Formula—Each tablet contains: Bismuth subnitrate, 5 grs.; Cerium oxalate, 1 gr.

Action and uses—A valuable combination in cases of intestinal irritation with vomiting from any cause.

Dose 1 to 2 tablets two or three times a day. The treatment in severe cases must be persisted in for several days.

TAB. BISMUTH AND SALOL.

Formula—Each tablet contains: Bismuth subnitrate, Salol, of each, 5 grs.

Dose 1 to 2 tablets.

TAB. BORIC ACID, 5 grs.

Action and uses—Antiseptic, disinfectant and deodorant. Used internally in cystitis, tuberculosis and diarrhea.

Dose 5 to 15 grains.

TAB. BRONCHIAL, LILLY.

Formula—Each tablet contains: Ext. Licorice, 1 gr.; Ammonium chloride, Oleoresin Cubeb, of each, ⅓ gr.; Ext. Hyoscyamus, ¼ gr.; Balsam Tolu, Seneka, of each, 1-5 gr.; Ipecac, 1-50 gr.

Action and uses—An excellent remedy for hoarseness, sore throat and irritation of the bronchial tubes. A tablet may be dissolved in the mouth as occasion requires.

TAB. CALOMEL AND SODA, NO. 1.

Formula—Each tablet contains: Calomel, Sodium bicarbonate, of each, 2½ grs.

Dose 1 to 2 tablets.

TAB. CALOMEL AND SODA, NO. 2.

Formula—Each tablet contains: Calomel, Sodium bicarbonate, of each, 2 grs.

Dose 1 to 2 tablets.

TAB. CAMPHOR MONOBROMATED, 2 grs.

Action and uses—See Pil. Camphor monobromated, page 141.

Dose 2 to 10 grains.

TAB. COCAINE, For preparing solutions.

Formula—Each tablet contains: Cocaine, 1½ grs.

Action and uses—A convenient form in which to carry the alkaloid for the extemporaneous preparation of solutions of cocaine. One tablet dissolved in one fluid dram of distilled water makes a 2% solution; two tablets in the same quantity of water makes a 4% solution. These tablets are put up in bottles of one hundred each, with blue label to distinguish them from tablet triturates.

TAB. CHLORODYNE.

Formula—Each tablet contains: Morphine hydrochlorate, 1-6 gr.; Ext. Cannabis Indica, ¼ gr.; Nitroglycerin, 1-300 gr.; Ext. Hyoscyamus, ½ gr.; Oleoresin Capsicum, Oil Peppermint, of each, 1-10 gr.

Action and uses—Anodyne, antispasmodic, sedative and diaphoretic.

Dose 1 tablet repeated every hour or so, if relief is not obtained by the first. No decided increase in the dose should be given even in severe cases except as directed by the physician.

TAB. CINCHONIDINE SULPHATE, 2 grs., 3 grs., 5 grs.
Action and uses See Pil. Cinchonidine sulphate, page 144.
Dose 2 to 15 grains.

TAB. CREOSOTE, BEECHWOOD, 1-4 m., 1-2 m., 1 m.
Action and uses—See Pil. Creosote, beechwood, page 147.
Dose 1-4 to 2 minims.

TAB. CYSTITIS, NO. 1, For Acid urine.
Formula—Each tablet contains: Boric acid, Potassium bicarbonate, of each, 2 grs.; Ext. Buchu, Ext. Couch grass, of each, 1 gr.; Ext. Corn silk, Ext. Hydrangea, of each, ½ gr.; Atropine sulphate, 1-500 gr.
Dose 1 to 2 tablets.

TAB. CYSTITIS, NO. 2, For Alkaline urine.
Formula—Each tablet contains: Benzoic acid, 3 grs.; Sodium biborate, 2 grs.; Ext. Buchu, Ext. Couch grass, of each, 1 gr.; Ext. Corn silk, Ext. Hydrangea, of each, ½ gr.; Atropine sulphate, 1-500 gr.
Dose 1 to 2 tablets.

TAB. DIARRHEA.
Formula—Each tablet contains: Bismuth subnitrate, 3 grs.; Pepsin saccharated, U. S., Aromatic chalk powder, of each, 2 grs.
Dose 1 to 2 tablets.

TAB. DIGESTIVE, AROMATIC, 5 grs.
Formula—Each tablet contains: Pepsin 1:3000, Pancreatin, of each, 1 gr.; Calcium lactophosphate, 2 grs.; Aromatics.
Dose 1 to 3 tablets.

TAB. DIURETIC.
Formula—Each tablet contains: Digitalis, 1 gr.; Potassium nitrate, 2 grs.; Ext. Buchu, Ext. Scoparius, of each, ½ gr.; Oil Juniper, 1 m.
Dose 1 to 2 tablets.

TAB. DOVER'S POWDER, 2 1-2 grs., 5 grs.
Action and uses—See Pil. Ipecac and Opium, No. 1 and No. 2, page 152.

TAB. DYSPEPSIA.
Formula—Each tablet contains: Bismuth subnitrate, 3 grs.; Pepsin 1:3000, Ginger, of each, 1 gr.
Dose 1 to 3 tablets.

TAB. FOUR CHLORIDES, Univ. Hosp. Pharm.
Formula—Each tablet contains: Quinine muriate, 1 gr.; Iron chloride ½ gr.; Corrosive sublimate, 1-48 gr., Arsenic chloride, 1-64 gr.
Action and uses—Tonic, antiperiodic and alterative.
Dose 1 to 2 tablets.

TAB. GONORRHEA.
Formula—Each tablet contains: Cubeb, Mass Copaiba, of each, 1 gr.; Iron sulphate exsic., Oil Sandalwood, Venice Turpentine, of each, ¼ m.; Oil Wintergreen, 1-10 m.
Action and uses—Tonic and alterative to the mucous membrane. A valuable prescription in obstinate gonorrhea and gleet.

TAB. HEADACHE CHOCOLATES, LILLY.
Formula—A palatable combination of Caffeine and Acetanilid with Chocolate.
Action and uses—Specially indicated in nervous sick headache, brain weariness, sciatica, neuralgia, acute rheumatism, whooping cough and bronchial irritation.
Dose 1 tablet dissolved slowly in the mouth, which may be repeated in half an hour if necessary.

WHEN ORDERING OR PRESCRIBING.

TAB. HYPOPHOSPHITES AND QUININE COMP. WITH STRYCHNINE.

Formula—Each tablet contains: Quinine hypophos., 1 gr.; Iron hypophos., Calcium hypophos., of each, ½ gr.; Sodium hypophos., Potassium hypophos., Manganese hypophos., of each, ¼ gr.; Strychnine hypophos., 1-64 gr.

Action and uses—Tonic and alterative to the nerve and brain tissue. Used in phthisis, scrofula, cachexy, debility from over mental exertion, in convalescence from exhausting diseases, etc.

Dose 1 to 2 tablets three times a day at meal time.

TAB. LACTATED PEPSIN, 5 grs.

Formula—This preparation combines the digestive properties of Pepsin, Pancreatin, Maltose, Diastase, Lactic acid and Hydrochloric acid.

Action and uses—Lactated pepsin is very beneficial in many forms of dyspepsia.

Dose 1 to 2 tablets three times a day after meals.

TAB. MANGANESE DIOXIDE, C. P., 2 grs., Manganese binoxide.

Action and uses—Tonic, alterative, emmenagogue. Used in syphilis, chlorosis, septicemia, scurvy, etc.

Dose 2 to 10 grains.

TAB. MIGRAINE.

Formula—Each tablet contains: Acetanilid, 2 grs.; Camphor monobromated, Caffeine citrate, of each, ½ gr.

Action and uses—Analgesic, hypnotic and anti-spasmodic.

Dose 1 to 2 tablets.

TAB. NEURALGIC BROWN-SEQUARD.

Formula—Each tablet contains: Ext. Hyoscyamus, Ext. Conium seed, of each, ⅝ gr.; Ext. Ignatia, Ext. Opium, of each, ½ gr.; Ext. Aconite leaves, ¼ gr.; Ext. Cannabis Indica, ½ gr.; Ext. stramonium, 1-3 gr.; Ext. Belladonna, 1-6 gr.

Action and uses—See Pil. Neuralgic Brown-Sequard, page 157.

Dose 1 tablet.

TAB. PEPSIN 1:3000, 5 grs.

Action and uses—A most reliable digestive. One tablet will dissolve 15000 grains coagulated albumen.

Dose 1 to 3 tablets.

TAB. PEPSIN 1:3000, AROMATIZED, 1 gr.

Formula—Each tablet contains: Pepsin combined with aromatics.

Action and uses—Digestive and stomachic.

Dose 1 tablet or more.

TAB. PEPSIN AND BISMUTH.

Formula—Each tablet contains: Pepsin saccharated, U. S., Bismuth subnitrate, of each, 3 grs.

Action and uses—Useful in many cases of dyspepsia, gastralgia, etc.

Dose 1 to 2 tablets.

TAB. PHENACETIN, 2 grs., 3 grs., 5 grs.

Dose 2 to 5 grains.

TAB. PHENACETIN AND SALOL.

Formula—Each tablet contains: Phenacetin, Salol, of each, 2½ grs.

Dose 1 to 3 tablets.

TAB. POTASSIUM BROMIDE, 2 grs., 5 grs., 10 grs.

Action and uses—Anti-epileptic, sedative, hypnotic. Used in epilepsy, neurasthenia, convulsions, delirium tremens, tetanus, strychnine and iodoform poisoning, syphilis, scrofula, etc.

Dose 2 to 60 grains. In tetanus or as an antidote to poison, up to half an ounce for a dose.

TAB. POTASSIUM CHLORATE, 5 grs.

Action and uses—An excellent remedy for sore throat, hoarseness, and irritation of the bronchial tubes. Also useful in mercurial salivation, croup and diphtheria.

Dose for a child, one-half tablet may be given every hour or two until relieved. **Adult dose, 1 to 2** in same time, allowing tablet to dissolve slowly in the mouth. It should never be given internally except when the stomach is full.

TAB. POTASSIUM IODIDE, 5 grs.

Action and uses—Alterative, emmenagogue. Solvent for uric acid. Used in pleuritis, rheumatism, syphilis, scrofula, aneurisms, scrofulous swellings, lead poisoning, etc., and in amenorrhea.

Dose 2 to 10 grains.

TAB. POTASSIUM PERMANGANATE, 1-2 gr., 1 gr., 2 grs.

Action and uses—See Pil. Potassium permanganate, page 162.

Dose 1-2 to 3 grains.

TAB. QUININE BISULPHATE, 1-2 gr., 1 gr., 2 grs., 3 grs., 4 grs., 5 grs.

Action and uses—See Pil. Quinine bisulphate, page 162.

Dose 1-2 to 10 grains.

TAB. QUININE SULPHATE, 1-2 gr., 1 gr., 2 grs., 3 grs., 4 grs., 5 grs.

Action and uses—See Pil. Quinine sulphate, page 162.

Dose 1-2 to 10 grains.

TAB. QUININE WITH CHOCOLATE, 1 gr., 2 grs.

Action and uses—A pleasant form for the administration of quinine, but not so active as the sulphate.

Dose 1 to 10 grains.

TAB. QUININE AND DOVER'S POWDER.

Formula—Each tablet contains: Quinine sulphate, Dover's powder, of each, 2½ grs.

Action and uses—Tonic and diaphoretic.

Dose 1 to 4 tablets.

TAB. SALICIN, 5 grs.

Action and uses—See Pil. Salicin, page 164.

Dose 5 to 15 grains.

TAB. SALICYLIC ACID, FROM OIL WINTERGREEN, 5 grs.

Action and uses—See Pil. Salicylic acid, page 165.

Dose 5 to 15 grains.

TAB. SALINE CHALYBEATE TONIC, FLINT.

Formula—Each tablet contains: Sodium chloride, 3 grs.; Calcium phosphate precip., ½ gr.; Potassium chloride, 3-20 gr.; Potassium sulphate, 1-10 gr.; Potassium carbonate, Calcium carbonate, Magnesium carbonate, Iron carbonate, of each, 1-20 gr.; Sodium carbonate, 3-5 gr.; Iron reduced, 9-20 gr.

Dose 1 to 2 tablets.

TAB. SALOL, 2 1-2 grs., 5 grs.
Action and uses—See Pil. Salol, page 165.
Dose 2 1-2 to 20 grains.

TAB. SAW PALMETTO COMP.
Formula—Each tablet contains: Ext. Saw Palmetto, 3 grs.; Ext. Corn silk, ½ gr.; Tincture Cantharides, Tincture Belladonna leaves, of each, 2 m.
Action and uses—This combination is especially valuable in cases of dribbling urine, especially of the aged when there seems to be want of power in the bladder, exerting its influence without impairment of any function. See also Fl. Ext. Saw Palmetto comp., page 104.
Dose 1 to 2 tablets.

TAB. SODA MINT.
Formula—Each tablet contains: Sodium bicarbonate, Ammonium bicarbonate, Oil Peppermint.
Action and uses—An agreeable stomachic and antacid. Especially useful in cases of seasickness, sick headache, heartburn, flatulence, indigestion, etc.
Dose for an adult, 1 to 2 tablets, repeated every 30 minutes until relieved. For a child, dissolve a tablet in a teaspoonful of water and give in teaspoonful doses, repeated according to age and degree of distress.

TAB. SODIUM BICARBONATE, 5 grs., 10 grs.
Action and uses—Useful in the treatment of acidity of the stomach, flatulence, indigestion, etc.
Dose one tablet every hour or two until relief is experienced.

TAB. SODIUM BROMIDE, 5 grs., 10 grs.
Action and uses—Similar to Tab. Potassium bromide, which see.

TAB. SODIUM SALICYLATE, 3 grs., 5 grs.
Action and uses—See Pil. Sodium salicylate, page 165.
Dose 3 to 20 grains.

TAB. SUN CHOLERA MIXTURE.
Formula—Each tablet represents ½ teaspoonful Sun cholera mixture.
Action and uses—A speedy cure for colic, diarrhea, cramp, pain in bowels, flatulence, cholera morbus, etc.
Dose, adult, 2 tablets every half hour until pain is relieved, then one every hour if needed. Children, one tablet every one or two hours as needed.

TAB. TONIC, AIKEN.
Formula—Each tablet contains: Quinine sulphate, 1 gr.; Iron by hydrogen, 2-3 gr.; Ext. Gentian, ½ gr.; Arsenous acid, Strychnine, of each, 1-50 gr.
Action and uses—See Pil. Tonic, Aikin, page 167.
Dose 1 tablet three times per day in chronic ague.

TAB. TRIPLE BROMIDES.
Formula—Each tablet contains: Sodium bromide, Potassium bromide, Ammonium bromide, of each, 2½ grs.
Action and uses—Generally the same as Tab. Potassium bromide, which see.
Dose 1 or more tablets.

TAB. TRIFOLIUM COMP.
Formula—Each tablet contains: Ext. Red Clover, Ext. Stillingia, Ext. Burdock, Ext. Poke root, of each, ½ gr.; Ext. Blue flag, ¼ gr.; Ext. Prickly ash bark, ⅛ gr.
Action and uses—Alterative.
Dose 1 to 3 tablets.

TAB. VAGINAL, WALLING.

Formula —Each tablet contains: Acetanilid, 5 grs.; Ext. White Oak bark, ½ gr.; Ext. Hyoscyamus, ¼ gr.

Action and uses —Proposed by Dr. W. H. Walling for local use in leucorrhea, inflammations, hyperesthesia, or any other condition requiring an antiseptic astringent and depletory for the vaginal tract. Cover the tablet with vaseline and insert into the vagina every other night.

TAB. VIBURNUM COMP.; UTERINE TONIC.

Formula —Each tablet contains: Ext. Black Haw, Ext. Cramp bark, of each, 1 gr.; Ext. Unicorn root, Ext. False Unicorn, Ext. Squaw vine, of each, ½ gr.; Caulophyllin, ½ gr.

Action and uses —Nervine and antispasmodic.

Dose 1 to 2 tablets.

ELI LILLY & COMPANY'S

SUGAR COATED

COMPRESSED TABLETS.

S. C. TAB. ALOES AND MASTICH.

Formula —Each tablet contains: Aloes, purified, 2 grs.; Mastich, ½ gr.; Red rose, ½ gr.

Action and uses —Used to quicken defecation. The action is principally upon the large intestine.

Dose 1 tablet before or after **dinner.**

S. C. TAB. CINCHONIDINE SULPHATE, 2 grs.

Action and uses —See Pil. Cinchonidine sulphate, page 144

Dose 1 to 6 tablets.

S. C. TAB. CODEINE, PINK, 1-4 gr.

Action and uses —See Pil. Codeine, page 145.

Dose 1 to 4 tablets.

S. C. TAB. MORPHINE SULPHATE, PINK, 1-8 gr., 1-4 gr.

Action and uses —See Pil. Morphine sulphate, page 156.

Dose 1 tablet.

S. C. TAB. PEPSIN 1:3000, 1 gr.

Action and uses —See Pepsin, U. S., page 232

Dose 1 tablet or more as required.

S. C. TAB. QUININE BISULPHATE, 1 gr., 2 grs., 3 grs., 4 grs., 5 grs.

Action and uses —See Pil. Quinine bisulphate, page 162.

Dose 1 to 10 grains.

S. C. TAB. QUININE SULPHATE, 1 gr., 2 grs., 3 grs., 4 grs., 5 grs.

Action and uses —See Pil. Quinine sulphate, page 162.

Dose 1 to 10 grains.

S. C. TAB. SUN CHOLERA; Brown.

Action and uses —See Compressed Tablets Sun cholera mixture, page 204

Dose 1 to 2 tablets.

STANDARDIZED FLUID EXTRACT
ERGOT, U. S.
(Claviceps purpurea,)

We invite the careful consideration of Physicians to our FLUID EXTRACT OF ERGOT. Methods and precautions dictated by progressive pharmacy are employed by us to supply a preparation to which we can safely apply the term

PERFECTION.

Physicians desiring a sample of our FLUID EXTRACT ERGOT will be promptly supplied by addressing

ELI LILLY & COMPANY.

EXT. ERGOTÆ FLD.; LILLY.

Prepared from best selected ERGOT of the most recent crop.

PROCESS OF MANUFACTURE—Fractional percolation without the employment of heat.

No ACID is used.

ALL CONSTITUENTS of medicinal value are present in the extract.

THE INERT OIL is absent.

LILLY'S IS THE ORIGINAL STANDARDIZED ERGOT.

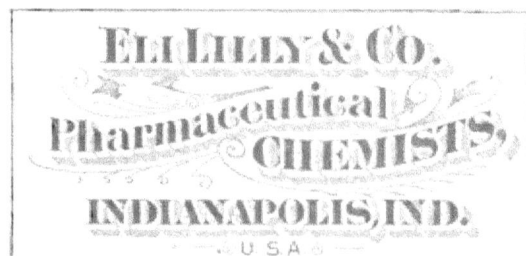

ELI LILLY & Co.
Pharmaceutical CHEMISTS,
INDIANAPOLIS, IND.
U S A

ELI LILLY & COMPANY'S

TABLET TRITURATES.

Very soluble, uniform, accurate and embody every desirable quality.

Tablets from special formulas quickly prepared when desired.

Therapeutical notes and doses are not given on this line of preparations as it practically duplicates the pill list and reference may be made to the list of pills, pages 132 to 168 for such information as may be desired.

TAB. TRIT. ACETANILID, 1 gr.

TAB. TRIT. ACETANILID COMP., DR. AULDE.
Formula—Each tablet contains: Acetanilid, 7-20 gr.; Caffeine, 1-20 gr.; Soda bicarbonate, 1-10 gr.

TAB. TRIT. ACONITINE, CRYSTALS, 1-500 gr., 1-200 gr.

TAB. TRIT. AGARICIN, 1-20 gr.

TAB. TRIT. ALOIN, 1-10 gr., 1-4 gr., 1-2 gr., 1 gr.

TAB. TRIT. ALOIN, BELLADONNA AND PODOPHYLLIN.
Formula—Each tablet contains: Aloin, Ext. Belladonna, Podophyllin, of each, ⅛ gr.

TAB. TRIT. ALOIN, BELLADONNA, PODOPHYLLIN AND NUX VOMICA.
Formula—Each tablet contains: Aloin, Ext. Belladonna, Podophyllin, Ext. Nux vomica, of each, 1-10 gr.

TAB. TRIT. ALOIN AND PODOPHYLLIN.
Formula—Each tablet contains: Aloin, Podophyllin, of each, ¼ gr.

TAB. TRIT. ALOIN, STRYCHNINE AND BELLADONNA, NO. 1.
Formula—Each tablet contain: Aloin, 1-5 gr.; Strychnine sulphate, 1-60 gr;. Ext. Belladonna, ⅛ gr.

TAB. TRIT. ALOIN, STRYCHNINE AND BELLADONNA, NO. 2.
Formula—Each tablet contains: Aloin, 1-5 gr.; Strychnine sulphate, 1-120 gr.; Ext. Belladonna, ⅛ gr.

TAB. TRIT. ALOIN, STRYCHNINE, BELLADONNA AND CASCARA.
Formula—Each tablet contains: Aloin, 1-5 gr.; Ext. Belladonna, ¼ gr.; Strychnine sulphate, 1-120 gr.; Ext. Cascara sagrada, ½ gr.

TAB. TRIT. ALOIN, STRYCHNINE, BELLADONNA AND IPECAC.
Formula—Each tablet contains: Aloin, 1-5 gr.; Strychnine sulphate, 1-60 gr.; Ext. Belladonna, ¼ gr.; Ipecac, 1-16 gr.

TAB. TRIT. ALOIN, STRYCHNINE, BELLADONNA AND PODO-PHYLLIN.
Formula—Each tablet contains: Aloin, Ext. Belladonna, Podophyllin, of each, ⅛ gr.; Strychnine, 1-60 gr.

TAB. TRIT. AMMONIUM MURIATE, 1 gr.

TAB. TRIT. AMMONIUM MURIATE, COMP., NO. 1.
Formula—Each tablet contains: Ammonium muriate, ¼ gr.; Cubeb, ⅛ gr.; Ext. Licorice, 1-10 gr.

TAB. TRIT. AMMONIUM MURIATE, COMP., NO. 2.
Formula—Each tablet contains: Ammonium muriate, ¼ gr.; Ext. Licorice, 1-10 gr.; Cubeb, ⅛ gr.; Potassium chloride, ½ gr.

TAB. TRIT. ANTISEPTIC, BERNAY, WHITE, For External Use.
Formula—Each tablet contains: Corrosive sublimate, 1⅜ grs.; Citric acid, 87-100 gr.

TAB. TRIT. ANTISEPTIC, BERNAY, BLUE; Supplied only when so specified. See Tab. Trit. Bernay, White.

TAB. TRIT. ARSENIC BROMIDE AND GOLD CHLORIDE, FLETCHER.
Formula—Each tablet contains: Arsenic bromide, 1-20 gr.; Gold chloride, 1-20 gr.

TAB. TRIT. ARSENIC SULPHIDE, 1-100 gr., 1-50 gr., 1-30 gr.

TAB. TRIT. ARSENOUS ACID, 1-200 gr., 1-150 gr., 1-100 gr., 1-60 gr., 1-50 gr., 1-40 gr., 1-30 gr., 1-20 gr.

TAB. TRIT. ATROPINE SULPHATE, 1-500 gr., 1-200 gr., 1-120 gr., 1-100 gr., 1-50 gr.

TAB. TRIT. BORIC ACID, 1-10 gr., 1-2 gr.

TAB. TRIT. BROWN MIXTURE, 1-2 teaspoonful, 1 teaspoonful.

TAB. TRIT. CACTUS GRAND, Fluid Extract, 3 m., 5 m.

TAB. TRIT. CAFFEINE, 1 gr.

TAB. TRIT. CAFFEINE CITRATE, 1-2 gr., 1 gr.

TAB. TRIT. CALCIUM SULPHIDE, 1-60 gr., 1-10 gr., 1-8 gr., 1-4 gr., 1-2 gr., 1 gr.

TAB. TRIT. CALOMEL, 1-50 gr., 1-40 gr., 1-30 gr., 1-20 gr., 1-12 gr., 1-10 gr., 1-8 gr., 1-6 gr., 1-5 gr., 1-4 gr., 1-3 gr., 1-2 gr., 1 gr., 2 grs., 3 grs.

TAB. TRIT. CALOMEL AND IPECAC, NO. 1.
Formula—Each tablet contains: Calomel, Ipecac, of each, ⅛ gr.

TAB. TRIT. CALOMEL AND IPECAC, NO. 2.
Formula—Each tablet contains: Calomel, Ipecac, of each, ¼ gr.

TAB. TRIT. CALOMEL, IPECAC AND SODA, NO. 1.
Formula—Each tablet contains: Calomel, 1 gr.; Ipecac, 1-10 gr.; Sodium bicarbonate, 1 gr.

TAB. TRIT. CALOMEL, IPECAC AND SODA NO. 2.
Formula—Each tablet contains: Calomel, 1-5 gr.; Ipecac, 1-10 gr.; Sodium bicarbonate, 1 gr.

TAB. TRIT. CALOMEL, PODOPHYLLIN AND SODA, NO. 1.
Formula—Each tablet contains: Calomel, Sodium bicarbonate, of each, ½ gr.; Podophyllin, 1-10 gr.

TAB. TRIT. CALOMEL, PODOPHYLLIN AND SODA, NO. 2.
Formula—Each tablet contains: Calomel, ¼ gr.; Podophyllin, 1-12 gr.; Sodium bicarbonate, ½ gr.

TAB. TRIT. CALOMEL AND SODA, NO. 1.
Formula—Each tablet contains: Calomel, Sodium bicarbonate, of each, ½ gr.

TAB. TRIT. CALOMEL AND SODA, NO. 2.
Formula—Each tablet contains: Calomel, 1-10 gr.; Sodium bicarbonate, 1 gr.

TAB. TRIT. CALOMEL AND SODA, NO. 3.
Formula—Each tablet contains: Calomel, ¼ gr.; Sodium bicarbonate, 1 gr.

TAB. TRIT. CALOMEL AND SODA, NO. 4.
Formula—Each tablet contains: Calomel, ½ gr.; Sodium bicarbonate, 1 gr.

TAB. TRIT. CALOMEL AND SODA, NO. 5.
Formula—Each tablet contains: Calomel, Sodium bicarbonate, of each, 1 gr.

TAB. TRIT. CALOMEL AND SODA, NO. 6.
Formula—Each tablet contains: Calomel, Sodium bicarbonate, of each, ¼ gr.

TAB. TRIT. CALOMEL AND SODA, NO. 7.
Formula—Each tablet contains: Calomel, ¼ gr.; Sodium bicarbonate, ½ gr.

TAB. TRIT. CALOMEL AND SODA, NO. 8.
Formula—Each tablet contains: Calomel, 1-20 gr.; Sodium bicarbonate, 1 gr.

TAB. TRIT. CALOMEL AND SODA, NO. 9.
Formula—Each tablet contains: Calomel, 1-6 gr.; Sodium bicarbonate, 1 gr.

TAB. TRIT. CALOMEL AND SODA, NO. 10.
Formula—Each tablet contains: Calomel, Sodium bicarbonate, of each, 1-5 gr.

TAB. TRIT. CALOMEL AND SODA, NO. 11.
Formula—Each tablet contains: Calomel, Sodium bicarbonate, of each, ⅛ gr.

TAB. TRIT. CAMPHOR MONOBROMATED, 1 gr.

TAB. TRIT. CAMPHOR, BELLADONNA AND QUININE; Rhinitis.
Formula—Each tablet contains: Camphor, Quinine sulphate, of each, ¼ gr.; Fl. Ext. Belladonna, ⅛ gr.

TAB. TRIT. CERIUM OXALATE, 1 gr.

TAB. TRIT. COCAINE HYDROCHLORATE, 1-16 gr., 1-10 gr., 1-8 gr., 1-6 gr., 1-4 gr.

TAB. TRIT. COCAINE HYDROCHLORATE, For preparing solutions; See Miscellaneous List, page 260

TAB. TRIT. CODEINE, 1-8 gr., 1-4 gr., 1-2 gr., 1 gr.

TAB. TRIT. COPPER ARSENITE, 1-5000 gr., 1-1000 gr., 1-500 gr., 1-200 gr., 1-100 gr.

TAB. TRIT. CORROSIVE SUBLIMATE, 1-1000 gr., 1-500 gr., 1-100 gr., 1-60 gr., 1-50 gr., 1-40 gr., 1-30 gr., 1-20 gr., 1-16 gr., 1-12 gr., 1-10 gr.

TAB. TRIT. DIARRHEA.
  Formula—Each tablet contains, Calomel, ½ gr.; Morphine sulphate, Capsicum, Camphor, of each, 1-16 gr.; Ipecac, 1-32 gr.

TAB. TRIT. DIGITALIN, PURE, 1-120 gr., 1-75 gr., 1-60 gr., 1-30 gr., 1-20 gr.

TAB. TRIT. DIGITALIS, FLUID EXTRACT, 1-2 m., 1 m.

TAB. TRIT. DIGITALIS, TINCTURE, 2 m., 5 m.

TAB. TRIT. DIGITALIS AND STROPHANTHUS; See Tab. Trit. Strophanthus comp.

TAB. TRIT. DOVER'S POWDER, 1-2 gr., 1 gr., 2 grs., 2 1-2 grs.

TAB. TRIT. ELATERIN, 1-40 gr., 1-20 gr., 1-10 gr.

TAB. TRIT. ELATERIUM, CLUTTERBUCK, 1-16 gr., 1-8 gr.

TAB. TRIT. FEVER, KENYON.
  Formula—Each tablet contains: Tr. Aconite, 1 m.; Morphine sulphate, 1-20 gr.; Tartar emetic, 1-50 gr.; Ipecac, ½ gr.

TAB. TRIT. FOWLER'S SOLUTION, 5 m.

TAB. TRIT. GELSEMIUM, TINCTURE, 1 m., 2 m.

TAB. TRIT. GOLD AND SODIUM CHLORIDE, 1-30 gr., 1-20 gr., 1-10 gr.

TAB. TRIT. HEART TONIC AND STIMULANT, DACOSTA; See Tab. Trit. Nitroglycerin comp.

TAB. TRIT. HEPATIC, KENYON.
  Formula—Each tablet contains: Euonymin, Ipecac, Calomel, of each, ½ gr.; Podophyllin, 1-20 gr.; Aloin, 1-12 gr.

TAB. TRIT. HYOSCINE HYDROBROMATE, 1-200 gr., 1-100 gr.

TAB. TRIT. HYOSCYAMINE, CRYSTALS, 1-200 gr., 1-100 gr.

TAB. TRIT. IRON ARSENATE, 1-8 gr.

TAB. TRIT. IRON AND ARSENIC.
  Formula—Each tablet contains: Iron by hydrogen, 1 gr.; Arsenous acid, 1-100 gr.

TAB. TRIT. IRON AND ARSENIC COMP.

Formula —Each tablet contains: Iron by hydrogen, 1 gr.; Arsenous acid, 1-100 gr.; Ignatia, 1-10 gr.

TAB. TRIT. IRON, ARSENIC AND STRYCHNINE, NO. 1.

Formula—Each tablet contains: Iron by hydrogen, 1 gr.; Arsenous acid, 1-100 gr.; Strychnine sulphate, 1-60 gr.

TAB. TRIT. IRON, ARSENIC AND STRYCHNINE, NO. 2.

Formula—Each tablet contains: Iron by hydrogen, 1 gr.; Arsenous acid, 1-50 gr., Strychnine sulphate, 1-60 gr.

TAB. TRIT. IRON, QUININE AND STRYCHNINE.

Formula—Each tablet contains: Iron by hydrogen, Quinine sulphate, of each, ½ gr.; Strychnine, 1-120 gr.

TAB. TRIT. IRON AND STRYCHNINE COMP.

Formula—Each tablet contains: Iron by hydrogen, Quinine sulphate, of each, ½ gr.; Arsenous acid, 1-100 gr.; Strychnine sulphate, 1-120 gr.

TAB. TRIT. LAXATIVE, CARMINATIVE.

Formula—Each tablet contains: Ext. Cascara sagrada, ½ gr.; Aloin, ⅛ gr.; Podophyllin, Oil Peppermint, of each, 1-10 gr.

TAB. TRIT. LITHIUM CARBONATE, 1 gr.

TAB. TRIT. MANGANESE BINOXIDE, C. P., 1-2 gr., 1 gr.

TAB. TRIT. MERCURY WITH CHALK, 1-10 gr., 1-5 gr., 1 gr., 2 grs.

TAB. TRIT. MERCURY BINIODIDE, 1-50 gr., 1-25 gr., 1-16 gr., 1-8 gr.

TAB. TRIT. MERCURY PROTIODIDE, 1-100 gr., 1-50 gr., 1-16 gr., 1-10 gr., 1-12 gr., 1-8 gr., 1-6 gr., 1-4 gr., 1-3 gr., 1-2 gr., 1 gr.

TAB. TRIT. MORPHINE SULPHATE, 1-50 gr., 1-20 gr., 1-16 gr., 1-10 gr., 1-8 gr., 1-6 gr., 1-5 gr., 1-4 gr., 1-2 gr.

TAB. TRIT. MORPHINE AND ATROPINE, NO. 1.

Formula—Each tablet contains: Morphine sulphate, ⅛ gr.; Atropine sulphate, 1-200 gr.

TAB. TRIT. MORPHINE AND ATROPINE, NO. 2.

Formula—Each tablet contains: Morphine sulphate, ¼ gr.; Atropine sulphate, 1-150 gr.

TAB. TRIT. MORPHINE AND ATROPINE, NO. 3.

Formula—Each tablet contains: Morphine sulphate, 1-6 gr., Atropine, sulphate, 1-180 gr.

TAB. TRIT. MORPHINE AND ATROPINE, NO. 4.

Formula—Each tablet contains: Morphine sulphate, ⅛ gr.; Atropine sulphate, 1-150 gr.

TAB. TRIT. MORPHINE AND ATROPINE, NO. 5.

Formula—Each tablet contains: Morphine sulphate, ¼ gr.; Atropine sulphate, 1-100 gr.

TAB. TRIT. NERVE TONIC, WESTBROOK.
  Formula—Each tablet contains: Zinc phosphide, 1-10 gr.; Ext. Nux vomica, ¼ gr.; Iron by hydrogen, 1 gr.

TAB. TRIT. NEURALGIC, KENYON.
  Formula—Each tablet contains: Zinc phosphide, 1-16 gr.; Strychnine sulphate, 1-60 gr.; Sodium arsenate, 1-20 gr.; Aconitine crystals, 1-400 gr.; Ext. Cannabis Indica, ½ gr.

TAB. TRIT. NITROGLYCERIN, 1-200 gr., 1-150 gr., 1-100 gr., 1-50 gr.

TAB. TRIT. NITROGLYCERIN, COMP., Heart Tonic and Stimulant, DACOSTA.
  Formula—Each tablet contains: Nitroglycerin, 1-100 gr.; Tr. Digitalis, 2 m.; Tr. Strophanthus, 2 m.; Tr. Belladonna, 2 m.

TAB. TRIT. NUX VOMICA, POWD., 1-30 gr., 1-10 gr., 1-8 gr., 1-4 gr., 1-2 gr., 1 gr.

TAB. TRIT. NUX VOMICA AND PEPSIN.
  Formula—Each tablet contains: Nux vomica, 1-100 gr.; Pepsin 1:3000, 1-10 gr.

TAB. TRIT. OPIUM, POWD., 1-4 gr., 1-2 gr., 1 gr.

TAB. TRIT. OPIUM, CAMPHORATED TINCTURE, 5 m., 10 m.

TAB. TRIT. OPIUM AND LEAD ACETATE.
  Formula—Each tablet contains: Opium, ½ gr.; Lead acetate, 1½ grs.

TAB. TRIT. PEPSIN 1:3000, 1-4 gr., 1-2 gr., 1 gr.

TAB. TRIT. PILOCARPINE HYDROCHLORATE, 1-8 gr.

TAB. TRIT. PODOPHYLLIN, 1-40 gr., 1-16 gr., 1-10 gr., 1-8 gr., 1-4 gr., 1-2 gr.

TAB. TRIT. POTASSIUM ARSENATE, 1-100 gr., 1-50 gr.

TAB. TRIT. POTASSIUM PERMANGANATE, See Compressed Tablet list, page 198

TAB. TRIT. QUININE SULPHATE, 1-2 gr., 1 gr.

TAB. TRIT. RHINITIS; See Tab. Trit. Camphor, Belladonna and Quinine.

TAB. TRIT. SACCHARIN, 1-2 gr.
  For use in sweetening beverages for diabetic patients. Full directions accompany each package.

TAB. TRIT. SALOL, 1-5 gr., 1-2 gr., 1 gr.

TAB. TRIT. SANTONIN, 1-2 gr., 1 gr.

TAB. TRIT. SANTONIN AND CALOMEL, NO. 1.
  Formula—Each tablet contains: Santonin, ½ gr.; Calomel, ½ gr.

TAB. TRIT. SANTONIN AND CALOMEL, NO. 2.
  Formula—Each tablet contains: Santonin, ¼ gr.; Calomel, ½ gr.

TAB. TRIT. SANTONIN AND CALOMEL, NO. 3.
Formula—Each tablet contains: Santonin, 1 gr.; Calomel, 1 gr.

TAB. TRIT. SANTONIN AND PODOPHYLLIN.
Formula—Each tablet contains: Santonin, ½ gr.; Podophyllin, 1-20 gr.

TAB. TRIT. SODIUM ARSENATE, 1-25 gr., 1-15 gr., 1-12 gr.

TAB. TRIT. SODIUM SALICYLATE, 1 gr.

TAB. TRIT. SPARTEINE SULPHATE, 1-2 gr.

TAB. TRIT. STROPHANTHUS, TINCTURE, 2 m.

TAB. TRIT. STROPHANTHUS COMP.
Formula—Each tablet contains: Tr. Strophanthus, 2 m.; Tr. Digitalis, 3 m.

TAB. TRIT. STRYCHNINE ARSENATE, 1-100 gr., 1-32 gr.

TAB. TRIT. STRYCHNINE NITRATE, 1-100 gr., 1-60 gr., 1-50 gr., 1-40 gr., 1-30 gr., 1-20 gr.

TAB. TRIT. STRYCHNINE SULPHATE, 1-100 gr., 1-60 gr., 1-50 gr., 1-40 gr., 1-32 gr., 1-30 gr., 1-20 gr., 1-16 gr.

TAB. TRIT. TONSILLITIS.
Formula—Each tablet contains: Tr. Aconite, 1-5 m.; Tr. Belladonna, Tr. Bryonia, of each, 1-10 m.; Mercury biniodide, 1-100 gr.

TAB. TRIT. TURPETH MINERAL, 1 gr.

TAB. TRIT. VERATRUM VIRIDE, TINCTURE, 1 m., 2 m.

TAB. TRIT. ZINC SULPHOCARBOLATE, 1 gr., 2 grs.

TAB. TRIT. ZINC PHOSPHIDE AND NUX VOMICA.
Formula—Each tablet contains: Zinc phosphide, 1-40 gr.; Nux vomica, ¼ gr.

TO PHYSICIANS AND DRUGGISTS.

Where Druggists do not have our preparations in stock we will always be glad to forward direct to physicians, by express, on receipt of price.

Druggists will find our preparations demanded by many physicians and acceptable to all. A very large proportion of druggists already have them. Those who have not may conveniently obtain supplies from any wholesale druggist or direct from the laboratory, the best plan being to regularly specify "Lilly" to the jobber with your drug orders.

ELI LILLY & COMPANY'S

HYPODERMIC TABLETS.

Perfect tablets for preparing solutions for hypodermic use must be instantly soluble, nonirritant and must perfectly preserve the medicament; these desirable properties we have succeeded in combining in our tablets.

They are packed in tubes of 25 tablets each, four tubes in a flat box, convenient for carrying or storing. They are also supplied in bottles of 100 tablets each.

HYPO. TAB. ACONITINE, CRYSTALS, 1-200 gr., 1-120 gr., 1-100 gr.

HYPO. TAB. APOMORPHINE HYDROCHLORATE, 1-120 gr., 1-50 gr., 1-20 gr., 1-10 gr.

HYPO. TAB. ATROPINE SULPHATE, 1-200 gr., 1-150 gr., 1-120 gr., 1-100 gr., 1-60 gr., 1-50 gr., 1-40 gr.

HYPO. TAB. CAFFEINE, 1-2 gr., 1-4 gr.

HYPO. TAB. COCAINE HYDROCHLORATE, 1-8 gr., 1-4 gr., 1-2 gr.

HYPO. TAB. CODEINE, 1-8 gr., 1-4 gr., 1-2 gr.

HYPO. TAB. CODEINE PHOSPHATE, 1-8 gr., 1-4 gr., 1-2 gr.

HYPO. TAB. CODEINE SULPHATE, 1-4 gr., 1-2 gr.

HYPO. TAB. CORROSIVE SUBLIMATE, 1-100 gr., 1-60 gr., 1-30 gr.

HYPO. TAB. DATURINE SULPHATE, 1-100 gr.

HYPO. TAB. DIGITALIN, PURE, 1-120 gr., 1-100 gr., 1-60 gr., 1-50 gr., 1-20 gr.

HYPO. TAB. HYOSCINE HYDROBROMATE, 1-100 gr., 1-50 gr.

HYPO. TAB. HYOSCYAMINE, CRYSTALS, 1-100 gr., 1-50 gr., 1-25 gr.

HYPO. TAB. MORPHINE HYDROCHLORATE, 1-4 gr.

HYPO. TAB. MORPHINE SULPHATE, 1-20 gr., 1-8 gr., 1-6 gr., 1-5 gr., 1-4 gr., 1-3 gr., 1-2 gr.

HYPO. TAB. MORPHINE AND ATROPINE, NO. 1.
Formula—Each tablet contains: Morphine sulphate, ¼ gr.; Atropine sulphate, 1-200 gr.

HYPO. TAB. MORPHINE AND ATROPINE, NO. 2.
Formula—Each tablet contains: Morphine sulphate, ¼ gr.; Atropine sulphate, 1-150 gr.

HYPO. TAB. MORPHINE AND ATROPINE, NO. 3.
Formula—Each tablet contains: Morphine sulphate, 1-6 gr.; Atropine sulphate, 1-180 gr.

HYPO. TAB. MORPHINE AND ATROPINE, NO. 4.

Formula—Each tablet contains: Morphine sulphate, ½ gr.; Atropine sulphate, 1-150 gr.

HYPO. TAB. MORPHINE AND ATROPINE, NO. 5.

Formula—Each tablet contains: Morphine sulphate, ¼ gr.; Atropine sulphate, 1-100 gr.

HYPO. TAB. MORPHINE AND ATROPINE, NO. 6.

Formula—Each tablet contains: Morphine sulphate, ½ gr.; Atropine sulphate, 1-100 gr.

HYPO. TAB. MORPHINE AND ATROPINE, NO. 7.

Formula—Each tablet contains: Morphine sulphate, ¼ gr.; Atropine sulphate, 1-200 gr.

HYPO. TAB. MORPHINE AND ATROPINE, NO. 8.

Formula—Each tablet contains: Morphine sulphate, ¼ gr.; Atropine sulphate, 1-100 gr.

HYPO. TAB. MORPHINE AND ATROPINE, NO. 9.

Formula—Each tablet contains: Morphine sulphate, 1-6 gr.; Atropine sulphate, 1-120 gr.

HYPO. TAB. MORPHINE AND ATROPINE, NO. 10.

Formula—Each tablet contains: Morphine sulphate, ½ gr.; Atropine sulphate, 1-120 gr.

HYPO. TAB. MORPHINE AND ATROPINE, NO. 11.

Formula—Each tablet contains: Morphine sulphate, ¼ gr.; Atropine sulphate, 1-50 gr.

HYPO. TAB. MORPHINE AND ATROPINE, NO. 12.

Formula—Each tablet contains: Morphine sulphate, ¼ gr.; Atropine sulphate, 1-60 gr.

HYPO. TAB. MORPHINE AND ATROPINE, NO. 13.

Formula—Each tablet contains: Morphine sulphate, ¼ gr.; Atropine sulphate, 1-120 gr.

HYPO. TAB. MORPHINE AND ATROPINE, NO. 14.

Formula—Each tablet contains: Morphine sulphate, 1-6 gr.; Atropine sulphate, 1-150 gr.

HYPO. TAB. MORPHINE AND ATROPINE, NO. 15.

Formula—Each tablet contains: Morphine sulphate, ⅓ gr.; Atropine sulphate, 1-120 gr.

HYPO. TAB. NITROGLYCERIN, 1-200 gr., 1-150 gr., 1-100 gr., 1-50 gr.

HYPO. TAB. NITROGLYCERIN AND STRYCHNINE.

Formula—Each tablet contains: Nitroglycerin, 1-100 gr.; Strychnine sulphate, 1-50 gr.

HYPO. TAB. PICROTOXIN, 1-50 gr.

HYPO. TAB. PILOCARPINE HYDROCHLORATE, 1-8 gr.

HYPO. TAB. STRYCHNINE NITRATE, 1-100 gr., 1-60 gr., 1-50 gr., 1-40 gr., 1-30 gr., 1-20 gr.

HYPO. TAB. STRYCHNINE SULPHATE, 1-150 gr., 1-120 gr., 1-100 gr., 1-60 gr., 1-50 gr., 1-40 gr., 1 32 gr., 1 30 gr., 1 20 gr.

ELI LILLY & COMPANY'S
VETERINARY
Hypodermic Tablets.

VET. HYP. TAB. ACONITINE CRYSTALS, 1-20 gr.

VET. HYP. TAB. ATROPINE SULPHATE, 1-4 gr., 1-2 gr.

VET. HYP. TAB. COCAINE HYDROCHLORATE, 1 gr., 3 grs.

VET. HYP. TAB. COLCHICINE, 1-4 gr.

VET. HYP. TAB. DIGITALIN, PURE, 1-4 gr.

VET. HYP. TAB. MORPHINE SULPHATE, 1-2 gr., 1 gr., 2 grs.

VET. HYP. TAB. MORPHINE AND ATROPINE.
Formula—Each tablet contains: Morphine sulphate, 1½ grs.; Atropine sulphate, ½ gr.

VET. HYP. TAB. PHYSOSTIGMINE SALICYLATE, 1-4 gr., 1-2 gr.

VET. HYP. TAB. PILOCARPINE HYDROCHLORATE, 1-2 gr.

VET. HYP. TAB. PILOCARPINE AND ESERINE.
Formula—Each tablet contains: Pilocarpine hydrochlorate, Eserine salicylate, of each, 1 gr.

VET. HYP. STRYCHNINE SULPHATE, 1-2 gr., 1 gr.

VET. HYP. TAB. VERATRINE HYDROCHLORATE, 1-4 gr.

VETERINARY PHYSICIANS
AND
SURGEONS

Are very large users of such of our remedies as are applicable to their practice. Especially are they interested in our line of standardized Fluid Extracts, Veterinary Hypodermic Tablets and also in our Veterinary Glycones which we prepare to special order as wanted. A full description of the action of Glycones; Lilly, will be found by reference to the index.

Attention is called to Formaseptol as a local antiseptic application and particularly also to the MOFFATT FORMALDEHYDE GENERATOR for rapid disinfection and purification of Veterinary Hospitals and stables.

ELI LILLY & COMPANY'S
Compressed Lozenges.

Our Compressed Medicated Lozenges are free from the large quantities of flour, starch and talc often employed. They contain only the medicament or flavor, pure sugar and a small proportion of cohesive material.

Remedies prepared in the form of Lozenges are too often regarded as simple confections. As a matter of fact however, they present many remedies in the most effective form, especially where it is desired to affect the throat and bronchials or to reach the stomach with such bulky powders as charcoal, bismuth, sulphur, etc.

LOZ. AMMONIUM CHLORIDE, U. S.
Action and uses—To allay irritation of the throat.
Dose 1 lozenge, dissolved in the mouth every three hours.

LOZ. AMMONIUM CHLORIDE AND LICORICE.
Formula—Each lozenge contains: Ammonium chloride, 2 grs.; Ext. Licorice, 8 grs.
Action and uses—Medicinally the same but more agreeable to the taste than Loz. Ammonium chloride, U. S.
Dose 1 lozenge every three hours.

LOZ. BISMUTH AND CHARCOAL.
Formula—Each tablet contains: Bismuth subnitrate, 2 grs.; Willow charcoal, 5 grs.
Action and uses—Valuable in gastric disturbance.
Dose 1 to 2 lozenges.

LOZ. BRONCHIAL, Formula A.
Formula—Each lozenge contains: Oleoresin Cubeb, Balsam Tolu, of each, 1-5 gr.; Oil Sassafras, 1-10 gr.; Ext. Licorice, 7 grs.
Action and uses—Demulcent and anodyne. Valuable in pectoral complaints.
Dose 1 lozenge as required.

LOZ. BRONCHIAL, Formula B.
Formula—Each lozenge contains: Ext. Licorice, 1 gr.; Balsam Tolu, Oil Sassafras, of each, 1-20 gr.; Cubeb, 3-10 gr.
Action and uses—Demulcent and anodyne. Valuable in pectoral complaints.
Dose 1 lozenge as required.

LOZ. BROWN MIXTURE.
Formula—Each lozenge contains: Ext. Licorice, 3 grs.; Opium, Benzoic acid, Camphor, Oil Anise, of each, 1-20 gr.; Tartar emetic, 1-40 gr.
Action and uses—A valuable and popular cough lozenge.
Dose 1 lozenge as required.

LOZ. BROWN MIXTURE AND AMMONIUM CHLORIDE.

Formula—Each lozenge contains: Brown mixture, 85 m., Ammonium chloride, 3 grs.

Action and uses—The addition of Ammonium chloride to the Brown mixture lozenge makes a very efficacious remedy in pharyngeal and laryngeal irritation.

Dose 1 lozenge dissolved in the mouth every three hours.

LOZ. CARBOLIC ACID, 1-2 gr.

Action and uses—Antiseptic and stimulant. Useful in scarlatina and diptheritic affections, also as an intestinal antiseptic, arresting fermentation and preventing eructations of gas.

Dose 1 lozenge four or five times daily.

LOZ. CHARCOAL, WILLOW, 5 grs., 10 grs.

Action and uses—Disinfectant and absorbent. Employed with advantage in diarrhea as an absorbent and in dyspepsia when accompanied with fetid breath and eructations.

Dose as required.

LOZ. CHARCOAL AND SODA MINT.

Formula—Each lozenge contains: Willow charcoal, Sodium bicarbonate, of each, 5 grs.; Ammonium carbonate, Oil Peppermint.

Action and uses—Disinfectant, absorbent and antacid.

Dose 1 to 2 lozenges.

LOZ. CHOCOLATE, WORM; See Loz. Santonin and Calomel, Chocolate.

LOZ. CORYZA; See Loz. Bronchial, Formula A.

LOZ. CUBEB, U. S.

Action and uses—Advantageously used in some cases of chronic cough and ulceration or chronic inflammation of the fauces.

Dose 1 lozenge as required.

LOZ. DIGESTIVE.

Formula—Each lozenge contains: Pepsin 1:3000, 1 gr.; Sulphur, ½ gr.; Oleoresin Ginger, 1-10 gr.

Dose 1 to 2 lozenges.

LOZ. ELM.

Formula—Each lozenge contains: Elm bark, 3 grs.

Action and uses—Demulcent.

Dose as required.

LOZ. GINGER, U. S.

Action and uses—Relieves gastric pains when due to flatulence.

Dose 1 lozenge as required.

LOZ. GINGER AND SODA.

Formula—Each lozenge contains: Tinct. Ginger, 10 m.; Sodium bicarbonate, 2 grs.

Action and uses—Stimulant and antacid. Use same as Loz. Ginger, U. S.

Dose 1 lozenge as required.

LOZ. GUAIAC.

Formula—Each lozenge contains: Resin Guaiac, 2 grs.

Action and uses—Nearly a specific for arresting crescent inflammation of the tonsils and useful in both acute and subacute inflammation of the pharynx and in acute follicular disease of the tonsils.

Dose 1 lozenge every two hours in acute inflammation; three times per day in chronic affections.

LOZ. EXT. LICORICE, 5 grs., 10 grs.
Action and uses—A useful demulcent. Allowed to dissolve in the mouth, it allays cough by healing the irritated membrane of the fauces.
Dose 1 lozenge as required.

LOZ. LICORICE POWDER COMP.
Formula—Each lozenge contains: Licorice powder, compound, U. S., 20 grs.
Action and uses—An agreeable and efficient laxative.
Dose 1 to 3 lozenges.

LOZ. LIME JUICE, GINGER AND PEPSIN.
Action and uses—Beneficial in debility of digestive apparatus. Relieves pains of indigestion, restores the appetite and removes dyspeptic symptoms.
Dose 1 to 3 lozenges.

LOZ. LIME JUICE AND PEPSIN.
Action and uses—Used in treatment of diseases of digestive organs. Aids digestion and relieves gastric pain.
Dose 1 to 3 lozenges.

LOZ. PECTORAL, JACKSON.
Formula—Each lozenge contains: Ext. Licorice, 2 grs.; Balsam Tolu, 1-5 gr.; Ipecac, Kermes mineral, of each, 1-15 gr.; Morphine hydrochlorate, Oil Wintergreen, of each, 1-20 gr.
Action and uses—Expectorant and anodyne. Allays cough.
Dose 1 to 3 lozenges. On account of the contained morphine, they should be used with especial care with children.

LOZ. PEPPERMINT, U. S.
Action and uses—Used in slight gastric or intestinal pains, nausea and flatulence.
Dose 1 to 3 lozenges.

LOZ. PEPSIN AND BISMUTH.
Formula—Each lozenge contains: Pepsin, saccharated, U. S., 2 grs.; Bismuth subnitrate, 3 grs.
Action and uses—Used in intestinal irritation and indigestion.
Dose 1 to 3 lozenges as required.

LOZ. PEPSIN, BISMUTH AND CHARCOAL.
Formula—Each lozenge contains: Pepsin, saccharated, U. S., 2 grs.; Bismuth subnitrate, Willow charcoal, of each, 3 grs.
Action and uses—An efficient remedy in dyspepsia and indigestion.
Dose 1 to 3 lozenges as required.

LOZ. PEPSIN, BISMUTH, CHARCOAL AND GINGER.
Formula—Each lozenge contains: Pepsin, saccharated, U. S., Willow charcoal, of each, 5 grs.; Bismuth subnitrate, 2 grs.; Tinct. Ginger, 2 m.
Action and uses—Used in cases of indigestion accompanied with intestinal irritation, eructations and pain.
Dose 1 to 3 lozenges.

LOZ. PEPSIN, BISMUTH AND GINGER.
Formula—Each lozenge contains: Pepsin, saccharated, U. S., 2 grs.; Bismuth subnitrate, 3 grs.; Ginger, 1 gr.
Action and uses—An efficient remedy in dyspepsia and indigestion, especially when accompanied with gastric and intestinal pains.
Dose 1 to 3 lozenges.

WHEN ORDERING OR PRESCRIBING.

LOZ. PEPSIN AND CHARCOAL.

Formula—Each lozenge contains: Pepsin, saccharated, U. S., Willow charcoal, of each, 5 grs.

Action and uses—Digestive, disinfectant and absorbent. Valuable in dyspepsia with fetid breath and eructations.

Dose 1 to 2 lozenges as required.

LOZ. PEPSIN, CHARCOAL, MAGNESIA AND GINGER.

Formula—Each lozenge contains: Pepsin, saccharated, U. S., Magnesia, of each, 2 grs.; Willow charcoal, 3 grs.; Ginger, 1 gr.

Action and uses—Similar to Loz. Pepsin and Charcoal but particularly applicable where there is acidity of the stomach and flatulence.

Dose 1 to 2 lozenges

LOZ. PEPSIN SACCHARATED, U. S., 5 grs.

Action and uses—A convenient form for the administration of Pepsin.

Dose 1 to 3 lozenges.

LOZ. POTASSIUM CHLORATE, U. S., LEMON.

Formula—Each lozenge contains: Potassium chlorate, 5 grs. They are also supplied, as required, flavored with Chocolate, Vanilla or Wintergreen.

Action and uses—Useful in sore throat.

Dose. If slowly dissolved in the mouth they may be used almost continuously but should not be given excessively to children.

LOZ. POTASSIUM CHLORATE AND AMMONIUM CHLORIDE.

Formula—Each lozenge contains: Potassium chlorate, Ammonium chloride, of each, 2½ grs.

Action and uses—Useful in ordinary sore throat, ulceration and bronchial irritation.

Dose 1 lozenge as required.

LOZ. POTASSIUM CHLORATE AND CUBEB.

Formula—Each lozenge contains: Potassium chlorate, 2 grs.; Oleoresin Cubeb, 1-5 gr.

Action and uses—Useful in sore throat with chronic cough and inflammation of the fauces.

Dose 1 to 2 lozenges as required.

LOZ. POTASSIUM CHLORATE AND GUAIAC.

Formula—Each lozenge contains: Potassium chlorate, 1 gr.; Resin Guaiac, 2 grs.; Ipecac, ½ gr.

Action and uses—Useful in acute and subacute inflammation of the pharynx and in acute follicular disease of the tonsils.

Dose 1 lozenge every hour or two in acute cases.

LOZ. SANTONIN, 1-2 gr.; 1 gr.; White or pink.

Action and uses—A pleasant and effective remedy for the expulsion of round worms.

Dose 1 or 2 lozenges according to the age of the child.

LOZ. SANTONIN AND CALOMEL, CHOCOLATE; Worm Lozenges.

Formula—Each lozenge contains: Santonin, Calomel, of each, ½ gr.

Action and uses—A pleasant and effective vermifuge.

Dose 1 to 2 lozenges.

LOZ. SANTONIN COMP., White or pink.

Formula—Each lozenge contains: Santonin, Calomel, of each, ½ gr.; Podophyllin, 1-20 gr.

Action and uses—Vermifuge and cathartic.

Dose 1 to 2 lozenges according to the age of the child.

LOZ. SANTONIN AND PODOPHYLLIN.

Formula—Each lozenge contains: Santonin, ½ gr.; Podophyllin, 1-20 gr.

Action and uses—Vermifuge and cathartic.

Dose 1 to 2 lozenges according to the age of the child.

LOZ. SULPHUR COMP.; SMITH.

Formula—Each lozenge contains: Sulphur, 5 grs.; Cream tartar, 2 grs.; Ext. Ipecac, 1-100 gr., Capsicum, 1-500 gr.; Arsenous acid, 1-1000 gr.; Calcium bisulphite, ⅛ gr.

Action and uses—Cooling laxative and alterative.

Dose 1 to 2 lozenges.

LOZ. SULPHUR AND POTASSIUM BITARTRATE.

Formula—Each lozenge contains: Sulphur, precipitated, 5 grs.; Potassium bitartrate, 2 grs.

Action and uses—Cooling laxative.

Dose 1 to 3 lozenges.

LOZ. WHITE PINE COMP.; Cough lozenges.

Formula—Each lozenge contains: White pine bark, Cherry bark, of each, 4 grs.; Balm Gilead buds, Spikenard, Sassafras, of each, ½ gr.; Bloodroot, ⅛ gr.; Veratrum, ⅛ gr.; Morphine sulphate, 1-100 gr.

Action and uses—A valuable expectorant. Useful in bronchial and pulmonary affections, readily relieving cough.

LOZ. WORM; See Loz. Santonin and Calomel.

PRUNICODEINE;

LILLY.

CONTAINS NO MORPHINE.

A SAFE AND RELIABLE REMEDY FOR ACUTE AND CHRONIC BRONCHIAL AFFECTIONS.

Dr. G. Kobler of Vienna, reports that at Prof. Von Schroetter's Medical Clinic, CODEINE was employed in the capacity of a *cough sedative* in seventy cases of *pulmonary* and *laryngeal phthisis.* The results were highly satisfactory and CODEINE has proved itself to be by far the best succedaneum for morphine as a cough sedative; it is far superior to extracts of hyoscyamus, cannabis indica, etc., both as regards certainty and safety of action, as well as freedom from untoward effects. CODEINE *does not affect intestinal peristalsis.* It is of special value in bronchial catarrh, as patients taking it not only cough less frequently, but expectorate more freely than when morphine is used. The many objections to the use of morphine has caused it to be largely displaced by CODEINE in the treatment of affections of the respiratory organs which are characterized by cough. Recognizing this tendency of the profession, in PRUNICODEINE, codeine is combined with Terpin Hydrate, Pinus Strobus, Prunus Virginianus and Sanguinaria. It has met with a very satisfactory reception by physicians generally and its continued use has induced a large demand for this valuable preparation.

ELI LILLY & COMPANY,

PHARMACEUTICAL CHEMISTS,

INDIANAPOLIS, IND.,

ELI LILLY & COMPANY'S.

ELASTIC FILLED
CAPSULES

present the most elegant and desirable form for the administration of those nauseous balsams and oils, the exhibition of which have heretofore given much trouble and annoyance.

CAPS. APIOL, 5 m.

Action and uses—Apiol in 5 minim doses is carminative, diuretic, diaphoretic and expectorant and stimulates the circulation. In doses of 15 minims it is emmenagogue and seems specially useful in the amenorrhea of anemia and when the discharge is fetid.

CAPS. CASTOR OIL, 10 m., 2 1-2 grams, 5 grams.
Dose 1 to 2 capsules as required.

CAPS. COD LIVER OIL, 10 m., 2 1-2 grams, 5 grams.
Dose 1 to 2 capsules as required.

CAPS. COD LIVER OIL AND CREASOTE; See Caps. Creasote and Cod liver oil.

CAPS. COPAIBA BALSAM, 10 m.
Dose 1 to 2 capsules.

CAPS. COPAIBA AND OIL CUBEB.
Formula—Each capsule contains: Copaiba, 7 m.; Oil Cubeb, 3 m.
Dose 1 to 2 capsules.

CAPS. COPAIBA AND OLEORESIN CUBEB.
Formula—Each capsule contains: Copaiba 7 m.; Oleoresin Cubeb, 3 m.
Dose 1 to 2 capsules.

CAPS. COPAIBA, CUBEB AND BUCHU.
Formula—Each capsule contains: Copaiba, 6 m.; Oleoresin Cubeb, 2 m.; Ext. Buchu, 2 grs.
Dose 1 to 2 capsules.

CAPS. COPAIBA CUBEB AND IRON.
Formula—Each capsule contains: Copaiba, 6 m.; Oleoresin Cubeb, 2 m.; Tincture Iron chloride, 2 m.
Dose 1 to 2 capsules.

CAPS. COPAIBA, CUBEB AND MATICO.
Formula—Each capsule contains: Copaiba, 6 m.; Oleoresin Cubeb, 3 m.; Oleoresin Matico, 1 m.
Dose 1 to 2 capsules.

CAPS. COPAIBA, CUBEB, MATICO AND SANDALWOOD.
Formula—Each capsule contains: Copaiba, Oleoresin Cubeb, Oil Sandalwood, of each, 3 m.; Oleoresin Matico, 1 m.
Dose 1 to 2 capsules.

CAPS. COPAIBA, CUBEB AND SANDALWOOD.

Formula—Each capsule contains: Copaiba, 6 m.; Oil Cubeb, Oil Sandalwood, of each, 2 m.

Dose 1 to 2 capsules.

CAPS. COPAIBA AND SANDALWOOD.

Formula—Each capsule contains: Copaiba, Oil Sandalwood, of each, 5 m

Dose 1 to 2 capsules.

CAPS. CREASOTE AND COD LIVER OIL, NO. 1.

Formula—Each capsule contains: Creasote, beechwood, 1 m.; Cod liver oil, 9 m.

Dose see Caps. Creasote and Cod Liver Oil, No. 2.

CAPS. CREASOTE AND COD LIVER OIL, NO. 2.

Formula—Each capsule contains: Creasote, beechwood, 2 m.; Cod liver oil, 8 m.

Action and uses—Chemically pure creasote from beechwood tar has been highly recommended for the cure of tuberculosis by such high authority as Dr. Julius Sonnenbroit, after an experience of several years in the treatment of a large number of cases. While many modes of administration have been suggested, the elastic filled capsule, containing two minims creasote and eight minims cod liver oil, is the least objectionable. "The average patient will not tolerate more than ten to 15 minims of creasote per day for any length of time and many will bear only two or three minims per day continuously administered. The best results are obtained where the maximum quantity is given which the patient will bear. It is very important that the treatment be uniform and uninterrupted."

Dose 1 capsule.

CAPS. CUBEB OIL, 10 m.

Dose 1 capsule.

CAPS. CUBEB OIL AND SANDALWOOD.

Formula—Each capsule contains: Oil Cubeb, Oil Sandalwood, of each, 5 m.

Dose 1 capsule.

CAPS. CUBEB OLEORESIN, 10 m.

Dose 1 capsule.

CAPS. CUBEB OLEORESIN AND SANDALWOOD.

Formula—Each capsule contains: Oleoresin Cubeb, Oil Sandalwood, of each, 5 m.

Dose 1 capsule.

CAPS. EUCALYPTUS OIL.

Formula—Each capsule contains: Oil Eucalyptus, Oil Sweet almonds, of each, 5 m.

Dose 1 capsule.

CAPS. MALE FERN AND KAMALA.

Formula—Each capsule contains: Oleoresin Male fern, 7 m.; Kamala, 4 grs.

Dose. The full dose for expulsion of tape worm is 3 to 4 capsules for an adult. The patient should live upon milk and a little bread for a day previous to taking the dose which should be given in the morning and repeated in two or three hours. At noon the usual meal may be eaten followed in the evening by a brisk cathartic if necessary.

CAPS. PALMESANTAL; LILLY.
  Formula—Each capsule represents: Saw Palmetto berries, 30 grs.; Oil Sandalwood, 2 m.
  Dose 1 to 2 capsules three times per day.

CAPS. PICHI.
  Formula—Each capsule represents: Pichi, 30 grs.
  Dose 1 capsule.

CAPS. SANDALWOOD OIL, 5 m., 10 m.
  Dose 1 capsule.

CAPS. WINTERGREEN OIL, 10 m.
  Dose 1 capsule.

LILLY'S LIQUID PEPSIN.

IMPROVED.

A MOST RELIABLE LIQUID DIGESTIVE.

For the treatment of pyrosis and other forms of dyspepsia in which the use of pepsin is indicated, and particularly in the diarrhea of infants during dentition, physicians will find this the most desirable form in which to exhibit this valuable remedy.

This preparation possesses in an exceptional degree the essential ingredient of the gastric juice, preserving it in a medium at once palatable and permanent.

One fluid dram will digest 1,500 grains coagulated albumen.

One fluid dram a (teaspoonful) will curd two pints of milk at 100° F. in a few minutes.

To prepare

JUNKET.

Take one-half pint of fresh milk, heated luke warm—not warmer than can be agreeably borne by the mouth; add one teaspoonful LILLY'S LIQUID PEPSIN, and stir just enough to mix. Let it stand till firmly curded; may be served plain or with grated nutmeg.

WHEY.

Curd warm milk with LILLY'S LIQUID PEPSIN as above directed; when firmly curdled beat up with a fork until all the curd is finely divided; now strain and the whey is ready for use.

Whey is highly nutritious fluid food, containing in solution the sugar and the salts (the mineral constituents) of the milk, and holding also in suspension a considerable portion of caseine and fat (cream) which pass through the strainer. It is peculiarly useful in many ailments, and always valuable as a means of variety in diet for the sick. It is frequently resorted to as a food for infants to tide over periods of indigestion, summer complaints, etc.

Price $1.00 per Pint Bottle.

ELI LILLY & COMPANY,

PHARMACEUTICAL CHEMISTS,

INDIANAPOLIS, INDIANA, U. S. A.

ELI LILLY & COMPANY'S

Solid and Powdered Extracts.

Our apparatus and processes for the production of solid and powdered extracts are such that evaporation is carried on at so low a temperature there is no appreciable loss of volatile principles. The resulting extracts therefore present the characteristic qualities of the drugs to an eminent degree. Where preparations are indicated as "standardized" the standard adopted will be found upon the label of each package.

In the case of SOLID EXTRACTS the containing jars bear our patented attachment for removing any adhering extract from the spatula, thus avoiding waste besides making it possible to keep the label and outside of the jar in a cleanly condition. All sizes are thus provided, excepting the one ounce jars.

For medicinal properties of solid and powdered extracts, refer to the fluid extract list, pages 5 to 130.

DOSAGE FOR ELI LILLY & COMPANY'S BRAND ONLY.

NAME OF EXTRACT	DOSE SOLID.	DOSE POWDERED.
Aconite leaves	1-2 to 1 gr	1-2 to 1 gr.
Aconite root standardized	1-8 to 1-2 gr	1-8 to 1-2 grs.
Aloes, aqueous	3 to 6 grs.	3 to 6 grs.
Apocynum; See Black Indian hemp.		
Arnica flowers	1 to 2 grs	1 to 2 grs.
Arnica root	3 to 5 grs.	
Bearsfoot	1 to 3 grs.	
Belladonna leaves, standardized	1-4 to 1-2 gr	1-4 to 1-2 gr.
Belladonna leaves, purely alcoholic, standardized	1-8 to 1-4 gr.	
Belladonna root, standardized	1-4 to 1-2 gr	1-4 to 1-2 gr.
Berberis aquifolium	2 to 4 grs	2 to 4 grs.
Bitter root	1-2 to 1 gr.	
Bittersweet	5 to 10 grs.	
Black ash bark	5 to 10 grs.	
Blackberry root		3 to 8 grs.
Black cohosh	5 to 10 grs	5 to 10 grs.
Black haw	5 to 10 grs	5 to 10 grs.
Black hellebore	3 to 5 grs	3 to 5 grs.
Black Indian hemp	1 to 3 grs	1 to 3 grs.
Black willow bark	5 to 10 grs.	
Black willow buds	5 to 10 grs.	
Bladderwrack	4 to 7 grs	4 to 7 grs.
Blessed thistle	4 to 8 grs.	
Bloodroot	1-2 to 1 gr.	1-2 to 1 gr.
Blue cohosh	2 to 5 grs	2 to 5 grs.
Blue flag	1 to 3 grs.	1 to 3 grs.
Boneset	3 to 10 grs	3 to 10 grs.
Buchu	5 to 10 grs	10 to 20 grs.
Buckthorn bark	5 to 15 grs.	
Bugleweed	5 to 10 grs.	
Burdock root	10 to 20 grs.	

NAME OF EXTRACT.	DOSE SOLID.	DOSE POWDERED.
Butternut	10 to 30 grs.	10 to 30 grs.
Calabar bean	1-16 to 1-8 gr.	
Calendula flowers	5 to 15 grs.	
Calumba; See Columbo.		
Canadian hemp; See Black Indian hemp.		
Cannabis Indica	1 to 10 grs	1 to 10 grs.
Capsicum	1-8 to 1-4 gr.	
Cascara amaraga	5 to 10 grs.	
Cascara sagrada	2 to 20 grs.	2 to 20 grs.
Cascarilla	4 to 6 grs	
Celery seed	4 to 8 grs.	
Chamomile Roman	2 to 8 grs.	
Chestnut leaves		3 to 8 grs.
Cimicifuga; See Black cohosh.		
Chimaphila; See Pipsissewa.		
Cinchona pale, standardized	5 to 20 grs.	
Cinchona red, standardized	3 to 10 gr.	
Cinchona yellow, standardized	5 to 15 grs.	5 to 15 grs.
Clover tops	5 to 10 grs.	
Coca leaves, standardized	4 to 12 grs.	
Colchicum root, standardized	1-2 to 1 gr.	1-2 to 1 gr.
Colchicum seed, standardized	1-2 to 1 gr.	1-2 to 1 gr.
Colocynth		1 to 2 grs.
Colocynth comp		5 to 20 grs.
Columbo	1 to 3 grs	1 to 3 grs.
Condurango		5 to 12 grs.
Conium fruit	1-4 to 1 gr	1-4 to 1 gr
Conium leaves	1-2 to 2 grs.	1-2 to 2 grs.
Cotton root bark	5 to 15 grs.	5 to 15 grs.
Couch grass	10 to 60 grs.	
Cramp bark		5 to 10 grs.
Cranesbill	4 to 8 grs	4 to 8 grs.
Cubeb	1 to 5 grs.	
Culver's root	5 to 15 grs.	5 to 15 grs.
Cypripedium; See Ladies' slipper.		
Damiana	5 to 15 grs	5 to 15 grs.
Dandelion	10 to 60 grs	10 to 60 grs.
Digitalis	1-8 to 1-2 gr	1-8 to 1-2 gr.
Dogwood	4 to 8 grs.	
Duboisia leaves	1-8 to 1-2 gr.	
Dulcamara; See Bittersweet.		
Elecampane	4 to 8 grs	4 to 8 grs.
Ergot		6 to 60 grs.
Ergot soluble in water	4 to 40 grs.	
Eriodyction; See Yerba santa.		
Eucalyptus	2 to 4 grs.	2 to 4 grs.
Euonymus, See Wahoo.		
Eupatorium; See Boneset.		
False bittersweet	4 to 8 grs.	
False unicorn	2 to 4 grs.	2 to 4 grs.
Foxglove; See Digitalis.		
Frangula; See Buckthorn bark.		
Fringetree bark	5 to 10 grs.	
Gelsemium, standardized	1-2 to 1 gr.	1-2 to 1 gr.
Gentian	5 to 15 grs.	5 to 15 grs.
Geranium; See Cranesbill.		

NAME OF EXTRACT	DOSE SOLID.	DOSE POWDERED.
Goldenseal	10 to 20 grs	10 to 20 grs.
Grindelia	10 to 20 grs	10 to 20 grs.
Guaiac		5 to 20 grs.
Guarana	5 to 10 grs	5 to 10 grs.
Hamamelis; See Witchhazel.		
Hemlock bark	5 to 10 grs	5 to 10 grs.
Henbane; See Hyoscyamus.		
Hop	5 to 15 grs	5 to 15 grs.
Horehound	6 to 12 grs.	
Hydrangea		10 to 20 grs.
Hydrastis; See Goldenseal.		
Hyoscyamus	1-2 to 1 gr	1-2 to 1 gr.
Ignatia bean	1-4 to 1 gr	1-4 to 1 gr.
Indian cannabis; See Cannabis Indica.		
Indigo		4 to 8 grs.
Ipecac, standardized	1-4 to 2 grs	1-4 to 2 grs.
Iris; See Blue flag.		
Jaborandi	3 to 6 grs.	3 to 6 grs.
Jalap	5 to 10 grs	5 to 10 grs.
Jamaica dogwood	4 to 8 grs	4 to 8 grs.
Juniper berries	5 to 20 grs.	
Kola nut	5 to 10 grs.	
Krameria; See Rhatany.		
Ladies' slipper	4 to 8 grs	4 to 8 grs.
Lappa; See Burdock.		
Leptandra; See Culver's root.		
Lettuce	5 to 10 grs	5 to 10 grs.
Licorice	10 to 20 grs.	
Life root	5 to 10 grs.	
Lobelia herb	1-4 to 1 gr	1-4 to 1 gr.
Male fern	15 to 60 grs.	
Mandrake	1 to 4 grs.	1 to 4 grs.
Mezereum	1-8 to 1-2 gr.	
Mistletoe		5 to 10 grs.
Musk root	1-2 to 1 gr.	
Myrrh		3 to 15 grs.
Nux vomica, standardized	1-8 to 1-2 gr	1-8 to 1-2 gr.
Opium, standardized	1-4 to 1 gr	1-4 to 1 gr.
Oxgall; See Miscellaneous Preparations, page 226.		
Pareira Brava		15 to 30 grs.
Physostigma; See Calabar bean.		
Phytolacca root; See Pokeroot.		
Pichi	2 to 10 grs	2 to 10 grs.
Pilocarpus; See Jaborandi.		
Pipsissewa	15 to 30 grs.	
Podophyllum; See Mandrake.		
Poison oak		1-2 to 2 grs.
Poke berries	4 to 8 grs.	
Poke root	6 to 12 grs	6 to 12 grs.
Prickly ash bark	2 to 5 grs	2 to 5 grs.
Pulsatilla	1-2 to 1 gr	1-2 to 1 gr.
Pumpkin seed	20 to 80 grs.	
Quassia	1-4 to 1-2 gr	1-4 to 1-2 gr.
Quebracho	2 to 8 grs	2 to 8 grs.
Queen of the meadow	5 to 10 grs	5 to 10 grs.
Red Clover blossoms; See Clover tops.		

NAME OF EXTRACT.	DOSE SOLID.	DOSE POWDERED.
Rhatany	2 to 10 grs	2 to 10 grs.
Rhubarb	2 to 15 grs	2 to 15 grs.
Rhus aromatica	1 to 6 grs.	
Rubus; See Blackberry root.		
Rumex; See Yellow dock.		
Sanguinaria; See Bloodroot.		
Sarsaparilla	5 to 10 grs	5 to 10 grs.
Sarsaparilla compound	5 to 10 grs.	
Savin		1-2 to 2 grs.
Saw Palmetto berries	6 to 12 grs.	
Scullcap	5 to 15 grs	5 to 15 grs.
Scutellaria; See Scullcap.		
Seneka		2 to 4 grs.
Senna	15 to 60 grs	15 to 60 grs.
Sheep laurel	2 to 4 grs.	
Sheep sorrel	5 to 10 grs.	
Squawvine	10 to 20 grs	10 to 20 grs.
Stargrass; See Unicorn root.		
Stillingia	1-2 to 4 grs	1-2 to 4 grs.
Stone root	1-2 to 2 grs	1-2 to 2 grs.
Stramonium leaves, standardized	1-8 to 1-2 gr	1-8 to 1-2 gr.
Stramonium seed, standardized	1-8 to 1-2 gr.	
Taraxacum; See Dandelion.		
Triticum; See Couchgrass.		
Unicorn root	1 to 3 grs	1 to 3 grs.
Uva Ursi	15 to 30 grs	15 to 30 grs.
Valerian	5 to 10 grs	5 to 10 grs.
Veratrum viride, standardized	1-4 to 1-2 gr	1-4 to 1 2 gr.
Vervain	5 to 10 grs.	
Viburnum prunifolium; See Black haw.		
Wahoo	5 to 10 grs	5 to 10 grs.
Warburg's tincture		2 to 12 grs.
Warburg's tincture, without aloes		2 to 12 grs.
Water pepper		5 to 10 grs.
White Indian hemp	1 to 4 grs.	
White oak bark	2 to 6 grs.	
Wild indigo	3 to 6 grs	3 to 6 grs.
Wild yam	5 to 10 grs	5 to 10 grs.
Witchhazel	5 to 10 grs	5 to 10 grs.
Wormwood	5 to 10 grs.	
Xanthoxylum; See Prickly ash.		
Yellow dock	5 to 10 grs	5 to 10 grs.
Yerba santa	6 to 15 grs.	

ELI LILLY & COMPANY'S
CONCENTRATIONS;
Eclectic Resinoids.

Concentrated preparations containing the valuable constituents of the drugs which they represent, freed from the greater portion of inert matter which usually accompanies them in other preparations. Our methods are adapted to each drug after careful study of its nature. For medicinal properties see corresponding drugs in Fluid Extract list, pages 3 to 159.

CONCENTRATION.	DRUG.	DOSE.
Aletrin	Unicorn root	1-2 to 2 grs.
Alnuin	Tag alder	3 to 6 grs.
Aloin	Aloes	1-10 to 2 grs.
Apocynin	Bitter root	1-2 to 1 gr.
Baptisin	Wild indigo	3 to 6 grs.
Barosmin	Buchu	5 to 10 grs.
Berberine, salts of; See page 224.		
Cascarin	Cascara sagrada	2 to 6 grs.
Chelonin	Balmony	3 to 6 grs.
Caulophyllin	Blue cohosh	2 to 4 grs.
Chimaphilin	Pipsissewa	2 to 5 grs.
Cimicifugin	Black cohosh	3 to 6 grs.
Cypripedin	Ladies' slipper	1-4 to 1-2 gr.
Digitalin	Foxglove	1-8 to 1-2 gr.
Dioscorein	Wild yam	3 to 5 grs.
Euonymin	Wahoo	2 to 4 grs.
Eupatorin	Boneset	1 to 4 grs.
Eupurpurin	Queen of the meadow	2 to 5 grs.
Gelsemin	Gelsemium	1-2 to 1 gr.
Geranin	Cranesbill	5 to 10 grs.
Gossypiin	Cotton root bark	1 1-2 to 3 grs.
Hamamelin	Whitchhazel	4 to 7 grs.
Helonin	False unicorn	2 to 3 grs.
Hydrastin	Goldenseal	4 to 8 grs.
Hydrastine and salts; See page 225.		
Hyoscyamin	Henbane	1-2 to 1 gr.
Inulain	Elecampane	3 to 6 grs.
Irisin	Blue flag	1 to 2 grs.
Jalapin	Jalap	2 to 4 grs.
Juglandin	Butternut	5 to 15 grs.
Leptandrin	Culver's root	2 to 8 grs.
Lobellin	Lobelia	1-2 to 2 grs.
Lycopin	Bugle weed	2 to 5 grs.
Macrotin; See Cimicifugin.		
Menispermin	Yellow parilla	1 to 5 grs.
Myricin	Bayberry	3 to 6 grs.
Phytollaccin	Poke root	3 to 6 grs.
Podophyllin	Mandrake	1-40 to 1 gr.
Populin	White poplar	1 1-2 to 3 grs.
Ptelin	Wafer ash	2 to 6 grs.
Sanguinarin	Blood root	1-2 to 1 gr.
Sanguinarine nitrate; See page 227.		
Scutellarin	Scullcap	3 to 6 grs.
Senecin	Life root	2 to 4 grs.
Trillin	Beth root	3 to 6 grs.
Virburnin	Cramp bark	3 to 6 grs.
Xanthoxylin	Prickly ash bark	2 to 8 grs.

WHEN ORDERING OR PRESCRIBING.

ELI LILLY & COMPANY'S

Miscellaneous Preparations.

ACETANILID POWDER; Lilly.

Pure acetanilid impalpably powdered for surgeons use. Dr. Eslamer, of the German Hospital, Philadelphia, used Acetanilid powder in all surgical cases for four months with happiest results. It is applied to chancroids, to syphilitic leg ulcers and to mucous patches. Simple ulcers following burns of the second degree healed promptly without pus.

ACETANILID COMP., SPECIAL, POWDER.

Formula—Acetanilid, 6 parts; Sodium bicarbonate, 2 parts; Ammonium chloride, Caffeine citrate, of each, 1 part.

Action and uses—See Compressed Tablets Acetanilid comp., special, page 178.

Dose 5 to 10 grains.

ACID SALICYLIC, c. p. from Oil Wintergreen.

Claimed to be greatly superior to the artificial acid for medicinal use.

ANALGESIC POWDER.

Formula—Acetanilid, 6 parts; Sodium bicarbonate, 4 parts; Caffeine citrate, 1 part.

Action and uses—See Compressed Tablets Analgesic, page 199.

Dose 5 to 10 grains.

BERBERINE HYDROCHLORATE; Lilly.
BERBERINE PHOSPHATE; Lilly.
BERBERINE SULPHATE; Lilly.

Salts of the yellow alkaloid of Hydrastis Canadensis. Found also in other plants.

Action and uses—The Berberine salts are antiperiodic, stomachic and tonic. Used in malarial affections, enlargement of the spleen, amenorrhea, anorexia, chronic intestinal catarrh, vomiting of pregnancy, etc. The phosphate is the most soluble salt.

Dose—Antiperiodic, 5 to 10 grains; stomachic and tonic, ½ to 1 grain.

BOROGLYCERIDE, 50% SOLUTION; Glyceritum boroglycerini, U. S.

Formula—Contains equal parts of true glyceryl borate and glycerin.

Action and uses—A valuable antiseptic and disinfectant; nonpoisonous and not irritating. Used for surgical dressings, promoting the healing of sores, wounds and suppurating surfaces. Being free from color and odor it presents palpable advantages over iodoform and other well known antiseptics.

Note.—True boroglyceride is soluble in 12 parts of water, the 50 per cent. solution therefore requiring 6 parts of water for solution, a lesser quantity of water will decompose the boroglyceride. Hence, should a solution be found which will dissolve in a lesser quantity than 6 parts of water it cannot possibly be a 50 per cent. solution of true boroglyceride.

CALOMEL SUGAR POWDER.

Formula—Calomel, 1 part; Milk sugar, 5 parts. Thus six grains represent 1 grain calomel.

It is maintained by many practitioners that calomel thoroughly triturated with pure milk sugar possesses a more energetic action than when undiluted. This article is prepared by prolonged trituration in power triturators.

In prescribing doses care should be taken to begin with about the same quantity of the calomel sugar powder as is usually given of calomel, increasing if necessary.

CHLORODYNE, Chandler's formula.

Formula—Each fluid ounce contains: Morphine sulphate, 4 grs.; Ext. Cannabis Indica, 8 grs.; Chloroform, 1 fluid dram; Oil Peppermint, 4 minims; Fluid Ext. Capsicum, 1 minim; Alcohol, Glycerin q. s. to make 1 fluid ounce.

Action and uses—Anodyne, antispasmodic, sedative and diaphoretic. This preparation produces all the desirable effects of opium, without the unpleasant after effects which so often follow the use of other opiates.

Dose for an adult is 20 drops; for children, 3 to 8 drops, according to age. The dose may be repeated every hour or so if relief is not obtained by the first. Any decided increase of the doses, even in severe cases, should only be given by the instruction of the physician.

COCAINE TABLETS, **for preparing solutions**; See Compressed Tablets Cocaine, page 200

ERGOTIN, BONJEAN.

Hydroalcoholic extract of Ergot.

Action and uses—Same as ergot.

Dose 3 to 10 grains.   Decomposes spontaneously in solution.

ERGOTIN, purified for hypodermic use.

This ergotin possesses all the valuable properties of ergot, absolutely free from inert matter and those principles proved to produce noxious effects. Admirably adapted to hypodermic use.

Dose 1 to 6 grains.

EUCALYPTUS AND THYMOL ANTISEPTIC.

Formula—Sodium borate, Benzoic acid, Boric acid, Thymol, Oil Eucalyptus, Oil Wintergreen, Oil Thyme, Oil Peppermint, Fluid Ext. Wild Indigo.

Action and uses—This valuable liquid antiseptic being nonpoisonous and acting without irritation, having a cooling and soothing effect, has a wide range of application both as an external and an internal remedy. It replaces iodoform and carbolic acid and may be substituted for either with confidence. It is a delightful addition to the bath and forms an elegant wash for the mouth. Used as a spray.

Internally the dose is 1 fluid dram three or four times daily.

HYDRASTINE; Lilly.   The white alkaloid of Hydrastis Canadensis.
HYDRASTINE HYDROCHLORATE; **Lilly.**
HYDRASTINE SULPHATE; **Lilly.**

The alkaloid Hydrastine is alterative, tonic and antiperiodic. Dose ⅓ to ½ grain. The hydrochlorate, soluble in water, is the salt generally used. It is astringent, alterative, tonic and hemostatic. Internally used in uterine hemorrhage, dyspepsia, hemorrhoids, etc. Dose ⅓ to 1 grain every two hours if necessary. Externally in gonorrhea, conjunctivitis leucorrhea, cervical erosions, acne, etc. As an astringent 1-10 to ½% solution; in diseases of the skin 1% ointment or lotion.

LIME JUICE AND PEPSIN.

An elegant and reliable digestive. One fluid dram digests, 1,500 grains coagulated albumen, by the official test.

Dose 1 to **4 fluid** drams.

LIQUID DIASTASE; Lilly.

Action and uses—An elegant preparation pleasant to the taste, readily digesting starchy foods. Of great value in the treatment of gastrointestinal dyspepsia, and for removing accumulation of flatus from stomach and bowels, accompanied by disagreeable eructations and intestinal pains.

Dose 1 to 2 teaspoonfuls after meals.

LOEFFLER'S SOLUTION, for the local treatment of diphtheria.

Made according to the formula of Prof. Loeffler, the discoverer of the diphtheria bacillus, and composed of Alcohol, 60%; Toluol, 36%, and

Solution ferric chloride, 4%. Menthol is added to deaden the pain caused by the application which is effected by means of pieces of wadding or as a spray, the affected parts being treated, at first every three or four hours. Of seventyone patients treated by this method from the outset, all were saved, while only one death occured out of twenty six cases treated after the second day of the attack.

OXGALL, PURIFIED, U. S.

Oxgall purified, U. S., powdered.

Action and uses—See Pil. Oxgall and Pil. Oxgall comp., page 158.

Dose 5 to 10 grains.

PANCREATIN, PURE; Lilly.

Properties—A concentrated preparation combining the various digestive ferments of the pancreatic secretions. It converts casein or other albuminous matter into grape sugar, curdles milk and emulsifies fats.

Five grains will thoroughly peptonize one pint of milk in at least one hour, if kept at a temperature of 110° F.

Dose 5 to 10 grains. It may be combined with pepsin in any proportion.

PANCREATIN, LIQUID; Lilly.

Formula—Each fluid dram represents 5 grs. Pancreatin, pure; Lilly, and will peptonize one pint of milk in at least one hour if kept at a temperature of 110° F.

Properties—See Pancreatin, pure; Lilly.

Dose 1 to 2 fluid drams.

PANCREATIN, SACCHARATED; Lilly.

Formula—Pancreatin pure; Lilly, 1 part; Sugar milk, 9 parts. Fifty grains of this preparation will peptonize one pint of milk in at least one hour if kept at a temperature of 110° F.

Properties—See Pancreatin pure; Lilly

Dose 30 to 120 grains.

PEPSIN U. S.; Powder, 1:3000.

This is strictly the official uniform preparation and meets every requirement of the Pharmacopœia, 1880. One grain will digest 3000 grains coagulated albumen by the U. S. test.

Dose 5 to 15 grains.

PEPSIN, U. S., Soluble scales, 1:3000.

This is strictly the official uniform preparation and meets every requirement of the Pharmacopœia, 1880. One grain will digest 3000 grains coagulated albumen by the U. S. test.

Dose 5 to 15 grains.

PEPSIN CONCENTRATED SOLUTION.

10 minims will digest 2,000 grains coagulated albumen.

A reliable and permanent article, useful in making the various liquid preparations of pepsin. Where it is desirable to make a preparation of the same strength of the N. F. pepsin elixirs, use 340 minims of this solution to each pint.

PEPSIN ESSENCE.

Possessing the valuable constituents of the gastric juice.

One teaspoonful will curd two pints of milk at 100° F. in a few minutes. To prepare

Junket—Take ½ pint of fresh milk, heated luke warm—not warmer than can be agreeably borne by the mouth; add one teaspoonful of Essence of Pepsin, and stir just enough to mix. Let it stand till firmly curded; may be served plain or with sugar and grated nutmeg.

Whey—Curd warm milk with Essence of Pepsin as above directed; when firmly curded beat up with a fork until the curd is finely divided; now strain and the whey is ready for use. Whey is highly nutritious fluid food, containing in solution the sugar and the mineral constituents of the milk, and holding also in suspension a considerable portion of casein and cream which passes through the strainer. It is peculiarly useful in many ailments, and always valuable as a means of variety in diet for the sick. It is frequently resorted to as a food for infants to tide over periods of indigestion, summer complaints, etc.

PEPSIN, LACTATED.

Formula—Each five grains contains: Pure pepsin, digestive power of 1:200, ½ gr.; Pancreatin, pure, ½ gr.; Lactid acid, Hydrochloric acid, Maltose and Diastase.

Action and uses—Lactated pepsin combining as it does the several digestive ferments has a wider range of application than simple pepsin. It is therefore preferable in cases where there is not only lack of digestion of the albuminoids but where starchy and fatty foods are not assimilated.

Dose 5 to 15 grains.

PEPSIN LIQUID, U. S., 1880.

Dose 1-2 to 2 fluid ounces.

PEPSIN, SACCHARATED, U. S.,

One grain will digest 300 grains coagulated albumen by the U. S. test.

SANGUINARINE NITRATE; Lilly.

Action and uses—Stimulant, tonic, expectorant, purgative, emetic. Used in dyspepsia, debility, colds, coughs and as an emetic. Soluble in water.

Dose 1-2 to 1-6 grain as an expectorant; 1-2 to 3-4 grain as an emetic. Given in solution.

SOLUTION BISMUTH AND HYDRASTIA.

Action and uses— A valuable local application in diseases of the eye, the nasal passages, and of mucous surfaces generally. Internally beneficial in diseases of the stomach or bowels. As an injection 1 part of solution to 4 parts of soft or distilled water. Absorbent cotton saturated with the undiluted solution may be used when desired. Internal doses, 10 to 30 minims in water, thrice daily.

SOLUTION HYPOPHOSPHITES COMP., without sugar.

Formula—Each fluid ounce contains: Calcium hypophosphite, Potassium hypophosphite, of each, 4 grs.; Iron hypophosphite, 2 grs.; Sodium hypophosphite, Manganese hypophosphite, Quinine hypophosphite, of each, 1 gr.; Strychnine hypophosphite, 1-32 gr.

Action and uses—A most valuable and efficient means of administering the hypophosphites. Being free from sugar it is useful in cases where the syrup would be inadmissable. As a general tonic and to replace waste this combination is perhaps unsurpassed. It is perfectly stable, free from salinity and astringency, does not derange the stomach and is well borne by the most delicate. It aids digestion, promotes nutrition and will be found invaluable for strengthing weakly constitutions suffering from languor and loss of appetite.

Dose 1 to 2 fluid drams at meal time. Children according to age.

PALMETTO CORDIAL; LILLY.

CORDIAL PALMETTO COMP.

Combining perfectly the therapeutic virtues of the fresh berries of *Serenœa Serrulata* and *Santalum Albnm.* For the treatment of diseases of

GENITO-URINARY SYSTEM.

Specially indicated in pre-senility, prostatic troubles, irritation of bladder and urethral inflammation.

See Page 194.

ELI LILLY & COMPANY,
Pharmaceutical Chemists,
INDIANAPOLIS, IND.

SPECIALTIES.

Elixir Purgans; Lilly................................See page 325

A palatable liquid cathartic composed of Rhamnus Purshiana, Euonymus atropurpureus, Cassia acutifolia purified, Iris versicolor, Hyoscyamus and aromatics. Booklet upon application.

Formaseptol; Lilly....................... .. ..See page 330.

A combination of Formaldehyde in liquid form with Cinnamol, Thymol, Eucalyptol, Menthol, Gaultheria, Sodium borate and Benzoic acid under the title, Formaseptol; Lilly. Presents advantages **over** any other liquid antiseptic now in use.

Glycones; Lilly. Infant and adult sizes...........See page 326.

An improved form of glycerin suppository, contain 95% pure glycerin. Send for booklet and sample.

Liquid Pepsin; Lilly....... ....See page 224.

One fluid dram will curd two pints of milk at 100° F. in a few minutes; the same quantity will peptonize 1500 grains coagulated albumen by the U. S. test.

Liquor Ferri; Lilly. ....See page 260.

A solution of an organic salt of iron, neutral, permanent, free from styptic taste compatible with bitter tonics, and does not derange the stomach when taken for a lengthy period. Contains the equivalent of 1% metallic iron.

Pil. Aphrodisiaca; Lilly............... ... .See page 324.

A food and tonic to the nervous system. **Extract Damiana**, Extract Nux vomica and Phosphorus, Oval in shape, pink in color. Send for booklet.

Prunicodeine; Lilly.... ....See page 221.

An elegant cough cordial, contains no morphine. Each fluid dram represents, Prunus Virginianus, 3 grs.; Pinus strobus, 2 grs.; Sanguinaria, ½ gr.; Terpin hydrate, ½ gr.; Codeine, ½ gr.

Succus Alterans; Lilly.. ....See page 311.

A powerful vegetable alterative, made prominent by Dr. J. Marion Sims. Formula and full particulars mailed to physicians and pharmacists upon application.

Yerbazin; Lilly...See page 327.

A perfect mask for the bitterness of Quinine, extremely palatable, and causes no chemical change in Quinine salts. Send for booklet.

BOTANICAL INDEX.

CONTAINING THE BOTANICAL NAMES AND SYNONYMS, AND COMMON
SYNONYMS OF DRUGS OCCURING IN THE FLUID
EXTRACT LIST, PAGES 5 TO 130.

For the convenience of our patrons and those having occasion to
consult our list we present the following index. The *left* column contains the botanical names, synonyms (with the authors' names or
their abbreviations), and the common synonyms; the *right* column
contains the names used in the list. The botanical synonyms in the
left column are indicated by an asterisk.

Abies Canadensis Michx.....................................Hemlock.
Acacia Catechu (Linn.) Willd................................Catechu.
Achillea Millefolium Linn....................................Yarrow.
Aconitum Napellus Linn.....................................Aconite.
*Aconitum vulgare D. C.....................................Aconite.
Acorus Calamus Linn.......................................Calamus.
Actæa alba (Linn.) Mill................................White cohosh.
Actæa racemosa Linn..................................Black cohosh.
*Actæa spicata var. alba Linn........................White cohosh.
Adiantum pedatum Linn..................................Maidenhair.
*Adonis vernalis Linn..............................Adonis vernalis.
Æsculus Hippocastanum Linn.........................Horse chestnut.
Agrimonia Eupatoria Walt..................................Agrimony.
*Agrimonia striata Michx..................................Agrimony.
Agropyrum repens (Linn.) Beauvois.....................Couch grass.
Ailanthus glandulosa Desf..................................Ailanthus.
Alder buckthorn..Buckthorn bark.
Aletris farinosa Linn....................................Unicorn root.
Alexandria senna..Senna.
Alkanna tinctoria Tausch..................................Alkanet.
Allium sativum Linn..Garlic.
Allspice...Pimenta.
*Alnus rugosa (Ehrh.) Koch..............................Tag alder.
Alnus serrulata Willd....................................Tag alder.
Aloe Perryi Baker..Aloes.
Aloe Socotrina, U. S..Aloes.
*Aloe succotrina Lam..Aloe.
Alpina officinarum Hance..................................Galangal.
Alstonia constricta F. v. Mueller...............Alstonia constricta.
Alstonia scholaris (Linn.) R. Brown.....................Dita bark.
Althæa officinalis Linn...........................Marshmallow root.
Ambrosia...Ragweed.
Ambrosia artemisiæfolia Linn..............................Ragweed.
American ash...American white ash.
American balm of Gilead..........................Balm of Gilead.
American beechnut.......................................Beech bark.
American cannabis....................................American hemp.
American gentian......................................Blue gentian.
American Greek valerian...............................Abscess root.
American mistletoe.......................................Mistletoe.
American mountain ash...............................Mountain ash.
American sanicle..Alum root.
American valerian..................................Ladies' slipper.
*Amomum Curcuma Jacq.....................................Turmeric.
Amomum Granum-paradisi Afzelius.................Grains of paradise.
*Amomum Melegueta Roscoe......................Grains of paradise.
Amomum repens Sonnerat.................................Cardamom.
Ampelopsis quinquefolia Michx........................American ivy.
*Amygdalus Persica Linn................................Peach leaves.
Anacyclus Pyrethrum (Linn.) D. C......................Pellitory.
*Anamirta Cocculus Wight & Arnott................Cocculus Indicus.
Anamirta paniculata Colebrook.....................Cocculus Indicus.
*Anchusa tinctoria Lam....................................Alkanet.
*Andromeda arborea Linn.............................Sourwood leaves.
*Andropogon saccharatus Roxb....................Broom corn seed.
*Anemone Hepatica Linn..................................Liverwort.
Anemone pratensis Linn..................................Pulsatilla.
Anemone Pulsatilla Linn................................Pulsatilla.
Anethum graveolens Linn......................................Dill.

Angelica atropurpurea Linn...Angelica.
Anise, common..Anise.
Anisum..Anise.
*Anona triloba Linn..Pawpaw seed.
Anthemis nobilis Linn...Chamomile.
*Anthemis Pyrethrum Linn...Pellitory.
Apium graveolens Linn...Celery seed.
Apium Petroselinum Linn...Parsley.
Apocynum androsæmifolium Linn...Bitter root.
Apocynum cannabinum Linn...Black Indian hemp.
Apple Peru..Stramonium.
Aralia hispida Vent..Dwarf elder.
Aralia nudicaulis Linn..American sarsaparilla.
Aralia racemosa Linn..Spikenard.
*Arbutus Uva Ursi Linn...Uva Ursi.
"Archangelica atropurpurea Hoffm.......................................Angelica.
Arctium Lappa Linn...Burdock.
*Arctium majus Schkuhr...Burdock.
Arctostaphylos glauca Lindley....................................Manzanita leaves.
Arctostaphylos Uva Ursi (Linn.) Sprengel....................Uva Ursi.
Areca Catechu Linn...Areca nut.
Arisæma triphyllum (Linn.) Torr...Indian turnip.
Aristolochia reticulata Nutt...Serpentaria.
Aristolochia Serpentaria Linn..Serpentaria.
Arnica montana Linn..Arnica.
*Artanthe elongata Miquel...Matico.
Artemisia Absinthium Linn...Wormwood.
Artemisia frigida Willd...Mountain sage.
*Artemisia maritima Linn., var. Stechmanniana Besser.............
                                Levant wormseed.
Artemisia pauciflora Weber..Levant wormseed.
Artemisia vulgaris Linn..Mugwort.
*Arum triphyllum Linn..Indian turnip.
*Asagræa officinalis Lindl...Cevadilla seed.
Asarum Canadense Linn...Canada snakeroot.
*Asclepias Cornuti Decaisne...Silkweed.
Asclepias incarnata Linn...................................White Indian hemp.
Asclepias Syriaca Linn...Silkweed.
*Asclepias Syriaca var. Illinœnsis Pers...Silkweed.
Asclepias tuberosa Linn...Pleurisy root.
Asimina triloba (Linn.) Dunal.................................Pawpaw seed.
Asparagus officinalis Linn...Asparagus.
Aspen...White popular bark.
*Aspidium Filix-mas Swartz..Male fern.
*Aspidium marginale Swartz..Male fern.
Aspidosperma Quebracho Schlecht............................Quebracho.
Astringent root...Cranesbill.
Atropa Belladonna Linn..Belladonna.
Aurantii Amari..Orange peel, bitter.
Aurantii Dulcis...Orange peel, sweet.
Australian fever bark....................................Alstonia constricta.
Australian fever tree..Eucalyptus.
Ava Kava..Kava Kava.
Avena sativa Linn..Avena sativa.
Balm..Lemon balm.
*Balsamodendron Myrrha Nees...Myrrh.
Balsam poplar..Balm of Gilead.
Balsam of Tolu...Tolu.
Balsam weed...Jewel weed.
*Banksia Abyssinica Bruce..Kousso.
Baptisia tinctoria (Linn.) R. Brown...............................Wild indigo.
Barosma betulina (Thunb.) Bartl. et Wendland...........Buchu.
Barosma crenulata (Linn.) Hooker.......................................Buchu.
Bay berry...Bay laurel.
Bean of St. Ignatius..Ignatia bean.
Bearberry..Manzanita leaves.
Bearberry..Uva Ursi.
Bearsbed...Hair cap moss.
Bedstraw...Cleavers.
*Benzoin Benzoin (Linn.) Coulter..Feverbush.
Benzoin odoriferum Nees...Feverbush.
Benzoin officinale Hayne..Benzoin.
Benzoinum..Benzoin.
Berberis aquifolium Pursh...Berberis aquifolium.
*Berberis nervosa Pursh..Berberis aquifolium.
*Berberis repens Lindley..Berberis aquifolium.
Berberis vulgaris Linn...Barberry bark.
Betelnut..Areca nut.

Betonica officinalis Linn........ .... Wood betony.
Betula rugosa Ehrh... Tag alder.
Bhang...Cannabis Indica.
*Bicuculla Canadensis (Goldie) Millsp .... Turkey corn.
*Bignonia Caroba Vellos............................ ....Caroba leaves.
*Bignonia Copaia Aublet................................ ...Caroba leaves.
*Bignonia sempervirens Linn.............................Gelsemium.
Bird pepper..Capsicum.
Birdseye................................... ....Adonis vernalis.
Birdsfoot violet........... .... Violet herb.
Birthroot.. Beth root.
Bitter apple...Colocynth.
Bitter cucumber..Colocynth.
Bitterstick..Chirata.
Bitter thistle... ....Blessed thistle.
Blackcherry..Belladonna.
Black larch..Tamarac bark.
Black mustard...Mustard seed.
Black root........ ....Culver's root.
Black snakeroot...Black cohosh.
Blooming spurge.......................Large flowering spurge.
Blue bells... Abscess root.
*Boldoa fragrans Ruiz et Pavon...................... .....Boldo leaves.
Bombay root... Galangal.
Bouncing Bet... .. Soapwort.
Boxwood..Dogwood.
Boybean ....Buckbean leaves.
*Brassica nigra Koch.......................................Mustard seed.
Brayera...Kousso.
*Bravera anthelmintica Kunth............................Kousso.
Brittlestem...Dwarf elder.
Broad leaved laurel..Mountain laurel.
Brookbean... ....Buckbean leaves.
Broom..Broom tops.
Broom corn grass............. ... .Broom corn seed.
Broom flowers..Broom tops.
Brunfelsia Hopeana (Hook.) Benth........................Manaca.
Bryonia alba Linn..White bryony.
*Buettneria florida (Linn.) Kearney...................Florida allspice.
Bugsbane ....Black cohosh.
Bullsfoot ....Coltsfoot.
Burning bush...Wahoo root bark.
*Bursa Bursa-Pastoris (Linn.) Weber..................... Shepherd's purse.
Butterfly-weed....................................Pleurisy root.
*Cactus grandiflorus Linn............................Cactus grandiflorus.
Calendula officinalis Linn............................. Calendula.
Calico bush..Mountain laurel.
*Callicocca Ipecacuanha Brotero......................... Ipecac.
Calumba ....Columbo.
Calycanthus...Florida allspice.
Calycanthus floridus Linn..............................Florida allspice.
*Camellia Thea Link....................................... Tea.
Canada fleabane...Fleabane.
Canada golden rod ....Solidago Canadensis.
Canadian hemp.......................................Black Indian hemp.
Cancer root...Beech drops.
Candleberry ....Bayberry.
Canker root.. ....Lionsfoot.
*Cannabis sativa Linn..................................Cannabis Indica.
Cannabis sativa Linn, var. Americana...............American hemp.
Cannabis sativa Linn, var. Indica.....................Cannabis Indica.
Cantharis...Cantharides.
Cantharis vesicatoria DeGeer............................Cantharides.
Capsella Bursa-Pastoris Moench.....................Shepherd's purse.
Capsicum fastigiatum Blume...........................Capsicum.
Carduus arvensis (Linn.) Robs........... ....Canada thistle.
Carolina allspice.......................................Florida allspice.
Carthamus tinctorius Willd.......................American saffron.
*Carum Carui Linn.......................................Caraway seed.
Carum Carvi Linn..Caraway seed.
Carum Petroselinum Bentham..........................Parsley.
*Caryophyllus aromatica Linn.............................Cloves.
Cassia acutifolia Delile..............................Senna.
Cassia angustifolia Vahl................................Senna.
*Cassia elongata Lem....................................Senna.
*Cassia lanceolata Nectoux.............................Senna.
*Castalia odorata (Dryand.) Woodv. & Wood........White pond lily.
Castanea dentata (Marsh.) Sudworth.................Chestnut leaves.

*Castanea sativa var. Americana **Watson &** Coulter.Chestnut leaves.
*Castanea vesca Gærtn..Chestnut leaves.
Catarrh root..Galangal.
Catchfly..Bitter root.
Catchweed...Cleavers.
Catsmint..Catnep.
Catswort..Catnep.
Caulophyllum...Blue cohosh.
Caulophyllum thalictroides (Linn.) **Michx**..............Blue cohosh.
Cayenne pepper.....................................Capsicum.
Ceanothus Americanus Linn.......................Jersey **tea.**
Celastrus scandens Linn.....................False bittersweet.
*Centaurea benedicta Linn........................Blessed thistle.
Cephaelis Ipecacuanha (Brotero) **A. Richard**.............Ipecac.
*Cerasus serotina Loiseleur.............................Cherry bark.
Cercis Canadensis Linn.................................Judas tree.
*Cereus grandiflorus Miller.....................Cactus grandiflorus.
*Cervispina cathartica Mœnch....................Buckthorn berries.
*Chamælirium Carolinianum Willd...............False unicorn root.
Chamælirium luteum (Linn.) Gray.............False unicorn root.
*Chamænerion angustifolium (Linn.) **Scop.**.........Willow herb.
*Chamomilla officinalis Koch...............German chamomile.
Checkerberry...Squaw vine.
Checkerberry...Winterberry.
Chelidonium majus Linn.......................Garden celandine.
*Chelone alba Pursh.....................................Balmony.
Chelone glabra Linn.......................................Balmony.
Chenopodium..................................American wormseed.
Chenopodium ambrosioides Linn., var. anthelminticum Gray
                               American wormseed.
Chenopodium anthelminticum **Linn**............American wormseed.
Chickentoe...Crawley root.
Chimaphila **umbellata (Linn.) Nutt**..................Pipsissewa.
Chinese anise..Star anise.
Chinese sumach...Ailanthus.
Chionanthus Virginica Linn.................Fringetree bark.
*Chironia angularis Linn........................Centaury.
Chittem bark..................................**Cascara** Sagrada.
Chocolate root.................................**Water** avens.
Chondodendron tomentosum **Ruiz et Pavon**..........Pareira brava.
Christmas rose.......................................Black hellebore.
*Chrysanthemum Chamomilla Meyer..........German chamomile.
Chrysanthemum Parthenium (Linn.) Pers...........Feverfew.
Churrus..Cannabis Indica.
Cicuta maculata Linn..............................Water hemlock.
*Cicuta virosa var. maculata **Coult. & Rose**..........Water hemlock.
Cimicifuga racemosa (Linn.) Nutt.............Black cohosh.
Cinchona Calisaya Weddell.......................Cinchona.
Cinchona officinalis Linn.......................Cinchona, pale.
Cinchona succirubra Pavon.......................Cinchona, red.
Cinnamomum, one or more Chinese species.............Cassia buds.
*Cinnamomum aromaticum Nees...............Cassia **buds.**
*Cinnamomum Cassia Blume...............Cassia buds.
Cinnamomum Zeylanicum Breyne..........Cinnamon, Ceylon.
*Cirsium arvense Scop.............................Canada thistle.
*Cistus Canadensis Linn..............................Frostwort.
Citrullus Colocynthis Schrader...............Colocynth.
Citrullus vulgaris Schrader...............Water melon seed.
Citrus Aurantium Linn.....................Orange peel, sweet.
Citrus Limonum Risso.......................Lemon peel.
Citrus vulgaris Risso......................Orange peel, bitter.
Claviceps purpurea (Fries) Tulasne..............Ergot.
Climbing bittersweet......................False bittersweet.
Clove garlic...Garlic.
*Cnicus arvensis Hoffm......................Canada thistle.
Cnicus benedictus Gærtn....................Blessed thistle.
Coakum..Poke.
*Cocculus **palmatus D. C.**...........................Columbo.
Cocklebur..Agrimony.
Coffea Arabica **Linn**..................................Coffee.
Cola..Kola nut.
Colchicum autumnale **Linn**........................Colchicum.
Colic root...Wild yam.
Collinsonia Canadensis **Linn**......................Stone root.
Common elder.....................................**Elder** flowers.
Commiphora Myrrha (Nees) Engler.................Myrrh.
Conium maculatum Linn.......................Conium.

Erigeron Canadensis Linn................................Fleabane.
Eriodictyon glutinosum Benth...........   ....Yerba santa.
Eryngium aquaticum Linn............................Water eryngo.
*Eryngium yuccaefolium Michx......... ....Water eryngo.
Erythroxylon Coca Linn.............................Coca leaves.
Eucalyptus globulus Lab.............................Eucalyptus.
Eugenia aromatica (Linn.) **Kuntze**....................Cloves.
*Eugenia caryophyllata **Thunb**.........................Cloves.
Eugenia Jamboiana **Linn**.........................**Jambul** seed.
*Eugenia Pimenta D. **C**............................Pimenta.
Euonymus atropurpureus **Jacq** ....Wahoo root bark.
Eupatorium.... ....Boneset.
Eupatorium perfoliatum Linn.........................Boneset.
Equisetum hyemale Linn.......................Equisetum hyemale.
Eupatorium purpureum Linn..................Queen of the meadow.
*Eupatorium trifoliatum Linn.................Queen of the meadow.
Euphorbia corollata Linn..................Large flowering spurge.
Euphorbia pilulifera Linn........ .. ..Euphorbia pilulifera.
*Euphrasia latifolia Linn.............................Eyebright.
Euphrasia officinalis Linn.............................Eyebright.
*Euryangium Sumbul Kauffman.......... ....Musk root.
*Exogonium Purga Benth...............................Jalap.
Fabiana imbricata Ruiz et Pavon.. ....Pichi.
Fagus atropunicea (Marsh.) Sudw.. ....Beech bark.
*Fagus ferruginea Ait.. ....Beech bark.
False alder..Black alder.
False hellebore..............................Adonis vernalis.
False valerian.....................................Life root.
False white cedar................................Arbor vitæ.
Ferula fœtida (Bunge) Regel.........................Asafœtida.
Ferula Sumbul (Kauffman) Hooker.... ....Musk root.
Field balm...Catnep.
Fishberry.......................................Cocculus Indicus.
Fiveleaved ivy................. ....American ivy.
Flag lily.   ...... ,,..............................Blue flag.
Flesh-colored Asclepias................... ......**White** Indian hemp.
Flower velure.....................................Coltsfoot.
Flytrap...Bitter root.
Fœniculum capillaceum Gilibert.......................Fennel seed.
*Fœniculum vulgare Gærta............................Fennel seed.
Foreign Indian hemp............................Cannabis Indica.
Foxglove...Digitalis.
*Franciscea uniflora **Don**............................Manaca.
Frangula.......................................Buckthorn bark.
*Frangula vulgaris Reich.........................Buckthorn bark.
Frankenia grandifolia Cham. **et Schlecht**............ Yerba reuma.
Frasera Carolinensis Walt...... .... American columbo.
*Frasera Walteri Michx.......................American columbo.
*Fraxinus alba Marsh.............. ....American white ash.
Fraxinus Americana Linn....................American white ash.
Fraxinus nigra Marsh...........................Black ash bark.
*Fraxinus sambucifolia Lam......................Black ash bark.
Fucus vesiculosus Linn..........................Bladderwrack.
Galipea Cusparia St. Hil......................Angustura bark.
*Galipea officinalis Hancock...................Angustura bark.
Galium Aparine Linn................................Cleavers.
Garcinia Mangostana Linn...........................Mango fruit.
Garden dill...Dill.
Garden lavender..............................Lavender flowers.
Garget...................................... ..   .. Poke.
Gaultheria procumbens Linn....................Wintergreen.
Gayfeather.................................Button snakeroot.
*Gelsemium **nitidum** Michx........................Gelsemium.
Gelsemium sempervirens (Linn.) Ait.................Gelsemium.
Gem fruit ....Coolwort.
Gentiana lutea Linn.................................Gentian.
Gentiana ochroleuca Friel....................Sampson snakeroot.
Gentiana puberula Michx........................Blue gentian.
*Gentiana quinqueflora Lam.................Fiveflowered gentian.
Gentiana quinquefolia Linn..................Fiveflowered gentian.
*Gentiana villosa Linn........................Sampson snakeroot.
Geranium..Cranesbill.
Geranium maculatum Linn...........................Cranesbill.
Geum rivale Linn..........................**Water** avens root.
Gill-over-the-ground ....Ground ivy.
Glycyrrhiza glabra Linn.............................Licorice.
*Glycyrrhiza glabra Linn. **var. glandulifera** (**Waldstein** & Kittaibel)
    Regel & Herder................................Licorice.

Iris Florentina Linn..Orris root.
Iris versicolor Linn.......................................Blue flag.
Jacaranda procera Sprengel..............................Caroba leaves.
Jack in the pulpit..Indian turnip.
Jacob's ladder..Abscess root.
James tea...Labrador tea.
Jamestownweed..Stramonium.
Jatamansi..Musk root.
*Jateorhiza Calumba Miers................................Columbo.
Jateorhiza Palmata (Lam.) Miers..........................Columbo.
Jesuit's bark..Cinchona.
Jimsonweed...Stramonium.
Job's tears..False gromwell.
Joepye weed..Boneset.
Juglans cinerea Linn.....................................Butternut bark.
Juglans nigra Linn.......................................Black walnut.
Juniperus communis Linn..................................Juniper berries.
Juniperus Sabina Linn....................................Savine.
*Juniperus Sabina var. procumbens Pursh..................Savine.

Kalmia angustifolia Linn.................................Sheep laurel.
Kalmia latifolia Linn....................................Mountain laurel.
Kameela..Kamala.
Knight's spur..Larkspur seed.
Knotgrass..Couch grass.
Kola acuminata R. Brown..................................Kola nut.
Kousso...Kousso.
Krameria Ixina Linn......................................Rhatany.
*Krameria tomentosa St. Hil..............................Rhatany.
Krameria triandra Ruiz et Pavon..........................Rhatany.

Lacinaria spicata (Linn.) Kuntze.........................Button snakeroot.
Lactuca sativa Linn......................................Lettuce.
Lactuca virosa Linn......................................Lactucarium.
Lambkill...Sheep laurel.
Lappa..Burdock.
*Lappa major Gærtn.......................................Burdock.
*Lappa minor Gærtn.......................................Burdock.
*Lappa officinalis Allioni...............................Burdock.
Larch..Tamarac bark.
*Larix Americana Michx...................................Tamarac bark.
Larix laricina (Duroi) Koch..............................Tamarac bark.
Lark's claw..Larkspur seed.
*Laurus Benzoin Hoatt....................................Benzoin.
*Laurus Benzoin Linn.....................................Feverbush.
*Laurus Cassia Ait.......................................Cassia buds.
*Laurus Cinnamomum Linn..................................Cinnamon, Ceylon.
*Laurus Sassafras Linn...................................Sassafras bark.
*Laurus variifolia Salisbury.............................Sassafras bark.
Lavandula officinalis Chaix..............................Lavender flowers.
*Lavandula vera D. C.....................................Lavender flowers.
Ledum Groenlandicum Œder.................................Labrador tea.
*Ledum latifolium Ait....................................Labrador tea.
*Leontice thalictroides Linn.............................Blue cohosh.
Leonurus cardiaca Linn...................................Motherwort.
Leopardsbane...Arnica.
Leptandra..Culver's root.
Leptandra Virginica (Linn.) Nutt.........................Culver's root.
*Leucanthemum Parthenium Godron..........................Feverfew.
Levisticum officinale Koch...............................Lovage.
*Liatris spicata Willd...................................Button snakeroot.
Lignum vitæ..Guaiac.
*Ligusticum Levisticum Linn..............................Lovage.
*Lindera Benzoin Blume...................................Feverbush.
Lippia dulcis Trev.......................................Lippia Mexicana.
Liquidambar styraciflua Linn.............................Sweet gum bark.
Liriodendron Tulipifera Linn.............................Tulip tree bark.
*Lithospermum Virginianum Linn...........................False gromwell.
Liver lily...Blue flag.
Lobelia inflata Linn.....................................Lobelia.
*Lonicera Marylandica Linn...............................Pink root.
Lycopus Virginicus Linn..................................Bugleweed.
Lyre tree..Tulip tree.
*Macropiper methysticum Miquel...........................Kava Kava.
Mad-dog scullcap...Scullcap.
Madweed..Scullcap.
Magnolia acuminata Linn..................................Cucumber tree.
*Magnolia glauca Linn....................................Magnolia bark.
Magnolia Virginiana Linn.................................Magnolia bark.

Oxydendron arboreum (Linn.) **D. C**................Sourwood leaves.
Pæonia officinalis Linn...........................Peony.
Pale touch-me-not................................Jewel weed.
Papaver somniferum Linn.........................Poppy head.
Pappoose root....................................Blue cohosh.
Para coto..Coto bark.
*Parthenocissus quinquefolia (Linn.) **Planch**........American ivy.
Partridgeberry...................................Squaw vine.
Pasque flower....................................Pulsatilla.
Passiflora incarnata Linn........................Passion flower.
Paullinia Cupana Kunth...........................Guarana.
*Paullinia sorbilis Martius......................Guarana.
Paul's betony....................................Bugleweed.
Paul's betony....................................Speedwell.
Peachwood..Logwood.
Pellitory of Spain...............................Pellitory.
Penthorum sedoides Linn..........................Virginia stone crop.
Pernambuco Jaborandi.............................Jaborandi.
*Persica vulgaris D. C...........................Peach leaves.
Peruvian bark....................................Cinchona.
Petroselinum sativum Hoffm.......................Parsley.
*Peucedanum graveolens Hiern.....................Dill.
Peumus Boldus Molina.............................Boldo leaves.
*Peumus fragrans Pers............................Boldo leaves.
Phoradendron flavescens (Pursh.) **Nutt**...........Mistletoe.
Physostigma......................................Calabar bean.
Physostigma venenosum **Balfour**..................Calabar bean.
Phytolacca decandra Linn.........................Poke.
Pickpocket.......................................Sheperd's purse.
Picræna excelsa (Swartz) Lindley.................Quassia.
Picramnia sp.?...................................Cascara amarga.
Pigeon berry.....................................Poke.
Pilocarpus Jaborandi Holmes......................Jaborandi.
Pilocarpus Selloanus Engler......................Jaborandi.
*Pimenta acris Wight.............................Bay laurel.
Pimenta officinalis Lindley......................Pimenta.
Pimpinella Anisum Linn...........................Anise seed.
Pimpinella Saxifraga Linn........................Saxifrage.
*Pimpinella Saxifraga Linn. var. major Koch......Saxifrage.
Pinus Canadensis Linn............................Hemlock bark.
*Pinus laricina Duroi............................Tamarac bark.
*Pinus pendula Ait...............................Tamarac bark.
Piper angustifolium Ruiz **et Pavon**...............Matico.
Piper Cubeba Linn. f.............................Cubeb.
*Piper elongatum Vahl............................Matico.
Piper methysticum Forster........................Kava Kava.
Piscidia Erythrina Jacq..........................Jamaica dogwood.
Plantago major Linn..............................Plantain leaves.
Pockwood...Guaiac.
Podophyllum peltatum Linn........................Mandrake.
Poison hemlock...................................Conium.
Polecatweed......................................Skunk cabbage.
Polemonium reptans Linn..........................Abscess root.
Polygala Senega Linn.............................Seneka.
*Polygonum acre H. B. K..........................Water pepper.
Polygonum Bistorta Linn..........................Bistort.
*Polygonum Hydropiper Michx......................Water pepper.
*Polygonum hydropiperoides Pursh.................Water pepper.
Polygonum punctatum Ell..........................Water pepper.
Polymnia Uvedalia Linn...........................Bearsfoot.
Polytrichum juniperinum Hedwig...................Haircap moss.
Populus balsamifera candicans (Ait.) Gray........Balm of Gilead.
*Populus candicans Ait...........................Balm of Gilead.
Populus tremuloides Michx........................White poplar bark.
Prenanthus alba Linn.............................Lionsfoot.
Prince's pine....................................Pipsissewa.
Prinos verticillatus **Linn**......................Black alder.
Privy..Privet.
Prunus Persicaria (Linn.) Seibold et Zuccarini...Peach leaves.
Prunus serotina Ehrh.............................Cherry bark.
*Prunus Virginiana Linn..........................Cherry bark.
Ptelea trifoliata Linn...........................Wafer ash.
Pterocarpus Marsupium Roxburg....................Kino.
Pterocarpus santalinus Linn. f...................**Red** saunders.
Pukeweed...Lobelia.
Punica Granatum Linn.............................**Pomegranate** root bark.
Purple angelica..................................Angelica.
Purple avens.....................................Water avens root.

Pussy willow..Black willow.
*Pyrola umbellata Linn.... ....Pipsissewa.
*Pyrus Americana D. C.... ....Mountain ash.
Quaking asp..White poplar bark.
*Quassia excelsa Swartz.... ....Quassia.
*Quassia Simaruba Linn. f............................Simaruba bark.
Queen's delight..Stillingia.
Queen's root..Stillingia.
Quercus alba Linn...........................White oak bark.
Quercus infectoria Oliver... ....Galls.
*Quercus lusitanica Lam............................see Galls.
*Quercus lusitanica Webb var. infectoria D. C............see Galls.
Quercus rubra Linn......................Red oak bark.
*Quercus tinctoria Bartram.....................Red oak bark.
Quickens......................................Couch grass.
Quillaja Saponaria Molina...........................Soap tree bark.
Raccoon berry..Mandrake.
Ragwort..Life root.
Rattleroot......r......................................Black cohosh.
Red bud...Judas tree.
Red centaury..American centaury.
Red clover ....Clover tops.
Red pepper..Capsicum.
Red puccoon..Blood root.
Red River snakeroot.....................................Serpentaria.
Red root ....Jersey tea.
Rhamnus cathartica Linn..........................Buckthorn berries.
Rhamnus Frangula Linn..........................Buckthorn bark.
Rhamnus Purshiana D. C.......................Cascara sagrada.
Rheum officinale Baillon...........................Rhubarb.
Rhus aromatica Ait.........................Rhus aromatica.
*Rhus Canadensis Marsh...........................Rhus aromatica.
Rhus glabra Linn....................................Sumach.
Rhus radicans Linn....................................Poison oak.
*Rhus toxicodendron radicans Marsh....................Poison oak.
Richweed...Stoneroot.
Ricinus communis Linn.........................Castor bean and leaves.
Rio Janeiro Jaborandi...................................Jaborandi.
Robin's rye...Haircap moss.
Rockfern..Maidenhair.
Rock rose..Frostwort.
Roman chamomile....................................Chamomile.
Rosebay ....Willow herb.
Roughroot...Button snakeroot.
Roundleaved dogwood.....................Green osier bark.
Roundleaved sundew..................................Sundew.
Round zedoary...Zedoary.
Rubus Canadensis Linn.................................Blackberry.
*Rubus Idæus Linn. var. strigosus Maxim..........Raspberry leaves.
Rubus strigosus Michx..............................Raspberry leaves.
Rubus trivialis Michx..................................Blackberry.
Rubus villosus Aiton..................................Blackberry.
Rumex Acetosella Linn.............................Sheep sorrel.
Rumex crispus Linn...................................Yellow dock.
*Rumex obtusifolius Linn.............................Yellow dock.
*Rumex sanguineus Linn.............................Yellow dock.
Ruta graveolens Linn....................................Rue.
*Sabal serrulata R. & S........................Saw palmetto berries.
Sabbatia angularis (Linn.) Pursh..............American centaury.
Safflower...American saffron.
Sage brush...'..Mountain sage.
Salix alba Linn.......................................White willow bark.
Salix nigra Marsh.....................................Black willow.
Salvia officinalis Linn..................................Sage.
Sambucus Canadensis Linn..........................Elder flowers.
Sambucus nigra Linn................................European elder.
Sanguinaria...Blood root.
Sanguinaria Canadensis Linn........................Blood root.
Santalum album Linn.................................Sandalwood.
Santal rubum...Red saunders.
Santonica...Levant wormseed.
Saponaria officinalis Linn...............................Soapwort.
*Sarothamnus scoparius Koch.........................Broom tops.
*Sarothamnus vulgaris Wimm.......................Broom tops.
*Sassafras officinale Nees et Eberm.................Sassafras bark.
Sassafras variifolium (Salisbury) O. Kuntze..... ....Sassafras bark.
Scarlet berry..Bittersweet.

*Scilla maritima Linn..Squill.
Schœnocaulon officinale Gray....................Cevadilla seed.
*Sclerotium Clavus D. C..Ergot.
Scoparius...Broom tops.
Scouring rush..............................Equisetum hyemale.
Scutellaria lateriflora Linn ....Scullcap.
Seaweed..Bladderwrack.
Seawrack...Bladderwrack.
Senecio aureus Linn......................................Life root.
*Senecio aureus Pursh......................................Senecio.
Senecio gracilis Pursh.....................................Senecio.
Seneka snakeroot...Seneka.
Serenœa serrulata (R. & S.) Hooker f......... Saw palmetto berries.
*Serratula spicata Linn........................Button snakeroot.
Sesamum Indicum Linn..............................Benne leaves.
*Sesamum orientale Linn..........................Benne leaves.
Sevenbarks...Hydrangea.
Shamrock..White clover.
Shrubby treefoil...Water ash.
Sierra salvia......................................Mountain sage.
Silphium laciniatum Linn...............................Rosinweed.
Simaba Cedron Planch...............................Cedron seed.
*Simaruba amara Aublet..........................Simaruba bark.
*Simaruba excelsa D. C................................Quassia.
Simaruba officinalis D. C.........................Simaruba bark.
Simpler's joy...Vervain.
Sinapis nigra (Linn.) Koch..........................Mustard seed.
Skunk bush.......................................Rhus aromatica.
Skunkweed.......................................Skunk cabbage.
Small spikenard.....................American sarsaparilla.
Smart weed..Water pepper.
Smilax lanceolata Linn...................Bamboo brier root.
Smilax medica Chamisso et Schlecht..................Sarsaparilla.
Smilax officinalis Kunth..............................Sarsaparilla.
*Smilax ovata Pursh...................... Bamboo brier root.
Smilax papyraceæ Duhamel, and other undetermined species ......
                                     Sarsaparilla.
Smooth sumach...Sumach.
Snakehead..Balmony.
Snakeweed..Serpentaria.
Snapping hazel.......................................Witch hazel.
Saapweed..Jewel weed.
Snargel...Serpentaria.
Socotrine aloes...Aloes.
Solanum Carolinense Linn ....Horse nettle.
Solanum Dulcamara Linn.............................Bittersweet.
*Solidago altissima Linn.................Solidago Canadensis.
Solidago Canadensis Linn......Solidago Canadensis.
Solidago odora Aiton....................................Golden rod.
Sophora tinctoria Linn..................................Wild indigo.
Sorbus Americana Marsh...........................Mountain ash.
*Sorbus microcarpa Pursh............................Mountain ash.
Sorghum saccharatum Persoon.................Broom corn seed.
Sorrel tree...Sourwood leaves.
Southern sarsaparilla.....................Bamboo brier root.
Spanish chamomile....................................Pellitory.
Spanish fly...Cantharides.
*Spathyema fœtida (Linn.) Raf........Skunk cabbage.
Spicebush..Fever bush.
Spicewood..Fever bush.
Spigelia Marylandica Linn..............................Pink root.
Spignet..Spikenard.
Spike lavender................................Lavender flowers.
Spindle tree...Wahoo.
Spirœa tomentosa Linn..................................Hardhack.
Spotted alder...Witch hazel.
Spotted hemlock...................................Water hemlock.
Spotted parsley....................................Water hemlock.
Squawbush...Cramp bark.
Squawmint..Pennyroyal.
Squawroot..Black cohosh.
Squaw root...Blue cohosh.
Stachys Betonica Benth...........................Wood betony.
Staffvine...False bittersweet.
*Staphisagria macrocarpa Spach..............Stavesacre seed.
Stargrass..Unicorn root.
Starwort......................................False unicorn root.
*Sterculia acuminata R. Brown........................Kola nut.

WHEN ORDERING OR PRESCRIBING.

*Uginea Scilla Steinheil..Squill.
Urtica dioica Linn..Nettle root.
Ustilago Maydis Leville........................Ustilago Maydis.
*Valeriana angustifolia Tausch.......................Valerian.
Valeriana officinalis Linn................................Valerian.
*Valeriana sambucifolia Mikan......................Valerian.
Velvet leaf...Pareira brava.
*Veratrum album var. viride Baker...............Veratrum viride.
*Veratrum luteum Linn.........................False unicorn root.
*Veratrum Sabadilla Schlecht....................Cevadilla seed.
Veratrum viride Alt..............................Veratrum viride.
Verbascum Thapsus Linn.......................Mullein leaves.
Verbena hastata Linn...................................Vervain.
*Verbena paniculata Lam................................Vervain.
Veronica officinalis Linn...............................Speedwell.
*Veronica Virginica Linn...........................Culver's root.
Viburnum Opulus Linn..............................Cramp bark.
Viburnum prunifolium Linn...........................Black haw.
Vine maple.......................................Yellow parilla.
Viola pedata Linn...................................Violet herb.
Viola tricolor Linn.....................................Pansy.
Violetbloom...Bittersweet.
Virginia creeper..................................American ivy.
Virginia snakeroot.................................Serpentaria.
*Viscum flavescens Pursh.............................Mistletoe.
*Vitis quinquefolia Lam............................American ivy.
Wake robin...................................**Indian turnip.**
Wake robin...**Bethroot.**
Waterflag..**Blueflag.**
Waxberry..**Bayberry.**
Waxmyrtle...**Bayberry.**
White baneberry............................**White cohosh.**
White flag..**Orris root.**
White saunders................................**Sandalwood.**
White walnut................................**Butternut bark.**
Whitewood..**Tulip tree.**
Wicky...**Sheep laurel.**
***Wigandia Californica Hook & Arn**............**Yerba santa.**
Wild bryony..................................**White bryony.**
Wild celandine.................................**Jewel weed.**
Wild cherry...................................**Cherry bark.**
Wild cinnamon..................................**Bay laurel.**
Wild cloves.....................................**Bay laurel.**
Wild ginger.............................**Canada snakeroot.**
Wild hops....................................**White bryony.**
Wild hydrangea ....**Hydrangea.**
Wild hyssop...**Vervain.**
Wild jessamine.................................**Gelsemium.**
Wild lemon.......................................**Mandrake.**
Wild mangosteen...............................**Mango fruit.**
Wild snowball.......................................Jersey tea.
Winterberry.......................................Black alder.
Winter bloom..................................Witch hazel.
Winter clover.....................................Squaw vine.
Wind root......................................Pleurisy root.
Wing seed..Wafer ash.
Wolfsbane...Aconite.
Woodbine...Gelsemium.
Woody nightshade..................................Bittersweet.
Xanthoxylum Americanum Miller...................**Prickly ash.**
*Xanthoxylum Carolinianum Lam...................Prickly ash.
Xanthoxylum Clava-Herculis Linn...................Prickly ash.
Yellow cinchona..............................Cinchona Calisaya.
Yellow gentian..............................American columbo.
Yellow jessamine..................................Gelsemium.
Yellow leaf cup....................................Bearsfoot.
Yellow puccoon...................................Golden seal.
Yellow root.......................................Golden seal.
Yellow wood.......................................Prickly ash.
Youthwort...Sundew.
Zanthoxylum......................................Prickly ash.
Zea Mays Linn.......................................Corn silk.
Zingiberis officinale Roscoe..........................Ginger.

INDEX OF DISEASES

WITH REMEDIES;

HAVING SPECIAL REFERENCE

TO THE USE OF

ELI LILLY & COMPANY'S

Pharmaceutical Preparations.

It is of course impossible in the scope of this work to enlarge upon the use of each remedy or its adaptation to peculiar phases of the disease under consideration in each case.

By referring, however, to the text connected with each class of preparations as Fluid Extracts, Pills, etc., much information will be found and suggestions for further research in the text books.

ABDOMINAL PLETHORA.
    Pills—Croton oil.—Elaterium. Clutterbuck and Saline cathartics in congestion of the portal circulation. In plethora of the abdominal viscera, Grape juice.—Saline waters. Light nutritious diet.

ABORTION.
    Fluid Extracts—Black cohosh.—Black haw.—Blue cohosh.—Cramp bark.—Ergot.—False unicorn root.—Opium, aqueous.—Unicorn root.
    Pills—Asafetida.—Gold chloride.
    Elixirs—Helonias comp.—Viburnum comp.
    Cordial—Helonias comp.

ABSCESS.
Succus Alterans; Lilly.
    Fluid Extract—Belladonna.
    Pills—Belladonna ext.—Calcium sulphide.
    Syrups—Calcium lactophosphate.—Hypophosphites comp.—Iron Quinine and Strychnine phosphates.
    Elastic Capsules—Cod liver oil.
    The cavity should be daily irrigated with FORMASEPTOL; Lilly, or it may be used as a dressing.

ACIDITY OF STOMACH.
    Fluid Extracts—Belladonna.—Nux vomica.—Pulsatilla.
    Pills—Antidyspepsia, Fothergill.—Antidyspeptic.—Bismuth subnitrate.—Digestive.—Nux vomica ext.—Oxgall.
    Tablets—Antidyspepsia.—Bismuth subgallate.—Bismuth subnitrate.—Dyspepsia.—Sodamint.—Sodium bicarbonate.
    Lozenges—Bismuth and Charcoal.—Carbolic acid.—Charcoal and Sodamint.—Ginger and Soda.—Pepsin and Bismuth.—Pepsin, Bismuth and Charcoal.—Pepsin, Bismuth, Charcoal and Ginger.—Pepsin, Bismuth and Ginger.—Pepsin and Charcoal.—Pepsin, Charcoal, Magnesia and Ginger.

WHEN ORDERING OR PRESCRIBING.

ACNE.
Succus Alterans; Lilly.

Fluid Extracts—Belladonna, locally.—Berberis aquifolium.—Ergot.

Pills—Arsenous acid.—Calcium sulphide.—Phosphorus.—Phosphorus comp.

Tablets—Antiseptic, alkaline, Seiler.—Antiseptic, external.

Lozenge—Sulphur comp.

Elixirs—Potassium bromide.—Phosphorus.—Phosphorus and Strychnine.

Syrup—Hypophosphites comp.

AGUE; See Intermittent fever.

ALBUMINURIA; See Bright's disease.

ALCOHOLISM.

Hypodermic Tablets—Strychnine nitrate, an absolute cure for dipsomania. Send for booklet on this subject to ELI LILLY & CO.

AMAUROSIS.

Fluid Extracts—Arnica.—Guaiac resin.—Nux vomica.—Rue.

Pills—Nux vomica ext.—Strychnine.

Tincture—Veratrum viride, brushed on the eyelids and temples twice daily. Use great care that it does not touch the conjunctiva.

AMENORRHEA.
Succus Alterans; Lilly.

Fluid Extracts—Aconite.—Black hellebore.—Black cohosh.—Blue cohosh.—Blue cohosh comp.—Cantharides.—Catnip.—Columbo.—Colocynth. Cotton root bark.—Ergot. False unicorn root.—Life root. Motherwort. Masterwort.—Mugwort.—Pennyroyal.—Pulsatilla, when the result of cold.—Rue.—Saffron.—Senecio.—Shepherd's purse. Squaw vine comp. Stavesacre. Tansy.—Unicorn root.—Ustilago maydis.—Vervain. Water pepper.

Pills—Aloes.—Aloes and Asafetida.—Aloes and Iron.—Aloes and Myrrh.—Emmenagogue, improved.—Emmenagogue, Mutter.—Emmenagogue, Rigaud.—Emmenagogue with Cotton root ext.—Ergotin.—Female. Amenorrhea.—Ferruginous, Blaud.—Iron carbonate.—Manganese binoxide.—Mercury biniodide.—Potassium permanganate.

Tablets—Potassium permanganate, highly recommended by Dr. Fordyce Barker.

ANEMIA.

Succus Alterans; Lilly, as a tonic, stimulates the appetite promotes assimilation and increases proportion of red corpuscles. Rapid increase of flesh reported in many cases.

Pills—Arsenous acid.—Ferruginous, Blaud.—Iron carbonate.—Iron citrate.—Iron compound.—Iron iodide.—Iron Quassia and Nux vomica. Phosphorus and Iron.—Iron, Quinine and Strychnine.—Iron Quinine and strychnine phosphates.—Phosphorus, Iron and Nux vomica.—Quinine compound.—Quinine and Iron.—Tonic, Atkens.

Elixirs—Calisaya and Iron.—Gentian and Iron chloride. Iron and Quinine phosphates.—Iron, Quinine and Strychnine phosphates.—Iron pyrophosphate.—Iron pyrophosphate, Quinine and Arsenic.—Iron pyrophosphate, Quinine and Strychnine.

Syrups—Hypophosphites compound.—Hypophosphites compound with Quinine and Strychnine.—Hypophosphites compound, Hematic.—Iron and Manganese hypophosphites.—Iron lactophosphate.

Elastic Filled Capsules—Cod liver oil.

ANEURISM.

Fluid Extracts—Digitalis.—Ergot.—Veratrum viride.

Pills—Iron iodide.—Potassium iodide.

ANGINA PECTORIS.

Fluid Extracts—Aconite.—Chamomile.—Digitalis.

Pills—Arsenous acid.—Cocaine hydrochlorate.—Morphine sulphate.—Opium.—Phosphorus.—Quinine when intermittent, or malaria is suspected.

APHONIA.
Lilly's Bronchial Tablets.
Pills—Atropine.

APHTHÆ.
Fluid Extracts—Golden seal.—Rhatany.
Pills—Quinine sulphate as a tonic.
Tablets—Bismuth.—Borax.—Boroglyceride, Lilly.—Potassium chlorate.—Potassium chlorate and Borax.

ARTHRITIS.
Fluid Extracts—Aconite.—Black cohosh.—Black haw.—Colchicum, with alkalies.
Pills—Arsenous acid.—Cinchonidine salicylate.—Potassium iodide.—Salicylic acid.
Elastic Filled Capsules—Cod liver oil.
Turkish baths—Massage.

ASTHMA.
Fluid Extracts—Aconite root.—Belladonna.—Cannabis Indica.—Conium. — Digitalis. — Eucalyptus. — Grindelia. — Hyoscyamus. — Opium, camphorated.—Ipecac.—Jaborandi.—Lobelia.—Musk root.—Nux vomica. — Quebracho. — Rosinweed. — skunk cabbage. — stramonium.—Sundew.—Yerba Santa.
Pills—Asiatic.—Atropine.—Camphor, Henbane and Valerian.—Camphor and Opium.—Cocaine hydrochlorate.—Morphia-atropia.—Morphine phine, Henbane and Camphor.—Morphine sulphate.—Pilocarpine hydrochlorate.—Strychnine.
Elixirs—Ammonium bromide.—Grindelia.—Potassium bromide.—Sodium bromide.

BILIOUSNESS.
Elixir Purgans, Lilly, reliably stimulates the liver without nausea or griping.
Fluid Extracts—Balmony.—Black alder.—Blue flag.—Boldo.—Colocynth.—Culver's root.—Dandelion.—Figwort.—Garden celandine.—Golden seal.—Ipecac.—Mandrake.—Prickly ash bark.—Stillingia.—Tamarac bark.—Wahoo.
Pills—Alterative.—Antibilious.—Blue mass.—Blue mass compound.—Calomel.—Calomel compound.—Cathartic compound, U. S.—Cathartic cholagogue.—Cathartic improved.—Cathartic vegetable.—Colocynth compound ext. and Blue mass.—Colocynth, Ipecac and Blue mass.—Hepatic.—Hepatic/eclectic.—Laxative/cole.—Leptandrin compound.—Liver granules.—Liver, improved vegetable.—Podophyllin.—Podophyllin and Berberine.—Podophyllin and Blue mass.—Podophyllin, Colocynth and Belladonna.—Podophyllin compound.—Podophyllin conc. compound, Eclectic.—Podophyllin and Leptandrin.—Rhubarb compound and Calomel.—Triplex.—Triplex, Francis.

BLADDER, CATARRH OF; See Cystitis.

BLADDER, IRRITABLE.
Fluid Extracts — Belladonna. — Bladderwrack. — Cantharides. — Couchgrass.—Cubeb.—Gelsemium.—Pareira brava.—Stavesacre.

BLADDER, PARALYSIS OF.
Fluid Extracts—Arnica.—Cannabis Indica.—Cantharides.—Ergot.—Nux vomica.
Pills—Strychnine.

BOILS.
Succus Alterans, Lilly, to purify the blood.
Pills—Calcium sulphide.

BONE, DISEASES OF.
Syrups—Calcium hypophosphite.—Calcium lactophosphate.—Calcium and Sodium hypophosphite.—Calcium, Sodium and Potassium hypophosphite.—Hypophosphites compound.—Phosphates compound.
Pills—Phosphorus.
Elastic Filled Capsules—Cod liver oil.

BREATH, FOUL.
- *Formaseptol; Lilly.*

Lozenges—Carbolic acid.—Charcoal.

Tablets—Potassium permanganate, 1 to 2 tablets in a glass of water as a mouth wash.

BRIGHT'S DISEASE.
Fluid Extracts—Broom tops.—Button snakeroot.—Cannabis Indica.—Cantharides.—Digitalis.—Ergot.—Hyoscyamus.—Jaborandi.—Pipsissewa.—Senega.

Pills—Cannabis Indica ext.—Copaiba.

Elixir—Gentian and Iron chloride.

Elastic Filled Capsules—Cod liver oil.

BRONCHITIS, ACUTE.
Prunicodeine; Lilly.

Fluid Extracts—Aconite root.—American Ivy.—Black cohosh.—Bloodroot.—Digitalis.—Eucalyptus.—Grindelia.—Ipecac.—Kava-kava.—Lobelia herb.—Poppy heads.—Skunk cabbage.—Spikenard.—Squill.—Squill compound.—Sundew.—Wild cherry.

Pills—Acetanilid.—Quinine sulphate.

Elixir—Grindelia.

Tablets—Bronchial; Lilly.—Ammonium chloride.

Lozenges—Ammonia, Jackson.—Ammonium chloride and Licorice, Brown Mixture.—Pectoral, Jackson.—White pine.—Wild cherry.—Wistar's.

Tincture—Opium, camphorated.

BRONCHITIS, CHRONIC.
Prunicodeine; Lilly.

Fluid Extracts—Cherry bark.—Cherry bark compound.—Cubeb.—Grindelia.—Ipecac.—Jersey tea.—Lobelia.—Muskroot.—Nux vomica.—Rosinweed.—Senega.—Skunk cabbage.—Squill.—Squill compound.—Sundew.—Virginia stonecrop.—Yerba santa.

Syrup—Hypophosphites compound with Quinine and Strychnine.

Tablets—Bronchial; Lilly.

Elastic Filled Capsules—Cod liver oil.

CALCULI, BILIARY.
Avoid starchy food, sweets and fats. Sodium phosphate persistently used. In the passage of the stone, which is extremely painful, Chlorodyne, Opium preparations or anesthetics to allay pain and spasms; also, the warm bath.

CALCULI, RENAL.
Fluid Extracts—Dwarf elder.—Gravelplant.—Haireap moss.—Hydrangea.—Queen of the meadow.—Stoneroot.—Uva Ursi.

Alkaline Mineral Waters—Vichy, Bethesda, etc.

CANCER.
Succus Alterans; Lilly, for constitutional treatment.

Fluid Extracts—Belladonna.—Conium.—Goldenseal.—Hyoscyamus.

Pills—Arsenous acid.—Asiatic.

Caustics—Chromic acid and Bromine for destruction of morbid growths—Iodoform and Salicylic acid to the surface of the sore.—Zinc chloride and Zinc sulphate, dried.

CATARRH, ACUTE, NASAL.
Fluid Extracts—Aconite root or Belladonna, in minimum doses, at intervals of half an hour to an hour or two. Fl. ext. Ipecac, in small doses alone, or with Fl. ext. Opium, aqueous or Fl. ext. Aconite.

Pills—Pilocarpine hydrochlorate.—Sodium salicylate.

CATARRH, BRONCHOPULMOMARY.

Prunicodeine; Lilly.

Fluid Extracts—Aconite.—Belladonna.—Bloodroot.—Cherry bark.—Cherry bark compound.— Eucalyptus.—Goldenseal. — Horebound.—Horehound compound.

Tablets—Bronchial; Lilly.

Lozenges—Ammonium chloride and Licorice.—Ammonia, Jackson.— Brown mixture.—Pectoral, Jackson.—White pine compound.—Wild cherry.—Wistar's.

Syrup—White pine compound.

CATARRH, CHRONIC NASAL.

Succus Alterans; Lilly, for constitutional treatment.

Fluid Extracts— Bloodroot. — Eucalyptus. — Goldenseal. — Horehound.—Horehound compound.—Ipecac.—Ipecac and senega.—Jersey tea. — Judas tree.— Lobelia.— Lobelia compound.— Marshmallow.—Mullein.—Pulsatilla.—Rosinweed.—Skunk cabbage.—Virginia stonecrop.—Yerba reuma.

Syrups— Horehound compound. — White pine compound. — Wild cherry.

Tablets—Potassium chlorate.—Ammonia chloride.

Lozenges— Ammonium chloride and Licorice.— Carbolic acid.—Cubeb.—Ipecac and Opium.—Licorice and Opium.—Pectoral, Jackson.—White pine compound.—Wistar's.—Wild cherry.

Elastic Filled Capsules—Cod liver oil.

CEREBRAL ANEMIA.

Pills—Coca, Phosphorus and Strychnine.—Ferruginous, Blaud.—Iron carbonate.—Iron citrate.—Iron by hydrogen.—Iron iodide.— Iron Quinine and Strychnine.—Phosphorus, Iron and Nux vomica.—Phosphorus, Iron, Quinine and Strychnine.—Tonic, Aiken.

Elixirs—Calisaya bark and Iron.—Calisaya bark, Iron and Strychnine.—Celery and Guarana.—Gentian and Iron chloride.—Iron pyrophosphate and Quinine.—Iron pyrophosphate, Quinine and Strychnine.

Syrups—Hypophosphites compound. — Hypophosphites compound with Quinine and Strychnine.—Hypophosphites compound, Hemstic.—Iron lactophosphate.—Iron and Manganese hypophosphites.

Wines—Beef and Iron.—Beef, Iron and Cinchona. Coca with hypophosphites.—Iron.—Iron bitter.

CEREBRAL CONGESTION.

Fluid Extracts—Aconite. — Belladonna.—Digitalis.—Ergot.—Gelsemium.—Veratrum viride.

Elixirs—Ammonium bromide.—Potassium bromide.—Sodium bromide.

Active cathartics—Blood letting.—Cold douche.

CEREBROSPINAL MENINGITIS.

Fluid Extracts—Aconite combined with Opium, aqueous, carried to arterial depression before exudation. Ergot or Gelsemium in period of congestion.

Pills—Quinine sulphate.

CHLOROSIS.

Succus Alterans; Lilly, as a tonic.

Fluid Extracts—Ergot.—Nux vomica.

Pills—Aloes and Iron. — Arsenous acid. — Asiatic. — Ferruginous, Blaud.—Iodoform and Iron.—Iron by hydrogen.—Iron carbonate.—Phosphorus, Iron and Nux vomica.—Phosphorus and Iron.—Phosphorus Iron and Quinine.— Phosphorus, Iron, Quinine and Strychnine.

Elixirs—Gentian and Iron chloride. Calisaya and Iron.—Iron pyrophosphate.—Iron pyrophosphate, Quinine and Strychnine.

CHOLERA AND CHOLERA MORBUS.

Lilly's Chlorodyne.—Tincture Opium Compound.

Fluid Extracts—Coto bark.—Cranesbill.—Ginger.—Goldenrod.—Pricklyash berries.—Wild yam.

Pills—Astringent. — Calomel. — Camphor and Opium. — Camphor, Opium and Tannin.—Opium and Lead acetate.

Syrup—Rhubarb and Potassium compound.

Tablets—Sun cholera.

CHOLERA INFANTUM.

Fluid Extracts—Blackberry.—Cranesbill.—Hemlock bark.—Minute doses of Ipecac in water.—Logwood.

Syrups—Rhubarb aromatic.—Rhubarb and Potassium compound.

Tincture—Opium, camphorated.

CHORDEE.

Fluid Extracts—Aconite.—Belladonna. — Cannabis Indica.— Cantharides, in minute doses.

Pills—Camphor monobromated.—Camphor and Opium.—Lupulin.—Lupulin and Camphor.—Morphine sulphate.—Morphatropia.

Elixir—Potassium bromide.

CHOREA.

Fluid Extracts—Belladonna. — Black cohosh.—Cannabis Indica.—Conium.—Gelsemium.—Hyoscyamus.— Ladies's slipper.— Lupulin.—Mistletoe.— Motherwort. — Mugwort. — Muskroot. — Nux vomica.—Opium, aqueous.—Scullcap.—Skunk cabbage.—Valerian.—Veratrum viride.

Pills—Arsenous acid.—Asiatic.—Asafetida.— Belladonna ext.—Cannabis Indica ext.—Ferruginous, Blaud. Iron carbonate for the condition of anemia and amenorrhea. Morphine sulphate.— Morphine valerianate.—Strychnine.—Zinc oxide.—Zinc phosphide **and** Nux vomica.—Zinc valerianate.

Elixirs—Potassium bromide.—Zinc valerianate.

Elastic Filled Capsules—Cod liver oil.

CIRRHOSIS OF LIVER.

Succus Alterans; Lilly.

Pills—Arsenous acid.—Asiatic.—Potassium iodide.—Iron iodide.—Iodoform and Iron.

Syrup—Hypophosphites compound.—Phosphates compound.

COLIC.

Cholorodyne; Lilly.

Fluid Extracts—Anise seed.—Asafetida for flatulent colic of infants.— Aromatic. Calamus.—Cardamon compound.—Caraway seed.—Catnep.— Coriander seed.— Ginger.—Lavender compound.—Opium, aqueous.—Spearmint.— Stone root.—Wild yam for bilious colic.

Pills—Asafetida.— Camphor and Opium.—Morphine sulphate.—Morphatropia.— Morphine valerianate.—Opium.

Tincture—Opium, camphorated.

COLIC, LEAD.

Magnesia sulphate to relieve constipation.—Sulphuric acid very dilute, in lemonade as a curative and prophylactic.—Iodides and bromides to cause excretion of lead.

CONSTIPATION.

Elixir Purgans; Lilly.

Glycones; Lilly, in all cases of impaction of the feces affords instant relief.

Fluid Extracts—Belladonna.—Buckthorn bark.— Butternut bark.—Calabar bean. Cascara sagrada.—Culver's root.— Dandelion.—Dandelion and Senna.—Fringetree bark.—Jalap.—Mandrake.—Nux vomica.—Rhubarb.—Senna compound.—Silkweed.—Wahoo.—Wild indigo.

Pills—Aloes.—Aloes and Mastich.—Aloes and **Nux** vomica.—Aloes, Nux vomica **and** Belladonna.—Aloin.—Aloin compound.—Aloin, Strychnine and Belladonna. — Anticonstipation. — Anticonstipation, Brundage. —Anticonstipation, Goss.— Anticonstipation, Palmer —Aperient, Bauer.—Aperient, Drysdale.—Apocynin compound.—A. S. B. and L; Lilly. Cathartic pills, as listed.—Cascara and Podophyllin.—Laxative, Cole.—Laxative, special, Fordyce Barker.—Leptandrin.—Leptandrin compound.—Podophyllin and Belladonna compound.—Podophyllin compound.—Rhubarb compound.

CONVALESCENCE.
Lilly's Liquid Pepsin.
Lilly's Calisaya Cordial.

Elixirs—Calisaya.—Calisaya and Iron.—Calisaya Iron and Bismuth.—Calisaya Iron and Strychnine.—Eucalyptus.—Gentian and Iron chloride.—Gentian Iron and Strychnine.—Iron pyrophosphate, Quinine and Strychnine.—Lactated pepsin.—Pepsin.—Pepsin and Bismuth.—Pepsin, Bismuth and Strychnine.—Pepsin and Strychnine.

Syrups—Hypophosphites compound, hematic.—Hypophosphites compound, with Quinine and Strychnine.

Wines—Coca.—Coca with Hypophosphites.—Beef and Iron.—Beef, Iron and Cinchona.—Iron, bitter.

Solution—Hypophosphites compound, without sugar.

COUGH.
Prunicodeine; Lilly.

Fluid Extracts—Aralia compound.—Belladonna.—Black cohosh.—Black cohosh compound.—Bloodroot.—Cannabis Indica.—Catnep.—Cherry bark.—Cherry bark compound.—Chestnut leaves.—Coltsfoot.—Comfrey.—Great laurel.—Grindelia.—Hyoscyamus.—Ipecac.—Ipecac and Senega.—Licorice.—Lobelia.—Lobelia compound.—Marshmallow.—Muskroot.—Opium, aqueous.—Poppy heads.—Rosinweed.—Senega. skunk cabbage.—Spikenard.—Squill.—Squill compound.—Stramonium.—Sundew.—Sunflower seed.—Tolu, soluble.—Water eryngo.—Yerba santa.

Syrups—Horehound compound.—Squill compound.—Wild cherry, to which Chlorodyne has been added.—White pine compound.

Tablets—Bronchial; Lilly.

Lozenges—Ammonium chloride and Licorice.—Licorice.—Licorice and Opium.—Morphine and Ipecac.—Pectoral, Jackson.—White pine compound.—Wild cherry.—Wistar's.

NOTE—As a base for extemporaneous cough mixtures there is no preparation equal to YERBAZIN; Lilly.

CROUP
Alum as emetic to dislodge false membrane and prevent its reformation. A teaspoonful of the powder in syrup every half hour until free emesis occurs.—Carbolic acid in spray.—Hydrogen dioxide, in spray.—Lactic acid applied locally to dissolve false membrane.—Lime water in spray.—Quinine in large doses.—Steam of slaking lime.—Wine of Ipecac as an emetic.

Water—Warm bath.—Hot compresses or fomentations to the throat.

CYSTITIS.
Fluid Extracts—Buchu.—Buchu compound.—Buchu and Pareira Brava.—Cantharides.—Corn silk.—Cubeb.—Eucalyptus.—Juniper berries.—Kava kava.—Manzanita.—Marshmallow.—Pareira Brava.—Pichi.—Pipsissewa.—Queen of the meadow.—Rhus aromatica.—Shepherd's purse.—Stoneroot.—Uva Ursi.—Yerba santa.

Pills—Copaiba.—Copaiba and Cubeb.—Copaiba compound.—Salicylic acid.

Elixirs—Buchu.—Buchu compound.—Buchu and Juniper compound.—Buchu and Pareira Brava.—Diuretic.

DEBILITY
Calisaya Cordial; Lilly.

Pills—Iron, Quinine and Strychnine phosphates.

Elixirs—Bark and Iron.—Calisaya.—Calisaya and Iron.—Calisaya, Iron and Strychnine.—Pepsin, Bismuth and Strychnine.—Gentian.—Gentian and Iron chloride.—Iron pyrophosphate, Quinine and Strychnine.

Syrup—Hypophosphites compound with Quinine and Strychnine.

Wines—Coca.—Coca with hypophosphites.—Beef and Iron.—Beef, Iron and Cinchona.—Iron, bitter.

Solution—Hypophosphites compound without sugar, see page 227.

DELIRIUM TREMENS.
Fluid Extracts—Belladonna when congestion of brain.—Cannabis Indica.—Capsicum.—Digitalis in cardiac depression.—Hyoscyamus.—Opium aqueous, cautiously.—Stramonium.

Pills—Quinine sulphate to restore digestion.—Zinc phosphide.

Elixirs—Ammonium, Potassium or Sodium bromide.—Ammonium valerianate.—Bromochloral compound.—Hypnotic.—Morphine valerianate.

DIABETES INSIPIDUS.

Fluid Extracts—Ergot.—Jaborandi.—Opium, aqueous.—Valerian.

Pills—Iron phosphate and Strychnine.—Potassium Iodide.

DIABETES MELLITUS.

Fluid Extracts—Ergot.—Jambul seed.

Pills—Arsenous acid.—Asiatic.— Codeine restrains the waste of sugar.—Gold chloride.—Sodium salicylate.

Elixirs—Potassium bromide.—Sodium salicylate.

Syrups—Calcium lactophosphate.—Phosphates, Chemical food.

Exclude starchy and saccharine food.—Milk and buttermilk are valuable in some cases.—Alkalies.—Alkaline mineral waters.

DIARRHEA.

Chlorodyne; Lilly.

Fluid Extracts — Avens.—Barberry. — Bayberry.—Belladonna. —Black alder.—Blackberry root.—Catechu.—Coto bark.—Cranesbill.—Ergot.—Galls, — Ginger.—Goldenrod — Hardhack.— Ipecac — Johnswort.— Judas tree.—Kino.—Logwood.—Muskroot.—Opium, aqueous.—Plantain leaves. — Poplar bark. — Pricklyash berries.— Rhatany.—Rhubarb.—Rhubarb, aromatic.—Rhubarb and Potassium compound.—Rhus aromatica.—Sheep laurel.— Squawvine.—Sumach.—Sumach berries.—Swamp dogwood.—Tag alder.—Trumpet plant.—White oak bark.—White pond lily.—Willow herb.—Yerba reuma.

Pills—Astringent.—Camphor and Opium.—Camphor, Opium and Tannin.—Opium and Lead acetate.

Lozenges—Alum and Kino.—Catechu—Ginger.—Pepsin, Bismuth and Ginger.—Rhatany.—Rhubarb and Magnesia.—Tannic acid, U. S.

Tinctures—Opium compound, Squibb's formula.—Opium camphorated.

DIPHTHERIA.

Besides such routine treatment as may be adopted there is no antiseptic more useful locally than FORMASEPTOL; Lilly. The air of the room and premises should be kept well disinfected with gaseous Formaldehyde by means of a Moffatt Generator so that the patient will constantly breathe the gas.

DROPSY.

Fluid Extracts — American ivy.— Broom tops.— Black Indian hemp. — Cantharides.—Colocynth.— Dwarf elder.— Digitalis.— Equisetum hyemale.—Hair cap moss.— Jaborandi.—Jalap.—Juniper berries.—Large flowering spurge.—Silkweed.—Squill.—Swamp dogwood.—White bryony.

Pills—Arsenous acid.—Asiatic.—Digitalis compound.—Elaterium.

Saline purgatives.

DYSENTERY.

Chlorodyne; Lilly.

Fluid Extracts—Aconite.—Avens root.—Barberry. Blackberry.—Coto bark.—Cranesbill.—Ergot.—Hardhack. —Hemlock bark.—Ipecac.—Jersey tea.—Johnswort.—Logwood.—Marsh rosemary.—Nux vomica.—Plantain leaves.—Rhubarb and Potassium compound.—Rhus aromatica.—Willow herb.—Witchhazel. —Yarrow.—Yerba reuma.

Pills—Astringent.—Bismuth and Nux vomica.—Silver nitrate.

Saline purgatives.

DYSMENORRHEA.

Fluid Extracts—Aconite.—Belladonna.—Black cohosh.—Blue cohosh.—Blue cohosh compound.—Cannabis Indica.—Cramp bark.—Cotton root bark.—Ergot. — Gelsemium.—Life root. — Pulsatilla.—Squawvine compound.—Sumbul.—Unicorn root.—Ustilago maydis.

Pills—Codeine.—Cohosh compound.—Ergotin and Cannabis Indica.—Female, amenorrhea.— Helonias compound.— Morphine sulphate.—Morphatropia.

Elixirs—Helonias compound.—Iron, Quinine and Strychnine phosphates.

DYSPEPSIA.

Lilly's Liquid Pepsin.—Pepsin, U. S.—Pepsin, saccharated, U. S.—Pepsin, lactated.

Pills—Antidyspepsia, Fothergill.—Antidyspeptic.—Bismuth and Nux vomica.—Digestive.—Iron, Quinine and Strychnine phosphates.

Elixirs—Pepsin.—Pepsin and Bismuth.—Pepsin, Bismuth and Strychnine.—Lactated Pepsin.—See list for other Pepsin combinations.

Tablets—Sodamint to relieve excess of acid.

Lozenges—Bismuth and Charcoal.—Charcoal.—Carbolic acid.—Pepsin.—Pepsin, Bismuth and Ginger.

DYSURIA—See Strangury.

ECZEMA.

Succus Alterans; Lilly.

Fluid Extracts—Blue flag, when patient is gouty.—Poison oak.—Violet herb.

Pills—Calcium sulphide.—Phosphorus.

Glycerole—Tannic acid, locally.

EMPHYSEMA.

Fluid Extracts—Grindelia.—Jaborandi—Lobelia herb. — Quebracho.—Senega.—Stramonium.

Pills—Arsenous acid or Asiatic long continued improves nutrition of lungs.—Strychnine, valuable respiratory stimulant.—Quinine sulphate.

Wine—Coca with hypophosphites.

Syrup—Hypophosphites compound with Quinine and Strychnine.—Phosphates, Iron, Quinine and Strychnine.

Elastic Filled Capsules—Cod liver oil.

EPILEPSY.

Fluid Extracts—Belladonna.—Calabar bean.—Cannabis Indica.—Cinchona.—Conium.—Digitalis.—Horsenettle.—Hyoscyamus.—Nux vomica.—Opium, aqueous.—Valerian.

Pills—Arsenous acid.—Asiatic.—Atropine.—Camphor, monobromated.—Camphor and Opium.—Camphor, Henbane and Valerian.—Cannabis Indica ext.—Morphine, Henbane and Camphor.—Silver nitrate.—Zinc oxide.—Zinc valerianate.

Elixirs—Potassium bromide when occuring in daytime.—Chloral for nocturnal variety.—Zinc valerianate.

EPISTAXIS.

Fluid Extracts—Aconite.—Arnica.—Belladonna.—Cranesbill.—Digitalis.—Ergot.—Ipecac.—Witchhazel.

Powdered alum.—Tannic acid.—Compression.

ERYSIPELAS.

Fluid Extracts—Aconite.—Belladonna.—Cinchona.—Jaborandi.—Poison oak.

Pills—Iron iodide.—Iron sulphate.—Quinine sulphate.—Salicylic acid.

Tincture—Iron chloride.

Locally—FORMASEPTOL, Lilly.—Carbolic acid.—Collodium.—Silver nitrate.

FEVERS.

Fluid Extracts—Aconite in simple inflammation and eruptive fevers. — Arnica. — Black cohosh.— Digitalis.— Eucalyptus.— Gelsemium.—Jaborandi.—Veratrum viride.

Pills—Acetanilid. — Cinchonidine salicylate. — Quinine sulphate. — Salicylic acid.

Acid drinks—Baths.—Liquor Ammonium acetate.

FLATULENCE.

Fluid Extracts—Anise seed.—Aromatic. — Calabar bean.—Calamus.—Cardamon compound.—Columbo.—Feverfew.—Ginger.—Lavender compound.—Nux vomica.—Peppermint.—Spearmint.—Valerian.

Pills—Asafetida.

Tablets—Sodamint.—Potassium bicarbonate.—Sodium bicarbonate.

Lozenges—Carbolic acid.—Charcoal.—Charcoal and Sodamint.—Ginger.—Peppermint.

GALL STONES; See Calculi, biliary.

GASTRALGIA.

> **Fluid Extracts**—Belladonna.—Ergot.—Opium, aqueous.—Nux vomica.—Pulsatilla.
>
> **Pills**—Bismuth and Nux vomica.—Morphine sulphate.—Sodium salicylate.
>
> **Elixirs**—Bismuth.—Bismuth and Strychnine.—Bismuth, Quinine and Strychnine.—Pepsin and Bismuth.—Pepsin, Bismuth, Iron, Quinine and Strychnine.
>
> **Tablets**—Sodamint.—Potassium bicarbonate.—Sodium bicarbonate.
>
> **Lozenges**—Bismuth and Ginger.—Pepsin and Bismuth.

GASTRITIS.

> **Fluid Extracts**—Cinchona.—Columbo.—Gentian.—Goldenseal.—Ipecac.—Nux vomica.—Pulsatilla.
>
> **Pills**—Arsenous acid.—Asiatica.—Bismuth and **Nux vomica**.—Opium and Lead acetates—Silver nitrate.
>
> **Elixirs**—Bismuth.—Bismuth and Strychnine.—Calisaya bark and Bismuth.—Calisaya bark, Bismuth and Strychnine.—Calisaya bark, Iron and Bismuth.—Calisaya bark, Pepsin and Bismuth.—Pepsin, Bismuth and Water ash.—Pepsin, Pancreatin and Bismuth.
>
> **Tablets**—Ammonium chloride.—Bismuth **subgallate**.—Digestive.—Dyspepsia.
>
> **Lozenges**—Bismuth and Charcoal.—Pepsin and Bismuth.—Pepsin, Bismuth and Ginger.

GLAND'S, ENLARGED.

> *Succus Alterans; Lilly.*
>
> **Pills**—Calcium sulphide.—Corrosive sublimate.—Iron iodide.—Iodoform and Iron.—Potassium iodide.

GLEET.

> **Fluid Extracts**—Buchu.—Buchu and Pareira brava.—Cantharides.—Judas tree as an injection.—Juniper berries.—Kavakava.—Manzanita.
>
> **Pills**—Blennorrhagic.—Copaiba.—Copaiba compound.—Sandalwood compound.—Gonorrhea.
>
> **Elastic Filled Capsules**—See list, pages 216, 217 and 218.

GONORRHEA.

> *Succus Alterans; Lilly.*
>
> **Fluid Extracts**—Aconite.—Buchu.—Cantharides.—Colocynth.—Colchicum.—Cannabis Indica.—Cubeb.—Eucalyptus.—Goldenseal non-alcoholic, as an injection.—Judas tree.—Kavakava.—Manzanita.—Sandalwood.—Sumach.—Veratrum viride.—Yerba reuma.
>
> **Pills**—Blennorrhagic.—Copaiba compound.—Copaiba **and Cubeb**.—Gonorrhea.
>
> **Elastic Filled Capsules**—Copaiba.—Copaiba and Cubeb.—Copaiba, Cubeb and Iron.—Copaiba, Cubeb and Matico.—Copaiba, Cubeb, Matico and Sandalwood.—Copaiba, Cubeb and Sandalwood.—Copaiba and Sandalwood.—Cubeb and Sandalwood.

GOUT.

> **Fluid Extracts**—Aconite.—Belladonna.—Bittersweet.—Colchicum.—Cinchona.—Guaiac.
>
> **Pills**—Arsenous acid.—Asiatic.—Iodoform.—Lupulin.—Potassium iodide.—Sodium salicylate.—Salicylic acid.—Strychnine.—Veratrine.
>
> **Elixir**—Lithium citrate.
>
> **Elastic Filled Capsules**—Cod **liver oil**.
>
> Farinaceous diet.—Acid fruits.

GRAVEL.

> **Fluid Extracts**—Corn silk.—Dwarf elder.—Gravel plant.—Haircap moss.—Hydrangea.—Juniper berries.—Queen of the meadow.—Stone root.—Uva Ursi.—Water eryngo.

HAY FEVER.
Pills—Arsenous acid.—Atropine.—Potassium iodide.
Elixirs—Grindelia.—Potassium bromide.
Ammonia cautiously inhaled.—Carbolic acid by inhalation.

HEADACHE.
Pills—Acetanilid.—Arsenous acid for throbbing pain in brow.—Cathartics when due to constipation.
Elixirs—Ammonium valerianate.—Bromochloral compound.—Celery and Guarana.—Chloral hydrate.—Guarana.—Hypnotic.—Morphine valerianate.—in sick headache, Potassium bromide.
Tablets—Acetanilid.—Acetanilid compound, special.—Acetanilid compound; Lilly.—Analgesic.—Migraine.
Aconite as an ointment when due to neuralgia.—Ammonium chloride when due to dysmenorrhea or amenorrhea.

HEARTBURN
Tablets—Sodamint.

HEART DISEASE.
Fluid Extracts—Aconite.—Black cohosh.—Cactus grandiflorus.—Digitalis in rapid action with low tension and valvular lesions.—Ergot where heart is dilated.—Hyoscyamus.—Lily of the valley.—Nux vomica.—Valerian.—Veratrum viride.
Pills—Arsenous acid.—Asiatic.—Atropine as an excitant.
Elixir—Potassium bromide for over action and simple hypertropy.

HEMATEMESIS.
Lilly's Ergotin Hypodermically.
Fluid Extracts—Cranesbill.—Ergot.—Ipecac.—Logwood.—Rhatany.—Witchhazel.
Alum.—Gallic acid.—Iced champagne.—Lead acetate.—Monsel's solution.—Tannic acid. Perfect rest.

HEMATURIA.
Lilly's Ergotin Hypodermically.
Fluid Extracts—Cannabis Indica.—Cranesbill.—Ergot.—Ipecac.—Matico.—Pipsissewa.—Rhatany.—Witchhazel.
Pills—Copaiba.—Quinine sulphate in intermittent trouble.
Alum.—Gallic acid.—Tannic acid.

HEMICRANIA; See Migraine.

HEMOPTYSIS.
Fluid Extracts—Aconite.—Arnica.—Digitalis.—Ergot, combined with Ipecac and Opium, aqueous, given in large doses.—Ipecac.—Witchhazel.
Alum.—Atropine hypodermically.—Ferric acetate.—Sodium chloride.—Turpentine.

HEMORRHAGE.
Fluid Extracts—Aconite.—Arnica.—Belladonna.—Cinchona.—Cranesbill.—Digitalis.—Ergot.—Ipecac.—Logwood.—Nux vomica.—Opium, aqueous.—Pipsissewa.—Rhatany.—White oak bark.—Witchhazel.
Syrup—Iron, Quinine and Strychnine phosphates.
Alum.—Gallic acid.—Lead acetate.—Iron perchloride, solution.—Monsel's solution.—Tannic acid.—Perfect rest.

HEMORRHAGE, UTERINE.
Ergotin; Lilly, Hypodermically.
Atropine sulphate; Lilly, Hypodermically.
Fluid Extracts—Black cohosh.—Digitalis.—Ergot in full doses.—Ipecac.—Nux vomica.
Astringents.—Electricity.—Hot water injections.—Monsel's solution

HEMORRHOIDS.

Elixir Purgans; Lilly, to procure soft and easy evacuations.—*Glycones; Lilly,* when troubled with fecal impaction.

Fluid Extracts—Belladonna.—Cranesbill.—Ergot.—Galls.—Opium, aqueous.—Rhatany.—White oak bark.

Carbolic acid injections. — Gallic acid. — Monsel's solution to arrest bleeding.—Tannic acid.—Thorough cleansing of the parts after each movement of the bowels by bathing.

HEPATIC DISEASES.

Elixir Purgans; Lilly, stimulates the flow of bile.

Fluid Extracts— Aconite in acute inflammation.— Blue flag.—Boldo.—Colchicum in congestion.—Colocynth.—Culver's root.—Dandelion.—Gentian.—Ipecac.—Nux vomica.—Wahoo.

Pills—Blue mass.—Blue mass compound.—Calomel.—Cathartic compound.— Cathartic, improved.-- Hepatic.—Hepatic, eclectic.—Phosphorus.

Ammonium chloride.—Sodium phosphate.

HOARSENESS.

Tablets—Bronchial.—Borax.—Potassium chlorate and Borax.

Lozenges—Alum and Kino.— Bronchial, formula A.—Bronchial, formula B.—Guaiac.—Catechu.

HYDROTHORAX.

Fluid Extracts—Bloodroot.— Broom tops. — Buchu. — Digitalis.—Jaborandi.—Juniper and Potassium acetate.

Pills—Elaterium, Clutterbuck.

Blister—Dry cupping.—Iodine.—Tincture Iron chloride.

HYPOCHONDRIASIS.

Fluid Extracts—Black cohosh.—Coca leaves.—Guarana.—Hyoscyamus.—Opium, aqueous.— Valerian.

Pills—Arsenous acid.—Asiatic.—Asafetida.—Cocaine.—Gold chloride.

Elixir—Potassium bromide.

Turkish baths.

HYSTERIA.

Fluid Extracts—Aconite.—Black cohosh.—Blue cohosh.—Cannabis Indica.—Catnep.—Coca.—Ergot.—Eucalyptus.—Ladies's lipper.—Lavender compound.— Motherwort.— Mugwort.— Muskroot.—Nux vomica.— Opium, aqueous.— Stavesacre.— Skunk cabbage. — Scullcap. — Scullcap compound.— Unicorn root.— Valerian.

Pills—Asafetida.— Asafetida compound. — Camphor, Henbane and Valerian.—Camphor, monobromated.—Camphor and Opium.—Coca, Phosphorus and Strychnine. — Lupulin and Camphor.— Morphine valerianate.—Morphine, Henbane and Camphor. Phosphorus and Iron.—Zinc phosphide and Nux vomica.— Zinc valerianate.

Elixirs—Ammonium valerianate.—Iron pyrophosphate, Quinine and Strychnine.—Potassium bromide.—Zinc valerianate.

Wine—Coca with hypophosphites.

Elastic Filled Capsules—Cod liver oil.

Electricity.—Cold or shower baths.

IMPOTENCE.

Pil. Aphrodisiaca; Lilly, send for booklet.

Fluid Extracts—Cannabis Indica.— Cantharides.— Coca leaves.—Damiana.— Ergot.—Sanguinaria.—Stillingia.

Pills—Coca, Phosphorus and Strychnine.—Phosphorus and Nux vomica.—Phosphorus and Iron.—Phosphorus, Iron and Nux vomica.—Phosphorus and Cannabis Indica.—Zinc phosphide and Nux vomica.

Wines—Coca.—Coca with hypophosphites.

INCONTINENCE OF URINE.

Fluid Extracts—Belladonna.—Couch grass.—Cantharides.—Cubeb.—Ergot—Hops.—Hyoscyamus.—Lupulin.—Pareira brava.

Pills—Iron iodide in anemic cases.—Lupulin.

Elixir—Potassium bromide.

Warm salt baths.

INDIGESTION; See Dyspepsia.

INFLAMMATION.

Fluid Extracts—Aconite in inflammation of respiratory organs.—Arnica.—Belladonna in some catarrhal inflammations.—Bryonia in pericarditis.—Digitalis as an arterial sedative to diminish blood supply to inflamed surfaces.—Ergot may abort incipient inflammation.—Gelsemium.—Jaborandi in acute bronchitis.—Veratrum viride.

Pills—Quinine and Dover's in incipient inflammation.

INFLUENZA.

Fluid Extracts—Aconite.— Black cohosh.— Bloodroot.— Cubeb.— Ipecac.

Pills—Acetanilid.—Antiseptic, intestinal.—Quinine sulphate.—Salicylic acid.—Sodium salicylate.—Strychnine.

Tablets—Acetanilid.— Acetanilid compound, special. — Acetanilid compound; Lilly.

INSOMNIA.

Fluid Extracts— Belladonna. — Cannabis Indica. - Chamomile.— Hops.—Hyoscyamus.—Muskroot.—Opium, aqueous.

Pills—Codeine.—Morphine sulphate.—Morphine valerianate.- Lupulin.

Elixir—Bromochloral compound. -Hypnotic. - Potassium bromide.

Wines—Coca.—Coca with hypophosphites.

Warm bath.

INTERMITTENT FEVER.

Fluid Extracts— Black pepper. -- Boldo. — Cinchona and compounds.—Centaury. Chirata.—Dogwood.—Eucalyptus. -Five flowered Gentian. Fringe tree bark. Grindelia.- Ignatia bean. -Poplar bark. - Quinine flower.—Tulip tree bark.

Pills - Arsenous acid.   Antimalarial, McCaw.   Antimalarial, Harper.—Antiperiodic.—Asiatic. - Calisaya bark alkaloids. Cinchonine sulphate.—Cinchonidine sulphate.—Cinchonidine, Iron and Strychnine.—Iron, Quinine and Strychnine.— Iron, Quinine and Strychnine phosphates.—Quinine sulphate. Quinine bisulphate. Quinine and Blue mass. Quinine and Capsicum. Quinine and Dover's.- Tonic, Aiken.—Tonic, Hematic. Tonic, Walker - Warburg's Tincture.—Warburg's Tincture, without aloes.

Elixirs—Calisaya bark and combinations.— Iron, Quinine and Strychnine phosphates. Iron pyrophosphate. Quinine and Strychnine.—Iron pyrophosphate, Quinine and Arsenic.

Tincture—Warburg's.—Warburg's, modified.-- Warburg's, without Aloes.

Yerbazin; Lilly, perfectly disguises the bitterness of Quinine.

JAUNDICE.

Elixir Purgans; Lilly, reliably stimulates the liver.

Fluid Extracts—Balmony.—Bayberry.- Bitter root.—Bittersweet.—Black alder.—Blue flag.—Boldo. — Boneset. — Colocynth. -- Culver's root. — Dandelion. — Figwort. — Garden celandine. — Goldenseal. — Ipecac.—Liverwort.—Mandrake.—Rhubarb.—Stillingia. - Wahoo.

Pills—Aloes.—Aloes, Nux vomica and Belladonna.—Aloin. Aloin compound.—Aloin, Strychnine and Belladonna. Alterative.—Antibilious.—A. S. B. and I.; Lilly.—Blue mass. Blue mass compound.—Calomel and Rhubarb.—Cathartic compound, U. S. - Cathartic, improved.—See formulas of other cathartic pills.—Cholagogue. Christopher.—Cook's.—Colocynth, Ipecac and Blue mass.—Leptandrin.—Leptandrin compound.—Liver, improved vegetable.—Liver granules.—Podophyllin. — Podophyllin and Blue mass. — Podophyllin compound. — Podophyllin compound, Eclectic. — Podophyllin and Berberine.—Podophyllin and Leptandrin.- Triplex.- Triplex, Francis.

Ammonium chloride in Fl. ext. Dandelion. - Sodium phosphate

JOINTS, AFFECTIONS OF.

Fluid Extracts Aconite for pains of inflammation.— Poison oak, internally and as a lotion in subacute stiffness after rheumatic fever.

Pills—Acetanilid for the pyrexia of polyarthritis.

Turpentine liniment for chronic enlargement.

LABOR.

Fluid Extracts—Cotton root bark.—Ergot.—Opium, aqueous.

Pills—Quinine sulphate.

Chloroform.—Chloral hydrate.

LACTATION.

Fluid Extracts—Belladonna arrests secretion of milk.—Jaborandi increases the secretion.

Syrup—Calcium lactophosphate, useful in debility of lactation.

LARYNGISMUS STRIDULUS.

Fluid Extracts Aconite.— Asafetida.— Belladonna.— Conium.— Ipecac.— Lobelia.—Valerian.

Pills Nitroglycerin.— Quinine sulphate in the interval may prevent attacks.

CHLOROFORM WILL STOP AN ATTACK AT ONCE, a few drops on a handkerchief sufficient.— Ammonia.— Chloral hydrate.— Ether.— Mustard.—Spinal sponging, cold.

LARYNGITIS.

Fluid Extracts—Aconite.— Belladonna.—Catechu.—Ipecac.

Pills— Ipecac and Opium.— Quinine and Dover's.

Lozenges—Cubeb, U. S.—Guaiac.

Alum.—Iodoform, locally.— Inhalation of vapor of hot water, containing Fl. exts. Opium, Hops or Hyoscyamus.

LEUCORRHEA.

Succus Alterans; Lilly, as a tonic.

Fluid Extracts Black walnut.— Black cohosh.—Ergot.— Goldenseal, nonalcoholic.— Jaudica tree.— Life everlasting.—Manzanita.— Matico.— Muskroot.—Pareira Brava.—Pulsatilla.— Rhus aromatica.— Stomach.—Viburnum stone crop.— White oak bark.— White pond lily.— Willow herb.—Yerba reuma.

Syrup—Calcium Lactophosphate.

Injections Formaldehyde; LILLY.— Alum, combined with Borax or Zinc sulphate.— Carbolic acid.— Fl. ext. Goldenseal, nonalcoholic, may be combined with Bismuth.—Iodoform and Tannin packed about the cervix.—Lead acetate.—Monsel's solution.

LOCOMOTOR ATAXIA.

Fluid Extracts—Belladonna.— Calabar bean.—Cannabis Indica.— Ergot.— Jaborandi.— Opium, aqueous.

Pills— Belladonna ext.— Cannabis Indica ext.— Gold and Sodium chloride.— Silver nitrate.— Phosphorus.

Elastic Filled Capsules—Cod liver oil.

Galvanism.

LUMBAGO.

Fluid Extracts— Belladonna.— Black cohosh.—Calabar bean.— Capsicum.— Veratrum viride.

Pills— Aconitine acid.— Ackfoe.— Belladonna ext.— Corrosive sublimate.— Morphine sulphate.— Potassium iodide.— Salicylic acid.

Belladonna plaster.— **Chloroform** liniment.— Galvanism.— Massage.— Warm bath.

LUPUS.

Succus Alterans; Lilly.

Pills—Copaiba.— Phosphorus.

Elastic Filled Capsules—Cod liver oil.

Locally—Chromic acid.—Carbolic acid.— Iodoform.—Nitric acid.—Zinc chloride.

MALARIA: See Intermittent and **Remittent Fevers.**

MANIA.

Fluid Extracts—Black cohosh.—Belladonna.—Cannabis **Indica.**—Digitalis.—Ergot.—Gelsemium.—**Hyoscyamus.**—Lupulin.—Opium, aqueous.—Stramonium.—Veratrum viride.

Pills—Camphor, monobromated.—Camphor and Opium.—Hyoscine hydrobromate.—Hyoscyamine, crystals.—Lupulin and Camphor.

Elixirs—Bromochloral **compound.**—Chloral **hydrate.**—**Hypnotic.**—Potassium bromide.

MEASLES.

Fluid Extracts—Aconite for the fever.—**Ipecac.—Jaborandi.**—Pleurisy root.—Pulsatilla.—Veratrum viride.

Low diet, no animal food.—Dark room, complete disuse of eyes.—Strict cleanliness.—Disinfection by gaseous Formaldehyde.

MELANCHOLIA.

Fluid Extracts—Black cohosh **in uterine despondency.—Cannabis** Indica.—Colchicum.—Valerian.

Pills—Cannabis Indica ext.—Camphor and Opium.—Camphor, monobromated.—Gold and Sodium chloride.—Phosphorus.

Elixirs—Bromochloral compound.—Chloral hydrate.—Hypnotic.—Potassium bromide.

MENORRHAGIA.

Fluid Extracts—Black cohosh.—Cannabis Indica.—Cotton root.—Digitalis.—Ergot.—Ipecac.—Kino.—Rhatany.—Rue.—Savin.—Witch-hazel.

Pills—Ergotin and Cannabis Indica.—Zinc phosphide.

Elixirs—Iron pyrophosphate, Quinine and Strychnine.—Potassium bromide.

Syrup—Calcium lactophosphate.

Hot water bag to the spine.

METRITIS, ACUTE.

Fluid Extract—Aconite for the fever.

Pills—Ergotin, Bonjean.

Hot water injections.—Bleeding.—Opium **in full doses.—Carbolic acid.**—Silver nitrate.—Saline laxatives.

METRORRHAGIA: See **Hemorrhage, uterine.**

MIGRAINE.

Fluid Extracts—Belladonna.—Bloodroot.—Cannabis Indica.—Coca.—Digitalis.—Ergot.—Eucalyptus.—Guarana.—Jamaica dogwood.—Nux vomica.—Valerian.

Pills—Acetanilid.—Migraine, No. 1.—Migraine, No. 2.—Nitroglycerin.

Tablets—Acetanilid.—Acetanilid compound, special.—Acetanilid compound, Lilly.—Analgesic.

Elixirs—Celery and Guarana.—Guarana.—Potassium bromide.

Wine—Coca.

Full doses of **Ammonium** chloride will frequently cut short the attack.

NAUSEA.

Fluid Extracts—Cocculus Indicus in cephalic nausea.—Columbo.—Ipecac in pregnancy.—Pulsatilla in dyspeptic nausea.

Lozenges—Peppermint.

Iced champagne.

NEURALGIA.

Fluid Extracts—Aconite where there is febrile excitement.—Belladonna.—Black cohosh.—Cannabis Indica.—Ergot.—Gelsemium in neuralgia of the fifth nerve, in ovarian neuralgia and in trifacial neuralgia.—Veratrum viride.

Pills—Acetanilid.—Arsenous acid.—Asiatic.—Neuralgic, Brown-Séquard.—Neuralgic, Gross.—Neuralgic, Gross, without Morphine.—Neuralgic, with Cinchonidine.—Nitroglycerin.—Phosphorus.—Phosphorus, Iron and Nux vomica.—Quinine Sulphate.—Sodium salicylate.—Zinc valerianate.

Elixir—Potassium bromide.

Ext. Aconite made into an ointment and applied locally.—Anesthetics.—Counter irritants.—Heat.—Mustard.

NIGHT SWEATS.
Fluid Extracts—Belladonna.—Ergot.
Pills—Agaricin.—Atropine.—Creasote, beechwood.
Wine—Coca with hypophosphites.
Aromatic sulphuric acid.

NYMPHOMANIA.
Pills—Camphor, monobromated.—Lupulin and Camphor.
Elixir—Potassium bromide.
Cold bath.—Mild diet.—Active exercise.

OBESITY.
Fluid Extract—Bladderwrack.
Elixir—Ammonium bromide.
Alkaline mineral waters.—Vegetable acids.—Potassium permanganate.

OZENA.
Formaseptol; Lilly.
Fluid Extract—Goldenseal, nonalcoholic, locally.
Glycerole—Tannic acid.

PARALYSIS.
Fluid Extracts — Arnica.— Belladonna. — Calabar bean. — Cantharides.—Cannabis Indica.—Cocculus Indicus.—Cinchona.—Ergot.—Ignatia.—Nux vomica.—Poison oak.
Pills—Phosphorus.—Phosphorus and **Strychnine**.—Strychnine.
Syrup—Calcium lactophosphate.
Elastic Filled Capsules—Cod liver oil.
Electricity.—Massage.

PERITONITIS.
Fluid Extracts—Aconite for the febrile movement.—Cocculus Indicus.—Opium, aqueous.—White Bryony.
Tablets—Acetanilid.
Chloral hydrate or Morphine sulphate hypodermically for restlessness.—Heat and poultices.—Ice bag to abdomen.—Quinine sulphate.

PHARYNGITIS.
Fluid Extracts—Aconite.—Belladonna.—Black cohosh.—Goldenseal.—Ipecac.
Lozenges—Alum and Kino.—Ammonium chloride.—Ammonia, Jackson.—Brown mixture and Ammonium chloride.—Capsicum.—Carbolic acid.—Catechu.—Guaiac.—Potassium chlorate and Ammonium chloride.—Tannic acid.

PHTHISIS.
Pranicodeine; Lilly, for the cough.
Fluid Extracts—Belladonna.—Cannabis Indica.—Cherry bark.—Eucalyptus.—Opium, aqueous.—Sundew.
Pills—Arsenous acid.—Asiatic.—Creasote, beechwood.
Syrups—Calcium and Sodium hypophosphites.—Calcium, Sodium and Potassium hypophosphites.—Calcium lactophosphate.—Hypophosphites compound.—Hypophosphites compound, hematic.—Hypophosphites compound with Quinine and Strychnine.
Wine—Coca with hypophosphites.
Elastic Filled Capsules—Cod liver oil.—Creasote and Cod liver oil.

PLEURISY.
Fluid Extracts—Aconite for the febrile stage.—White Bryony in second stage. — Digitalis.— Jaborandi.— Large flowering spurge.—Opium, aqueous.—Pleurisy root.—Squill.—Veratrum viride.
Pills—Quinine sulphate.
Elastic Filled Capsules—Cod liver oil.
Counter irritation.—Leeching.—Potassium iodide.—Tartar emetic.

PNEUMONIA.

Fluid Extracts — Aconite. — Belladonna. — Digitalis. — Ipecac. — Opium, aqueous. — Senega. — Serpentaria for liquefaction of the exudation. — Veratrum viride.

Tartar Emetic or Ammonium carbonate.

Quinine sulphate in large doses during congestion, and in small tonic doses when depression comes on, in solution or suspended in Yerbazin; Lilly. Pills should not be given in such cases.

Blisters at onset to promote resolution.

PSORIASIS.

Succus Alterans; Lilly.

Pills — Arsenous acid. — Asiatic. — Calcium sulphide. — Phosphorus.

Syrup — Hypophosphites compound.

Elastic Filled Capsules — Cod liver oil.

Saline purgatives. — Sulphur.

PTYALISM.

Fluid Extract — Belladonna.

Vegetable astringents.

PUERPERAL CONVULSIONS.

Fluid Extracts — Aconite. — Belladonna. — Veratrum viride.

Elixir — Potassium bromide.

Hypodermic Tablet — Pilocarpine, hydrochlorate.

Anesthetics, especially Chloroform for temporary relief. — Bloodletting in cerebral congestion. — Chloral hydrate. — Morphine sulphate, hypodermically.

PUERPERAL FEVER.

Fluid Extracts — Opium, aqueous, in wakefulness or delirium. — Stramonium. — Veratrum viride.

Tablets — Potassium permanganate.

Quinine sulphate. — Quinine and Dover's or Cinchonidine salicylate in large doses. Should not be given in pills but suspended in Yerbazin; Lilly. Fordyce Barker recommends, Warburg's tincture, half a fluid ounce every four hours till fever abates, then in doses diminished to 1 or 2 fluid drams until convalescence. — Carbolic acid. — Turpentine.

PYROSIS.

Lilly's Liquid Pepsin is a reliable remedy. Half a wineglassful in sweetened water taken during each meal is the best. It may be sipped as a glass of wine. The use of the remedy should be continued for a month or more, and repeated as often as there appears any return of the trouble.

Elixir — Bismuth.

Sodium sulphite.

REMITTENT FEVER.

Fluid Extracts — Aconite. — Gelsemium. — Ipecac. — Opium, aqueous. — Quassia in convalescence. — Serpentaria.

Tablets — Acetanilid.

Tincture — Warburg's in small doses.

Quinine sulphate. — Cinchonidine salicylate **suspended in** Yerbazin; Lilly, is preferable to pills in such cases.

Acids. — Cold drinks. — Laxatives. — Sponging **with tepid water.**

RHEUMATISM, ACUTE.

Fluid Extracts — Aconite for the fever. — Arnica. — Black cohosh. — Belladonna. — Bittersweet. — Colchicum. — Conium. — Digitalis. — Jaborandi. — Opium, aqueous. — Poison **oak.** — Veratrum viride. — White Bryony.

Pills — Corrosive sublimate. — Cinchonidine salicylate. — Iodoform and Iron. — Potassium iodide. — Quinine sulphate. — Quinine and Dover's. — Rheumatic, without Mercury. — Salicylic acid.

Elixirs — Rheumatic. — Salicylic acid. — Salicylic acid compound. — Sodium salicylate.

Lime juice. — Sponging with cold water. — Stimulating liniments. — Galvanism.

RHEUMATISM, CHRONIC.

Succus Alterans; Lilly has proven of great value in many cases. It should be given in full doses.

Fluid Extracts—Black cohosh.—Belladonna.- Colchicum.—Coto bark.—Guaiac.— Kavakava.— Mezereum.— Pipsissewa.- Prickly ash bark.—Poke berries.—Poke root.—Soapwort.—Yellow parilla.

Pills—Antirheumatic.—Cinchonidine salicylate.—Quinine sulphate.—Rheumatic.- Rheumatic without Mercury.- Salicylic acid.

Elixirs—Lithia citrate.— Rheumatic — Salicylic acid compound.—Sodium salicylate.

Alkaline mineral waters.— Sulphurous waters and baths.— Turkish bath.

RICKETTS; Rachitis.

Succus Alterans; Lilly.

Pills—Iron iodide. Phosphorus.—Quinine sulphate.

Syrups Calcium lactophosphate.- Iron iodide. Phosphates compound, Chemical food.

Elastic Filled Capsules—Cod liver oil.

Food rich in phosphates, oil and lime.—Sponging, cold or salt water.—Full animal diet.

RUBEOLA; See Measles.

SCABIES.

Succus Alterans; Lilly.

Fluid Extract—Stavesacre seed 2 parts, mixed with simple ointment 7 parts, apply locally.

Pills—Calcium sulphide.— Corrosive sublimate.— Potassium iodide.

Alkaline baths.—Green soap.—Sulphur baths.

SCARLET FEVER.

Fluid Extracts—Aconite for the fever and local inflammation.—Belladonna when eruption is imperfect and heart's action depressed.—Digitalis as an antipyretic and diuretic.

Antiseptics for Spraying the Throat—Formasept rol, Lilly.—Carbolic acid.— Chlorine water.—Hydrochloric acid.— Potassium chlorate.—Resorcin.—Sodium benzoate.

Ammonium carbonate as stimulant to depressed circulation.—Oil inunctions to diminish irritation of skin and lessen temperature.—Quinine as a tonic and antipyretic should be given, suspended in Yerbazin; Lilly; pills not admissible.

SCIATICA.

Fluid Extracts—Belladonna.—Black cohosh.—Guaiac.—Nux vomica.—Poison oak.—Veratrum viride.

Pills—Acetanilid.—Nitroglycerin.—Potassium iodide.—Salicylic acid.

Elastic Filled Capsules—Cod liver oil.

Atropine, Cocaine or Morphine, subcutaneously, separately or combined.—Acupuncture.- Blisters.— Chloroform deeply injected in old cases.—Counter irritation.—Galvanism.—Turkish baths.

SCROFULA.

Succus Alterans; Lilly, now so generally used in hospitals and private practice, is the most valuable remedy in the treatment of scrofula.

Fluid Extracts—American ivy. American sarsaparilla.—Berberis aquifolium.— Bitter root. — Bittersweet.— Black walnut.— Burdock root.—Burdock seed.—Button snakeroot.- Clover tops.—False bittersweet.—Figwort. Garden celandine.—Plantain leaves.—Poke root.—Prickly ash bark.— Sarsaparilla. sarsaparilla compound.— Sheep laurel. Soapwort.—Stillingia.— Stillingia compound.— Tag alder.—Turkey corn.— Twin leaf. White pond lily.—Water eryngo.—Yellow dock.— Yellow dock compound.—Yellow parilla.

Pills –Calcium sulphide.—Iron iodide.—Iodoform and iron.—Iodoform and Mercury.—Mercury protiodide.

Elixir—Cordyalis compound.

Syrups—Calcium lactophosphate.—Hypophosphites compound with Quinine and Strychnine.- Iron iodide.—Iron and Manganese hypophosphites.—Phosphates compound, Chemical food.

Elastic Filled Capsules—Cod liver oil.

SEA SICKNESS.

Atropine and Morphine, separately or combined, subcutaneously.—Amyl nitrite by inhalation.—Bitters, such as Columbo or Nux vomica.—Chloral hydrate before nausea sets in.—Chloroform, a few drops by the stomach frequently.—Champagne, iced, in small quantity.—Elixir Ammonium bromide.

SKIN DISEASES.

Succus Alterans; Lilly, of great value in all cases.

Fluid Extract—Jaborandi when skin secretions are deficient.

Pills—Arsenous acid, or Asiatic in chronic scaly skin diseases.—Calcium sulphide in scrofulous sores often seen upon children.—Quinine sulphate where depression of vital forces exist.

Carbolic acid locally in acute and chronic affections.—Iodides when caused by metallic poisons.—Mineral acids when caused by indigestion.—Oils and fats by inunction.

SORE THROAT; See Laryngitis, Pharyngitis, etc.

SPERMATORRHEA.

Pil. Aphrodisiaca; Lilly.

Fluid Extracts—Belladonna.—Black cohosh.—Coca.—Cantharides.—Damiana.—Digitalis.—Ergot when genitals are relaxed and erections feeble.—Gelsemium.—Nux vomica.

Pills—Coca, Phosphorus and Strychnine.—Camphor, monobromated, when a genital sedative is indicated.—Lupulin.—Lupulin and Camphor.—Phosphorus, Iron and Strychnine where anemia is a marked feature.

Locally—Fl. ext. Goldenseal, nonalcoholic.—Silver nitrate.—Mineral and vegetable astringents.

SPLEEN, ENLARGED.

Fluid Extracts—Belladonna.—Ergot.—Grindelia.

Pills—Arsenous acid.—Asiatic.—Quinine sulphate.—Quinine and Arsenic.

Elixir—Potassium bromide.

STERILITY.

Pil. Aphrodisiaca; Lilly.

Succus Alterans; Lilly, when dependent on syphilis.

Pills—Coca, Phosphorus and Strychnine.—Gold and Sodium chloride.—Phosphorus combinations.

Wine—Coca and hypophosphites.

STOMATITIS.

Fluid Extracts—Blackberry.—Cranesbill.—Eucalyptus.—Goldenseal, nonalcoholic.—Rhatany.

Tablets—Borax.—Potassium chlorate and Borax.—Potassium chlorate.

Brandy and water. Bismuth subnitrate freely applied.—Hydrochloric acid applied directly to the ulcers.—Potassium chlorate in solution.

STRANGURY.

Fluid Extracts—Aconite root.—Belladonna.—Cannabis Indica.—Cantharides.—Equisetum hyemale.—Ergot.—Gelsemium.—Opium, aqueous.—Pipsissewa.—Uva Ursi.—Veratrum viride.

Pills—Camphor and Opium.

Elixir—Potassium bromide.

Spirit Nitrous ether.—Turpentine.

SYPHILIS.

Succus Alterans; Lilly, has been successfully used in the principal hospitals of the United States, as well as by a very large number of private practitioners and has received the unqualified endorsement of leading members of the medical profession.
See page 311.

TETANUS.

Fluid Extracts—Aconite.—Belladonna.—Calabar bean.—Cannabis Indica.—Cantharides.—Cinchona.—Conium.—Gelsemium.—Hyoscyamus.—Jaborandi.—Nux vomica.

Pills—Atropine.—Belladonna ext.—Cannabis Indica ext.—Hyoscyamine crystals.—Hyoscyamus ext.—Hyoscine hydrobromate.—Jaborandi ext.—Nux vomica ext.—Morphine sulphate.—Quinine sulphate.—Strychnine.

Elixirs—Bromochloral compound.—Chloral hydrate.—Hypnotic.—Potassium bromide.

Amyl nitrate.—Chloroform.—Ether.—Electricity.—Ice bag.—Purgatives.—Tobacco.

TONSILITIS.

Fluid Extracts—Aconite when accompanied by fever.—Belladonna.—Guaiac in full doses said to abort the attack.

Pills—Calomel in small doses to reduce inflammation.—Quinine sulphate in large doses at the outset may abort the attack.

Tablets—Potassium chlorate.

Lozenges—Alum and Kino.—Capsicum.—Guaiac.

TOOTHACHE.

Fluid Extracts—Gelsemium.—Jamaica dogwood.—Opium, aqueous.—Prickly ash berries.—Stavesacre.

Chlorodyne on cotton.—Carbolic acid.—Creasote.—Morphine sulphate.—Oil Cloves.—Resorcin.—Saturated solution Sodium carbonate held in the mouth.—Solution of Alum in Nitrous ether.—Tannin dissolved in Ether.

TYPHOID FEVER.   Aconite

Fluid Extracts—Arnica.—Belladonna.—Cinchona.—Digitalis.—Ergot.—Ipecac.—Serpentaria.—Veratrum viride.—Wild indigo.

Wine—Coca in convalescence.

A milk diet usually most suitable.—Acetanilid as an antipyretic.—Calomel in ten grain doses during the first week or ten days.—Muriatic acid to reduce fever and restrain diarrhea.—Tincture Iodine compound lessens violence and shortens duration.—Quinine in large doses, either in solution or suspended in Yerbazin; Lilly. Pills should not not be given.—Bismuth subnitrate—Carbolic acid with Iodine.—Cold baths.—Fowler's solution with Tincture Opium to restrain diarrhea.—Ice.—Resorcin.—Salicylic acid.—Silver nitrate.

TYPHUS FEVER.   Aconite

Fluid Extracts—Arnica.—Belladonna.—Digitalis.—Guarana.—Hyoscyamus.—Opium, aqueous.—Rhatany.—Serpentaria.

Acetanilid.—Chloral hydrate.—Camphor.—Coffee.—Purgatives.—Nutritious diet.

ULCERS.

Succus Alterans; Lilly, in full doses persistently.

FORMASEPTOL; Lilly, locally as an antiseptic wash and dressing.

Locally—Alum, dried, feeble escharotic, destroys unhealthy granulations.—Copper sulphate.—Nitric acid, powerful escharotic to destroy unhealthy tissues and change character of surface.—Potassium chlorate in powder in epithelioma.—Silver nitrate.—Vienna paste.—Zinc sulphate, dried, valuable caustic, easily managed.—Zinc chloride, much more powerful, penetrating and more painful.

UREMIA.

Fluid Extracts—Colchicum.—Digitalis for procuring free action of kidneys.—Jaborandi, active diuretic, but contraindicated where the heart is weak or fatty.

Vapor and hot water pack to promote free diaphoresis.

Saline or hydragogue cathartics.—Morphine sulphate, hypodermically for convulsions.—Chloroform.—Chloral hydrate.

URTICARIA.

Acetanilid internally.—Nitric acid as a dilute wash.—Tincture Benzoin compound painted on the skin for the itching.—Sodium salicylate pills 2½ grs. each, every half hour, effective.—Colchicum in gouty cases.—Warm baths.

VOMITING.

Fluid Extracts—Blue flag.—Coca.—Cocculus Indicus.—Columbo.—Ipecac.—Nux vomica.—Opium, aqueous.—Serpentaria.—Veratrum viride.

Elixir—Potassium bromide.

Bismuth subnitrate.—Chloroform, a few drops.—Chloral hydrate.—Calomel, minute doses in cholera infantum.—Cerium oxalate in pregnancy.—Carbolic acid.—Effervescent alkaline drinks.—Fowler's solution.—Hydrocyanic acid.—Ice.—Iced champagne or brandy in small quantity frequently.—Ipecac in **very** small doses.—Milk and lime water.—Pepsin.

WHOOPING COUGH.

Fluid Extracts—Chestnut leaves in syrup.—Lobelia.

Elixirs—Ammonium bromide.—Potassium bromide.

Alum where there is copious bronchial secretion.—Asafetida.—Carbolic acid.—Chlorodyne.—Hydrocyanic acid dilute.

WORMS.

Fluid Extracts—Ailanthus.—American wormseed.—Kamala.—Male fern.—Pink root.—Pink root and Senna.—Pomegranate bark.—Pumpkin seed.—Quassia.—Valerian for convulsions.

Lozenges—Santonin.—Santonin and Calomel.—Santonin compound.—Santonin and Podophyllin.—Worm.

Elastic Filled Capsules—Male **fern** and **Kamala** especially for tape worm, see page 247.

"THE IDEAL FERRUGINOUS TONIC."

LIQUOR FERRI; Lilly,

AN ORGANOFERRIC COMPOUND.

LILLY'S IRON contains no albumen or nitrogenous substance whatever, being a new discovery and entirely different from any iron compound heretofore produced.

This preparation represents, in its fixed **proportion, one per cent.** of metallic iron in neutral combination.

The iron is combined with an organic radical **in** a very peculiar and characteristic condition. While permanent under all ordinary circumstances, it is instantly changed by the digestive process when taken into the stomach, the iron being virtually presented for assimilation in a nascent state.

It is neutral, being neither acid nor alkaline.

It does not derange the digestive functions even when taken regularly for a lengthy period, and is rapidly assimilated.

It is permanent in all temperatures.

It is agreeable and free from styptic taste.

It is compatible with the bitter tonics, such as cinchona, gentian and columbo, the fluid extracts of either of which may be added in proper proportion when required.

It is in all respects the ideal ferruginous tonic **so long desired by** physicians and so long sought for by chemists.

DOSE—For an adult, ½ to **1** teaspoonful **during or after meals** for children, less in proportion **to age.**

Price, $1.00 per Pint Bottle.

TABLE OF DOSES.

We have endeavored to make this table as complete as space would permit, giving not only the remedies in general use but also many of those which have not as yet found their way into general favor.

All remedies treated of elsewhere in this book are omitted from the table. For instance, crude drugs seldom or never given in substance are omitted and the doses of their respective preparations must be sought under the head of the corresponding fluid extract; also the doses of preparations contained in our list such as pills, granules, elixirs, syrups, wines, tinctures, cordials, solid and powdered extracts, concentrations, tablets, miscellaneous preparations, etc. will be found in the place where such preparations are treated, see Index.

The doses in the table are expressed in terms of both the Apothecaries' and Metric systems, the aim being, not to give exact equivalents but such metric quantities as as can be conveniently and safely used in calculating prescriptions.

All doses given, unless otherwise specified, are for adults; smaller doses being calculated according to the following rule:

RULE FOR DOSES BY AGE.

The proportionate dose for any age under adult life is represented by the number of the next birthday divided by 24 i. e. for one year, $\frac{2}{24}=\frac{1}{12}$; for two years, $\frac{3}{24}=\frac{1}{8}$, etc.

REMEDIES.	Apothecaries'.	Metric.	
Absinthin	1½ — 4 grs.	0.1 — 0.25	gm.
Acetal	2 — 3 fl. drs	8.0 — 12.0	c.c.
Acetanilid	2 — 10 grs.	0.12 — 0.6	gm.
monobrom. (asepsin.)	1 — 8 grs.	0.06 — 0.5	gm.
Acetone	5—15 m.	0.3 — 1.0	c.c.
Acetyl-phenyl-hydrazine	¾ — 1 gr.	0.015 — 0.06	gm.
Acetyl-tannin	3— 8 grs.	0.2 — 0.5	gm.
Acid acetic, dil.	1— 2 fl. drs.	4.0 — 8.0	c.c.
agaricic	¼—½ gr.	0.01 — 0.03	gm.
anisic	5—15 grs.	0.3 — 1.0	gm.
arsenous	1/100—¼ gr.	0.0006 — 0.005	gm.
benzoic	10—25 grs.	0.6 — 1.6	gm.
boric	5—15 grs.	0.3 — 1.0	gm.
camphoric	8—30 grs.	0.5 — 2.0	gm.
carbolic	¼ — 2 grs.	0.015 — 0.12	gm.
cathartic	4 — 6 grs.	0.25 — 0.4	gm.
cinnamic (by injection)	¼ — ¾ grs.	0.015 — 0.045	gm.
citric	10—30 grs.	0.6 — 2.0	gm.
cubebic	5—10 grs.	0.3 — 0.6	gm.
dibromogallic	10—30 grs.	0.6 — 2.0	gm.
di-ioto-salicylic	8—20 grs.	0.5 — 1.3	gm.
embelic	3— 6 grs.	0.2 — 0.4	gm.

Remedies.	Doses. Apothecaries'.	Doses. Metric.
Acid filicic	8—15 grs.	0.5 — 1.0 gm.
gallic	5—15 grs.	0.3 — 1.0 gm.
gynocardic	½—3 grs.	0.03 — 0.2 gm.
hydriodic	15—30 m.	1.0 — 2.0 c. c.
hydrobrom. dil.	20—120 m.	1.3 — 8.0 c.c.
hydrochlor., dil.	3—10 m.	0.2 — 0.6 c.c.
hydrocinnamic	10—20 m.	0.6 — 1.3 c.c.
hydrocyanic	1—5 m.	0.06 — 0.3 c.c.
hydrofluoric, dil.	20—30 m.	1.0 — 2.0 c.c.
hypophosphorous, dil	10—30 m.	0.6 — 2.0 c.c.
isovaleric	3—4 m.	0.2 — 0.25 c.c.
lactic	15—30 m.	1.0 — 2.0 c.c.
mono-iodo-salicylic	5—10 grs.	0.3 — 0.6 gm.
nitric, dil	3—15 m.	0.2 — 1.0 c.c.
nitrohydrochlor	1—8 m.	0.06 — 0.5 c.c.
nitrohydrochlor. dilute	5—20 m.	0.3 — 1.3 c.c.
oxalic	½—1 gr.	0.03 — 0.06 gm.
oxynaphtoic (alpha)	1½—3 grs.	0.1 — 0.2 gm.
para-cresotic	2—20 grs.	0.12 — 1.3 gm.
phenyl-acetic	10—15 m.	0.6 — 1.0 c.c.
phosphoric, dil.	5—30 m.	0.3 — 2.0 c.c.
picric	½—3 grs.	0.03 — 0.2 gm.
pyridine-tricarbonic	10 grs.	0.6 gm.
salicylic	2—15 grs.	0.12 — 1.0 gm.
santoninic	1—5 grs.	0.06 — 0.3 gm.
sclerotic (ergotic)	½—1 gr.	0.03 — 0.06 gm.
succinic	5—15 grs.	0.3 — 1.0 gm.
sulphanilic	10—20 grs.	0.6 — 1.3 gm.
sulphuric arom	5—15 m.	0.3 — 1.0 c.c.
sulphuric dilute	5—15 m.	0.3 — 1.0 c.c.
sulphurous	5—60 m.	0.3 — 4.0 c.c.
tannic	1—20 grs.	0.06 — 1.3 gm.
tannic albuminated	1—20 grs.	0.06 — 1.3 gm.
tartaric	10—30 grs.	0-6 — 2.0 gm.
valerianic	2—10 drops.	0.1 — 0.4 c.c.
Aconitine, cryst.	1/500—1/100 gr.	0.00012 — 0.0006 gm.
Adonidin	1/16—¼ gr.	0.004 — 0.015 gm.
Agaric (white)	15—30 grs.	1.0 — 2.0 gm.
Agaricin	1/6—1 gr.	0.01 — 0.06 gm.
Agathin	2—8 grs.	0.12 — 0.5 gm.
Alantol	¼ m.	0.01 c.c.
Alcohol	1—4 fl. drs.	4.0 — 15.0 gm.
Allyl tribromide	5—10 m.	0.3 — 0.6 c.c.
Aloes, purified	1—5 grs.	0.06 — 0.3 c.c.
Aloin	1/10—2 grs.	0.006 — 0.12 gm.
Alphol	8—15 grs.	0.5 — 1.0 gm.
Alum	10—20 grs.	0.6 — 1.3 gm.
Aluminum acetate	5—10 grs.	0.3 — 0.6 gm.
Ammoniac	10—30 grs.	0.6 — 2.0 gm.
Ammonium acetate	15—30 grs.	1.0 — 2.0 gm.
arsenate	1/20 gr.	0.003 gm.
benzoate	5—15 grs.	0.3 — 1.0 gm.
bisulphite	10—30 grs.	0.6 — 2.0 gm.
borate	10—20 grs.	0.6 — 1.3 gm.
bromide	10—30 grs.	0.6 — 2.0 gm.
camphorate	1—3 grs.	0.06 — 0.2 gm.
carbolate	2—6 grs.	0.12 — 0.4 gm.
carbonate	5—10 grs.	0.3 — 0.6 gm.
chloride	1—20 grs.	0.06 — 1.3 gm.
embelate	3—6 grs.	0.2 — 0.4 gm.
fluoride	1/24—1/6 gr.	0.0025 — 0.01 gm.
formate	5 grs.	0.3 gm.
glycero-phosphate	3—4 grs.	0.2 — 0.25 gm.
hypophosphite	10—30 grs.	0.6 — 2.0 gm.
hyposulphite	5—30 grs.	0.3 — 2.0 gm.
iodide	2—10 grs.	0.12 — 0.6 gm.
phosphate	10—20 grs.	0.6 — 1.3 gm.
picrate	¼—½ gr.	0.015 — 0.03 gm.
salicylate	2—10 grs.	0.12 — 0.06 gm.
sulphate	10—20 grs.	0.6 — 1.3 gm.
sulphite	5—20 grs.	0.3 — 1.3 gm.
sulphocarbolate	1—5 grs.	0.06 — 0.3 gm.
tartrate	5—30 grs.	0.3 — 2.0 gm.
valerianate	1—6 grs.	0.06 — 0.4 gm.

Remedies.	Doses.			
	Apothecaries'.		Metric.	
Amylamine hydrochlor	7—15	grs.	0.5 — 1.0	gm.
Amylene hydrate	60—90	m.	4.0 — 6.0	c.c.
Amyl nitrite { internally	¼—1	m.	0.015 — 0.06	c.c.
Amyl nitrite { by inhalation	2—5	m.	0.12 — 0.3	c.c.
Anemonin	1/10—1	gr.	0.006 — 0.06	gm.
Aniline sulphate	¾—1½	grs.	0.05 — 0.1	gm.
Antimony et pot. tart. { diaph.	1/16—¼	gr.	0.004 — 0.015	gm.
Antimony et pot. tart. { emetic	1—2	grs.	0.06 — 0.12	gm.
arsenate	1/50	gr.	0.0012	gm.
iodide	¼—1	gr.	0.015 — 0.06	gm.
oxide	1—3	grs.	0.06 — 0.2	gm.
sulphide (black)	5—15	grs.	0.3 — 1.0	gm.
sulphide (penta)	1/6—1½	grs.	0.01 — 0.1	gm.
sulphurated	1—5	grs.	0.06 — 0.3	gm.
Antipyrin	5—15	grs.	0.3 — 1.0	gm.
Apiol (camphor)	5—15	grs.	0.3 — 1.0	gm.
Apiol (liquid)	3—10	grs.	0.2 — 0.6	gm.
Apocodeine	3—4	grs.	0.2 — 0.25	gm.
Apomorph. hydro. { internally	1/10—1/6	gr.	0.006 — 0.01	gm.
Apomorph. hydro. { hypoder'ly	1/20—1/10	gr.	0.003 — 0.006	gm.
Arbutin	3—5	grs.	0.2 — 0.3	gm.
Arsenic bromide	1/50—1/10	gr.	0.0012 — 0.006	gm.
chloride	1/60—1/15	gr.	0.001 — 0.004	gm.
iodide	1/50—1/10	gr.	0.0012 — 0.006	gm.
sulphide	1/100—1/10	gr.	0.0006 — 0.006	gm.
Asafetida	2—12	grs.	0.12 — 0.8	gm.
Asaprol	8—15	grs.	0.5 — 1.0	gm.
Asparagin	5—10	grs.	0.3 — 0.6	gm.
Aspidospermine { (amorph.)	1—2	grs.	0.06 — 0.12	gm.
Aspidospermine { (cryst.)	⅓—1	gr.	0.02 — 0.06	gm.
Atropine	1/300—1/60	gr.	0.0002 — 0.001	gm.
sulphate	1/120—1/60	gr.	0.0005 — 0.001	gm.
Avenine (alkaloid)	1/120—1/64	gr.	0.0005 — 0.001	gm.
Balsam gurjun	8—60	m.	0.5 — 4.0	c. c.
peru	10—25	m.	0.6 — 1.6	c. c.
Baptisin (pure)	½—5	grs.	0.03 — 0.3	gm.
Barium chloride	1/10—½	grs.	0.006 — 0.03	gm.
sulphide	½—1	gr.	0.03 — 0.06	gm.
Bobeerine and salts	1/12—1½	grs.	0.005 — 0.1	gm.
Benzacetine	8—15	grs.	0.5 — 1.0	gm.
Benzanilid	10—15	grs.	0.6 — 1.0	gm.
Benzene (benzol)	5—10	drops.	0.3 — 0.6	c.c.
Benzin (petrol. ether)	5—10	drops.	0.3 — 0.6	c.c.
Benzosol	5—15	grs.	0.3 — 1.0	gm.
Berberine and salts { antiper.	8—15	grs.	0.5 — 1.0	gm.
Berberine and salts { tonic	½—1	gr.	0.03 — 0.06	gm.
Betol (naphto-salol)	4—8	grs.	0.25 — 0.5	gm.
Bismuth ammon. cit	1—5	grs.	0.06 — 0.3	gm.
phosphate	2—20	grs.	0.3 — 1.3	gm.
salicylate	5—20	grs.	0.3 — 1.3	gm.
subcarb	5—30	grs.	0.3 — 2.0	gm.
subgallate	5—20	grs.	0.3 — 1.3	gm.
subiodide	1½—3	grs.	0.1 — 0.2	gm.
subnitrate	5—30	grs.	0.3 — 2.0	gm.
Blue mass—see mass of Mercury				
Boldine (alkaloid)	1/30—1/10	gr.	0.002 — 0.006	gm.
Boldo-glucin (boldin)	1—3	grs.	0.06 — 0.2	gm.
Boroglycerin (solid)	30—90	grs.	2.0 — 6.0	gm.
Bromal hydrate	3—15	grs.	0.2 — 1.0	gm.
Bromalin	30—60	grs.	2.0 — 4.0	gm.
Bromanide	10—15	grs.	0.6 — 1.0	gm.
Bromoform	5—20	m.	0.3 — 1.3	c. c.
Brucine	1/12—½	gr.	0.005 — 0.03	gm.
Bryonin	⅙—⅓	gr.	0.01 — 0.02	gm.
Butyl-chloral hydrate	5—20	grs.	0.3 — 1.3	gm.
Cacsium and ammon. bromide	15—45	grs.	1.0 — 3.0	gm.
Caffeine	1—5	grs.	0.06 — 0.3	gm.
and sod. benzoate	2—10	grs.	0.12 — 0.6	gm.
and sod. cinnamate	2—6	grs.	0.12 — 0.4	gm.
and sod. hydrobrom	2—10	grs.	0.12 — 0.6	gm.
citrated	2—10	grs.	0.12 — 0.6	gm.
citrated efferves	60—120	grs.	4.0 — 8.0	gm.
iodide	2—4	grs.	0.12 — 0.25	gm.
Calcium benzoate	10—30	grs.	0.6 — 2.0	gm.

REMEDIES.	DOSES. Apothecaries'.		DOSES. Metric.	
Calcium borate....(for children)	1—5	grs.	0.06 — 0.3	gm.
bromide	5—60	grs.	0.3 — 4.0	gm.
carbolate	2—5	grs.	0.12 — 0.3	gm.
carb., precip	5—20	grs.	0.3 — 1.3	gm.
chloride	10—20	grs.	0.6 — 1.3	gm.
glycero-phosphate	2—5	grs.	0.12 — 0.3	gm.
hippurate	5—15	grs.	0.3 — 1.0	gm.
hypophosphite	10—30	grs.	0.6 — 2.0	gm.
hyposulphite	3—10	grs.	0.2 — 0.6	gm.
iodide	1—3	grs.	0.06 — 0.2	gm.
lactate	3—10	grs.	0.2 — 0.6	gm.
lactophosphate	3—10	grs.	0.2 — 0.6	gm.
permanganate	¼—2	grs.	0.075 — 0.12	gm.
phosphate dibasic	8—20	grs.	0.5 — 1.3	gm.
phosphate precip	2—10	grs.	0.12 0.6	gm.
quinovate	⅕—½	gr.	0.012 — 0.03	gm.
saccharate	10—30	grs.	0.6 — 2.0	gm.
salicylate	8—20	grs.	0.5 — 1.3	gm.
santoninate	½—1½	grs.	0.03 — 0.1	gm.
sulphide, crude	1/20—3	grs.	0.003 — 0.2	gm.
sulphite	1/10—5	grs.	0.006 — 0.3	gm.
sulphocarbolate	5—15	grs.	0.3 — 1.0	gm.
Calomel—*see Mercurous chloride, mild.*				
Camphor	2—10	grs.	0.12 — 0.6	gm.
carbolated	5—10	m.	0.3 — 0.6	c. c.
monobromated	1—10	grs.	0.06 — 0.6	gm.
salicylated	1—5	grs.	0.06 — 0.3	gm.
Canada Turp. (Balsam Fir.)	5—30	grs.	0.3 — 2.0	gm.
Cannabindon	½—1	m.	0.02 — 0.06	c. c.
Cannabine (alkaloid)	1½—4	grs.	0.1 — 0.25	gm.
Cannabinon	½—1½	grs.	0.03 — 0.1	gm.
Cannabin tannate	5—10	grs.	0.3 — 0.6	gm.
Capsicum	5—10	grs.	0.3 — 0.6	gm.
Carbon disulphide	½—1	m.	0.03 — 0.06	c. c.
Carlsbad salt, true	½—1	oz.	15.0 — 30.0	gm.
Carpaine hydrochlor.	1/20—1/10	gr.	0.003 — 0.006	gm.
Cerberin	1/240—1/64	gr.	0.00025— 0.001	gm.
Cerium nitrate	1—3	grs.	0.06 — 0.2	gm.
oxalate	1—10	grs.	0.06 — 0.6	gm.
Cetrarin (bitter prin)	1½—3	grs.	0.1 — 0.2	gm.
Charcoal	20—60	grs.	1.3 — 4.0	gm.
Chinoidin	1—20	grs.	0.06 — 1.3	gm.
Chinolin tartrate	5—20	grs.	0.3 — 1.3	gm.
Chloralamid	10—45	grs.	0.6 — 3.0	gm.
Chloral-ammonia	15—30	grs.	1.0 — 2.0	gm.
caffeine	3—6	grs.	0.2 — 0.4	gm.
hydrate	5—20	grs.	0.3 — 1.3	gm.
Chloralimide	15—45	grs.	1.0 — 3.0	gm.
Chloralose	3—12	grs.	0.2 — 0.8	gm.
Chloral-urethane	10—45	grs.	0.6 — 3.0	gm.
Chlorodyne	5—20	m.	0.3 — 1.3	c. c.
Chloroform	2—20	m.	0.12 — 1.3	c. c.
Chrysarobin	⅛—10	grs.	0.008 — 0.6	gm.
Cinchonidine salicylate	2—10	grs.	0.12 — 0.6	gm.
Cinchonine and salts	1—30	grs.	0.06 — 2.0	gm.
Citrophen	15	grs.	1.0	gm.
Citrullin	⅙—⅓	gr.	0.01 — 0.02	gm.
Cobalt and pot. nitrate	¼—½	gr.	0.015 — 0.03	gm.
Cocaine cantharidate (by injec.)	1/50—1/40	gr.	0.0012 — 0.0015	gm.
carbolate	1/12—⅙	gr.	0.005 — 0.01	gm.
hydrochlor	1/10—½	gr.	0.006 — 0.03	gm.
nitrate	¼—¾	gr.	0.015 — 0.045	gm.
Cochineal ....(for an infant)	⅓	gr.	— 0.02	gm.
Codeine	1/16—1	gr.	0.004 — 0.06	gm.
phosphate	1½—2	grs.	0.1 — 0.12	gm.
Confection of rose	10—60	grs.	0.6 — 4.0	gm.
senna	1—2	drs.	4.0 — 8.0	gm.
Colchicein	1/120—1/64	gr.	0.0005 — 0.001	gm.
Colchicine	1/120—1/64	gr.	0.0005 — 0.001	gm.
tannate	1/64—1/16	gr.	0.001 — 0.004	gm.
Colocynthin	⅙—⅔	gr.	0.01 — 0.04	gm.
Columbin (bit. princ)	½—1	gr.	0.03 — 0.06	gm.
Condurangin	1/10—¼	gr.	0.006 — 0.015	gm.
Coniine salts	1/30—1/12	gr.	0.002 — 0.005	gm.

Remedies.	Doses.					
	Apothecaries'.		Metric.			
Convallamarin.	1/4— 2	grs.	0.015	—	0.12	gm.
Convallarin.	2— 4	grs.	0.12	—	0.25	gm.
Convolvulin.	1— 3	grs.	0.06	—	0.2	gm.
Copaiba	10—60	m.	0.6	—	4.0	c. c.
Copper acetate.	1/8— 1/4	gr.	0.008	—	0.015	gm.
ammoniated	1/6— 1	gr.	0.01	—	0.06	gm.
and ammon. **sulphate**	1/2— 2	grs.	0.03	—	0.12	gm.
arsenate	1/32— 1/8	gr.	0.002	—	0.008	gm.
arsenite	1/100	gr.			0.0006	gm.
nitrate	1/12— 1/6	gr.	0.005	—	0.01	gm.
oxide (black)	3/4—1 1/2	grs.	0.05	—	0.1	gm.
phosphate	1/8— 1/2	gr.	0.008	—	0.03	gm.
sulphate { emetic	2— 5	grs.	0.12	—	0.3	gm.
sulphate { tonic	1/6— 1/2	gr.	0.01	—	0.03	gm.
Cornutine	1/20— 1/6	gr.	0.003	—	0.01	gm.
Coronillin	1—2 1/2	grs.	0.06	—	0.15	gm.
Corrosive sublimate—*see Mercuric* ***chloride,*** *corrosive.*						
Cotoin.	1— 4	grs.	0.06	—	0.25	gm.
Creatin.	1 1/2	grs.			0.1	gm.
Creatinine	1 1/2	grs.			0.1	gm.
Creolin	3— 5	m.	0.2	—	0.3	c. c.
Creosal	8—15	grs.	0.5	—	1.0	gm.
Cresalol **(para-)**	5—15	grs.	0.3	—	1.0	gm.
Creasote	1/4— 2	m.	0.015	—	0.12	c. c.
carbonate	10—20	m.	0.6	—	1.3	c. c.
Cresol (meta-).	1— 3	m.	0.06	—	0.2	c. c.
Croton chloral	5—20	grs.	0.3	—	1.3	gm.
Cupro-hemol	1 1/2—2 1/2	grs.	0.1	—	0.15	gm.
Curare	1/20— 1/6	gr.	0.003	—	0.01	gm.
Curarine { hypodermic	1/200— 1/80	gr.	0.0003	—	0.0008	gm.
Curarine { internal	1/100— 1/40	gr.	0.0006	—	0.0015	gm.
Cytisine hydrochlor	1/20— 1/12	gr.	0.003	—	0.005	gm.
Daturine (true) and salts	1/250— 1/64	gr.	0.00025	—	0.001	gm.
Decoction of cetraria	2— 4	fl. ozs.	60.0	—	120.0	c. c.
Delphinine	1/60— 1/12	gr.	0.001	—	0.005	gm.
Diastase	3/4— 3	grs.	0.05	—	0.2	gm.
Digitalein	1/64— 1/32	gr.	0.001	—	0.002	gm.
Digitalin (French)	1/250—1/100	gr.	0.00025	—	0.0006	gm.
Digitalin (German)	1/100— 1/30	gr.	0.0006	—	0.002	gm.
Digitoxin	1/250—1/120	gr.	0.00025	—	0.0005	gm.
Diuretin	10—15	grs.	0.6	—	1.0	gm.
Donovan's solution	2— 8	m.	0.12	—	0.5	c. c.
Duboisine sulphate	1/100— 1/60	gr.	0.0006	—	0.001	gm.
Elaterin	1/20— 1/10	gr.	0.003	—	0.006	gm.
Elaterium	1/16— 1/2	gr.	0.004	—	0.03	gm.
Emetine { emetic	1/16— 1/8	gr.	0.004	—	0.008	gm.
Emetine { expect.	1/120— 1/60	gr.	0.0005	—	0.001	gm.
Emulsion of almond	2— 4	fl. drs.	8.0	—	15.0	c. c.
ammoniac.	2— 8	fl. drs.	8.0	—	30.0	c. c.
asafetida	1— 2	fl. ozs.	30.0	—	60.0	c.c.
chloroform	1— 8	fl. drs.	4.0	—	30.0	c. c.
Erythrophleine hydrochlorate	1/32— 1/16	gr.	0.002	—	0.004	gm.
Eserine and salts	1/200— 1/32	gr.	0.0003	—	0.002	gm.
Ether	10—60	m.	0.6	—	4.0	c. c.
acetic	10—30	m.	0.6	—	2.0	c. c.
formic	1— 2	fl. drs.	4.0	—	8.0	c. c.
hydriodic	5—16	m.	0.3	—	1.0	c. c.
hydrobromic	10—60	m.	0.6	—	4.0	c. c.
isovalerianic	1— 2	m.	0.06	—	0.12	c. c.
lactic	8—16	m.	0.5	—	1.0	c. c.
Ethoxy-caffeine	4	grs			0.25	gm.
Ethylene bromide	1— 2	m.	0.06	—	0.12	c. c.
Eucalyptene hydrochlor	24	grs.			1.5	gm.
Eucalyptol	3—10	m.	0.2	—	0.6	c. c.
Eugenol	8—30	m.	0.5	—	2.0	c. c.
Euonymin **(pure)**	1/2— 3	grs.	0.03	—	0.2	gm.
Euphorin	8—16	grs.	0.5	—	1.0	gm.
Europhen (by injection)	1/2—1 1/2	grs.	0.03	—	0.1	gm.
Exalgin	1— 5	grs.	0.06	—	0.3	gm.
Ferratin	4— 8	grs.	0.25	—	0.5	gm.
Ferric hydrate	30—60	grs.	2.0	—	4.0	gm.
Ferric hyd. with magnesia	1	oz.			30.0	gm.
Ferro-hemol	8	grs.			0.5	gm.
Ferropyrine	8—15	grs.	0.5	—	1.0	gm.

Remedies.	Doses.					
	Apothecaries'.		*Metric.*			
Formanilid	2—4	grs.	0.12	—	0.25	gm.
Fowler's solution....	2—8	m.	0.12	—	0.5	c.c.
Fuchsine (rosanilin).....	½—3	grs.	0.03	—	0.2	gm.
Gadinol (morrhuol)..	5—16	m.	0.3	—	1.0	c. c.
Galbanum. ...	10—20	grs.	0.6	—	1.3	gm.
Gallobromal....	10—30	grs.	0.6	—	2.0	gm.
Gamboge.........	2—5	grs.	0.12	—	0.3	gm.
Geissospermine...	8—30	grs.	0.5	—	2.0	gm.
Gelsemining and salts....	1/120—1/30	gr.	0.0005	—	0.002	gm.
Glycerin..........	1—2	fl. drs.	4.0	—	8.0	c.c.
Glycerite of carbolic acid.	5—10	m.	0.3	—	0.6	c.c.
gallic acid..	20—60	m.	1.3	—	4.0	c.c.
tannic acid.........	10—60	m.	0.6	—	4.0	c.c.
Glycyrrhizin ammon.....	5—15	grs.	0.3	—	1.0	gm.
Gold and pot. bromide ..	1/6—2/3	gr.	0.01	—	0.04	gm.
and sodium chloride.	1/40—1/10	gr.	0.0015	—	0.006	gm.
arsenite.	1/60—1/12	gr.	0.001	—	0.005	gm.
chloride.	1/40—1/10	gr.	0.0015	—	0.006	gm.
iodide	1/64—1/8	gr.	0.001	—	0.008	gm.
monobromide..	1/20—1/5	gr.	0.003	—	0.012	gm.
monocyanide............	1/15—1/4	gr.	0.004	—	0.015	gm.
oxide......................	1/20—1/4	gr.	0.003	—	0.015	gm.
tricyanide................	1/20—1/10	gr.	0.003	—	0.006	gm.
Gualacol.....................	1—15	m.	0.06	—	1.0	c.c.
benzoate....................	5—15	grs.	0.3	—	1.0	gm.
biniodide..................	2—15	grs.	0.12	—	1.0	gm.
carbonate...................	3—8	grs.	0.2	—	0.5	gm.
phosphate	2—15	grs.	0.12	—	1.0	gm.
salol........................	15—20	grs.	1.0	—	1.3	gm.
Guaranine......................	1—5	grs.	0.06	—	0.3	gm.
Gyno-cyan-auridzarin..........	1/2000—1/300	gr.	0.00003	—	0.0002	gm.
Hashishin (Séc)................	1/8—1/4	gr.	0.008	—	0.015	gm.
Helenin (alant camphor).......	1/6—1/3	gr.	0.01	—	0.02	gm.
Heliotropin (piperonal).........	15	grs.			1.0	gm.
Helleborein.....................	1/16—1/3	gr.	0.004	—	0.02	gm.
Hematin-albumen..............	1—4	drs.	4.0	—	15.0	gm.
Hemo-gallol....................	4—8	grs.	0.25	—	0.5	gm.
Hemoglobin...........	15—45	grs.	1.0	—	3.0	gm.
Hemol	2—8	grs.	0.12	—	0.5	gm.
Hexamethylene-tetramine.. ...	90	grs.	per diem		6.0	gm.
Homatropine and salts.	1/120—1/60	gr.	0.0005	—	0.001	gm.
Honey of rose	1—2	drs.	4.0	—	8.0	c. c.
Hydracetin.	¼—1	gr.	0.015	—	0.06	gm.
Hydrastine and salts.....	¼—½	gr.	0.015	—	0.03	gm.
Hydrastinine hydrochlor.......	¼—½	gr.	0.015	—	0.03	gm.
Hydrogen peroxide (3% sol.)....	½—1	fl. dr.	2.0	—	4.0	c. c.
Hydrohydrastinine hydrochlor.	⅓—½	gr.	0.02	—	0.03	gm.
Hydroquinone................	5—15	grs.	0.3	—	1.0	gm.
Hyoscine hydrobrom. } ordinarily	1/400—1/100	gr.	0.00015	—	0.0006	gm.
} for insane	1/50	gr.			0.0012	gm.
Hyoscyamine and salts.. } ordinarily	1/120—1/60	gr.	0.0005	—	0.001	gm.
} for insane	⅛—¼	gr.	0.008	—	0.015	gm.
Hypnal.	15—30	grs.	1.0	—	2.0	gm.
Hypnone..	5—10	m.	0.3	—	0.6	c.c.
Ichthyol..................	5—20	grs.	0.3	—	1.3	gm.
Ilicin (fr. Ilex aquifol.)..	2—5	grs.	0.12	—	0.3	gm.
Ingluvin.	10—30	grs.	0.6	—	2.0	gm.
Iodine.	½—1	gr.	0.03	—	0.06	gm.
chloride	⅛—¼	gr.	0.008	—	0.015	gm.
Iodized starch....	3—10	grs.	0.2	—	0.6	gm.
Iodo-caffeine......	5—8	grs.	0.3	—	0.5	gm.
Iodoform	1—3	grs.	0.06	—	0.2	gm.
Iodol	½—5	grs.	0.03	—	0.3	gm.
Iodo-pyrin..	6—20	grs.	0.4	—	1.3	gm.
Iodo-theine.	2—8	grs.	0.12	—	0.5	gm.
Iron acetate.	3—10	grs.	0.2	—	0.6	gm.
albuminate........	3—10	grs.	0.2	—	0.6	gm.
ammonio-chloride	4—12	grs.	0.25	—	0.8	gm.
and ammon. cit	2—5	grs.	0.12	—	0.3	gm.
and ammon. sulphate.	5—15	grs.	0.3	—	1.0	gm.
and ammon. tartrate....	5—20	grs.	0.3	—	1.3	gm.
and mag. sulph....	5—10	grs.	0.3	—	0.6	gm.
and mangan. sulph	1—2	grs.	0.06	—	0.12	gm.
and quin. arsenate	1/16—⅛	gr.	0.004	—	0.008	gm.

REMEDIES.	Apothecaries'.	Metric.		
Iron and quin. arsenite.	$\frac{1}{16}$— $\frac{1}{8}$	gr.	0.004 — 0.008	gm.
and quin. chloride...	1½— 3	grs.	0.1 — 0.2	gm.
and quin. citrate...........	1 — 5	grs.	0.06 — 0.3	gm.
and quin. cit. with strych...	¼— 2	grs.	0.015 — 0.12	gm.
and quin. hypophosphite...	2 –10	grs.	0.12 — 0.6	gm.
and quin. peptonate........	1— 5	grs.	0.06 — 0.3	gm.
and quin. valerianate......	2–10	grs.	0.12 — 0.6	gm.
and sod. oxalate............	3—15	grs.	0.2 — 1.0	gm.
and sod. pyrophosphate....	3—15	grs.	0.2 — 1.0	gm.
and sod. tartrate...........	10—30	grs.	0.6 — 2.0	gm.
and strych. citrate..........	1— 3	grs.	0.06 — 0.2	gm.
arsenate	$\frac{1}{12}$— ¼	gr.	0.003 — 0.015	gm.
bromide (ferric)	$\frac{1}{3}$— 1	m.	0.02 — 0.06	c. c.
bromide (ferrous)...........	1— 5	grs.	0.06 — 0.3	gm.
bromo-iodide.............	½— 2	grs.	0.03 — 0.12	gm.
carbonate (green)...........	5—15	grs.	0.3 — 1.0	gm.
carb. saccharated..........	2—10	grs.	0.12 — 0.6	gm.
citrate...	2— 5	grs.	0.12 — 0.3	gm.
dialyzed....................	10—30	m.	0.6 — 2.0	c. c.
ferrocyanide...............	2— 5	grs.	0.12 — 0.3	gm.
glycero-phosphate..........	2	grs.	0.12	gm.
hypophosphite............	5—10	grs.	0.3 — 0.6	gm.
iodide	1— 3	grs.	0.06 — 0.2	gm.
iodide **saccharated**..........	5—25	grs.	0.3 — 1.5	gm.
lactate...................	1— 3	grs.	0.06 — 0.2	gm.
lacto-albuminate...........	1— 5	grs.	0.06 — 0.3	gm.
lacto-phosphate............	1— 5	grs.	0.06 — 0.3	gm.
malate....................	1— 5	grs.	0.06 — 0.3	gm.
oxalate (ferrous)..........	2— 6	grs.	0.12 — 0.4	gm.
oxide (magnetic)...........	5 —20	grs.	0.3 — 1.3	gm.
peptonate	2— 8	grs.	0.12 — 0.5	gm.
phosphate, soluble.........	5—10	grs.	0.3 — 0.6	gm.
phospho-sarcolactate........	8	grs.	0.5	gm.
picrate....................	¼— 1	gr.	0.015 — 0.06	gm.
protochloride.............	2— 3	grs.	0.12 — 0.2	gm.
pyrophos. precip...........	2 - 5	grs.	0.12 — 0.3	gm.
pyrophos. soluble....	2— 5	grs.	0.12 — 0.3	gm.
reduced	¼— 6	grs.	0.015 — 0.4	gm.
saccharate.................	8—30	grs.	0.5 — 2.0	gm.
salicylate	3—10	grs.	0.2 — 0.6	gm.
santonate......	¼— 1	gr.	0.015 — 0.06	gm.
subcarbonate...............	5—30	grs.	0.3 — 2.0	gm.
subsulphate................	2— 5	grs.	0.12 — 0.3	gm.
succinate.................	60	grs.	4.0	gm.
sulphate, dried.............	½— 2	grs.	0.03 — 0.12	gm.
tannate..................	3— 5	grs.	0.2 — 0.3	gm.
valerianate	1— 3	grs.	0.06 — 0.2	gm.
Iron-casein...........	2— 5	grs.	0.12 — 0.3	gm.
Juice, belladonna	3—10	m.	0.2 — 0.6	c. c.
conium	20—60	m.	1.3 — 4.0	c. c.
digitalis	3—10	m.	0.2 — 0.6	c. c.
hyoscyamus................	30—60	m.	2.0 — 4.0	c. c.
lime	1 — 2	fl. ozs.	30.0 — 60.0	c. c.
scoparius....	1— 2	fl. drs.	4.0 — 8.0	c. c.
taraxacum..	1— 4	fl. drs.	4.0 — 15.0	c. c.
Koussein (Brayerin) in 4 doses..	15—30	grs.	1.0 — 2.0	gm.
Kairin	3—30	grs.	0.2 — 2.0	gm.
Lactophenin	8—15	grs.	0.5 — 1.0	gm.
Lactucine....	1— 5	grs.	0.06 — 0.3	gm.
Lantanine...................	2 — 8	grs.	0.12 — 0.5	gm.
Lead acetate...............	½— 5	grs.	0.03 — 0.3	gm.
iodide..................	$\frac{1}{8}$— ¼	gr.	0.008 — 0.012	gm.
Lemon juice................	½— 4	fl. ozs.	15.0 — 120.0	c. c.
Lime chlorinated.	3— 6	grs.	0.2 — 0.4	gm.
sulphurated	$\frac{1}{12}$— 3	grs.	0.005 — 0.2	gm.
water,...................	½— 2	fl. ozs.	15.0 — 60.0	gm
Lithium acetate...........	8—24	grs.	0.5 — 1.5	gm.
and **caffeine** sulphonate.....	15	grs.	1.0	gm.
and pot. **tartrate**	30—60	grs.	2.0 — 4.0	gm.
and sod. **benzoate**	10—30	grs.	0.6 — 2.0	gm.
benzoate.................	5 —30	grs.	0.3 — 2.0	gm.
bromide.................	5—20	grs.	0.3 — 1.3	gm.
carbonate...	2—15	grs.	0.12 — 1.0	gm.
citrate	5 —30	grs.	0.3 — 2.0	gm.

REMEDIES.	DOSES. Apothecaries'.		Metric.		
Lithium citrate effervescent	60—120	grs.	4.0	— 8.0	gm.
dithiosalicylate	3—10	grs.	0.2	— 0.6	gm.
glycero-phosphate	2— 5	grs.	0.12	— 0.3	gm.
guaiacate	1— 5	grs.	0.06	— 0.3	gm.
hippurate	5—20	grs.	0.3	— 1.3	gm.
iodide	1— 5	grs.	0.06	— 0.3	gm.
phosphate	10—30	grs.	0.6	— 2.0	gm.
salicylate	5—60	grs.	0.3	— 4.0	gm.
sulphate	10—30	grs.	0.6	— 2.0	gm.
valerianate	5—15	grs.	0.3	— 1.0	gm.
Lobeline hydrobromate	⅛— 1	gr.	0.008	— 0.06	gm.
sulphate	⅛— 2	grs.	0.008	— 0.12	gm.
Lupulin	5—15	grs.	0.3	— 1.0	gm.
Lycetol	4— 8	grs.	0.25	— 0.5	gm.
Lysidine	15—30	grs.	1.0	— 2.0	gm.
Magnesia	10—60	grs.	0.6	— 4.0	gm.
Magnesium acetate	5—60	grs.	0.3	— 4.0	gm.
benzoate	3—20	grs.	0.2	— 1.3	gm.
bisulphate	5—20	grs.	0.3	— 1.3	gm.
borate	5—20	grs.	0.3	— 1.3	gm.
bromide	10—20	grs.	0.6	— 1.3	gm.
carbonate	10—60	grs.	0.6	— 4.0	gm.
chloride	½— 1	oz.	15.0	— 30.0	gm.
citrate	30—120	grs.	2.0	— 8.0	gm.
citrate effervescent	¼— 1	oz.	4.0	— 30.0	gm.
copaivate	10—20	grs.	0.6	— 1.3	gm.
ergotate	⅔— 1	gr.	0.04	— 0.06	gm.
glycero-phosphate	2— 5	grs.	0.12	— 0.3	gm.
gynocardate	15—60	grs.	1.0	— 4.0	gm.
hydrate	60—120	grs.	4.0	— 8.0	gm.
hypophosphite	10—20	grs.	0.6	— 1.3	gm.
iodide	2—10	grs.	0.12	— 0.6	gm.
lactate	15—45	grs.	1.0	— 3.0	gm.
lactophosphate	3—15	grs.	0.2	— 1.0	gm.
malate	30—120	grs.	2.0	— 8.0	gm.
phosphate (acid)	10—30	grs.	0.6	— 2.0	gm.
phosphite	5—20	grs.	0.3	— 1.3	gm.
salicylate	15—120	grs.	1.0	— 8.0	gm.
silicate	1— 4	drs.	4.0	— 15.0	gm.
sulphate	¼— 1	oz.	4.0	— 30.0	gm.
sulphite	10—60	grs.	0.6	— 4.0	gm.
tartrate	8—15	grs.	0.5	— 1.0	gm.
Malakin	15	grs.		1.0	gm.
Manganese and iron lactate	1— 5	grs.	0.06	— 0.3	gm.
arsenate	1/10— 1/5	gr.	0.002	— 0.012	gm.
bromide	1— 8	grs.	0.06	— 0.5	gm.
carbonate	8—40	grs.	0.5	— 2.6	gm.
citrate	1— 3	grs.	0.06	— 0.2	gm.
dioxide	½—10	grs.	0.03	— 0.6	gm.
glycero-phosphate	1— 2	grs.	0.06	— 0.12	gm.
hypophosphite	10—20	grs.	0.6	— 1.3	gm.
iodide	1— 3	grs.	0.06	— 0.2	gm.
lactate	1— 5	grs.	0.06	— 0.3	gm.
lacto-phosphate	1— 5	grs.	0.06	— 0.3	gm.
protoxide	2—10	grs.	0.12	— 0.6	gm.
peptonate	20—60	grs.	1.3	— 4.0	gm.
salicylate	2—10	grs.	0.12	— 0.6	gm.
sulphate	2— 5	grs.	0.12	— 0.3	gm.
sulphite	5—20	grs.	0.3	— 1.3	gm.
sulphocarbolate	3—15	grs.	0.2	— 1.0	gm.
Manna	1— 2	ozs.	30.0	— 60.0	gm.
Mannit	6— 8	drs.	20.0	— 30.0	gm.
Mass of copaiba	3—15	grs.	0.2	— 1.0	gm.
ferrous carbonate (Vallet's)	2— 5	grs.	0.12	— 0.3	gm.
mercury (blue mass) alt.	½— 3	grs.	0.03	— 0.2	gm.
mercury (blue mass) purg.	5—20	grs.	0.3	— 1.3	gm.
Menispermine	1— 5	grs.	0.06	— 0.3	gm.
Menthol	½— 3	grs.	0.03	— 0.2	gm.
Mercuric amido-propionate	1/12— ⅙	gr.	0.005	— 0.01	gm.
asparaginate	1/50— 1/16	gr.	0.0012	— 0.004	gm.
benzoate	1/32— 1/10	gr.	0.002	— 0.006	gm.
bromide	1/16— ¼	gr	0.004	— 0.015	gm.
chloride, corrosive	1/100— ¼	gr.	0.0006	— 0.015	gm.
chloride, peptonized	½—1½	grs.	0.03	— 0.1	gm.

REMEDIES.	Apothecaries'		Metric.		
Mercuric cyanide	1/80 — 1/10	gr.	0.0008 — 0.006		gm.
iodide, **red**	1/40 — 1/4	gr.	0.0015 — 0.015		gm.
nitrate	1/60 — 1/8	gr.	0.001 — 0.008		gm.
oxide, red	1/50 — 1/10	gr.	0.0012 — 0.006		gm.
phenolate	1/3 — 1/2	gr.	0.02 — 0.03		gm.
salicylate (basic)	1/3 — 1	gr.	0.02 — 0.06		gm.
subsulph., yellow	2 — 5	grs.	0.12 — 0.3		gm.
succinimide	1/5	gr.	0.012		gm.
sulphide, black	3—15	grs.	0.2 — 1.0		gm.
Mercur-iodo-hemol	2— 5	grs.	0.12 — 0.3		gm.
Mercurous bromide	1/8 — 1/4	gr.	0.008 — 0.015		gm.
chloride, mild (alt. / purg.)	1/2 — 1	gr.	0.03 — 0.06		gm.
	3—15	grs.	0.2 — 1.0		gm.
iodide, **yellow**	1/20 — 1	gr.	0.003 — 0.06		gm.
nitrate	1/30 — 1/4	gr.	0.002 — 0.015		gm.
tannate	1 — 3	grs.	0.06 — 0.2		gm.
Mercury and antim. sulphide	2— 4	grs.	0.12 — 0.25		gm.
and arsenic iodide	1/60 — 1/30	gr.	0.001 — 0.002		gm.
and pot. hyposulphite	1/5 — 1/2	gr.	0.012 — 0.02		gm.
gallate	1 1/2 — 3	grs.	0.1 — 0.2		gm.
naphtolate	1/2 — 1	gr.	0.03 — 0.06		gm.
nitrate, ammoniated	1/4 — 3	grs.	0.015 — 0.2		gm.
thymol-acetate	1 — 1 1/2	grs.	0.06 — 0.1		gm.
with chalk	1/2 —10	grs.	0.03 — 0.6		gm.
Metaldehyde	2— 8	grs.	0.12 — 0.5		gm.
Methacetin	3— 5	grs.	0.2 — 0.3		gm.
Meth-oxy-caffeine	4	grs.	0.25		gm.
Methylal	4— 5	m.	0.25 — 0.3		c. c.
Methylene blue	1— 3	grs.	0.06 — 0.2		gm.
Methyl salicylate	5—10	m.	0.3 — 0.6		c. c.
Mixture, chalk	4	fl. drs.	15.0		c. c.
glycyrrhiza comp.	1— 8	fl. drs.	4.0 — 30.0		c. c.
iron comp.	2— 4	fl. drs.	8.0 — 15.0		c. c.
Monesin	1/10 — 1/2	gr.	0.006 — 0.03		gm.
Morphine	1/20 — 1/2	gr.	0.003 — 0.03		gm.
sulphate	1/20 — 1/2	gr.	0.003 — 0.03		gm.
valerianate	1/8 — 1/2	gr.	0.008 — 0.03		gm.
Muscarine	1/8 — 2	grs.	0.008 — 0.12		gm.
nitrate	1/10 — 3/4	gr.	0.006 — 0.05		gm.
Musk	2—10	grs.	0.12 — 0.6		gm.
Mussæin	1— 2	ozs.	30.0 — 60.0		gm.
Mustard (as an emetic)	2— 4	drs.	8.0 — 15.0		gm.
Myrrh	10—30	grs.	0.6 — 2.0		gm.
Myrtol	1— 2	m.	0.06 — 0.12		c. c.
Napelline	1/5 — 1/2	gr.	0.01 — 0.03		gm.
Naphtalin	3—15	grs.	0.2 — 1.0		gm.
Naphtol (beta-)	3— 8	grs.	0.2 — 0.5		gm.
benzoate	4— 8	grs.	0.25 — 0.5		gm.
camphorated	2— 5	m.	0.12 — 0.3		c. c.
Narceine	1/3 — 3/4	gr.	0.02 — 0.05		gm.
Narcotine hydrochlor.	2—10	grs.	0.12 — 0.6		gm.
Naregamine	2—15	grs.	0.12 — 1.0		gm.
Neurodin	5—24	grs.	0.3 — 1.5		gm.
Nickel bromide	5—10	grs.	0.3 — 0.6		gm.
sulphate	1/2 — 3	grs.	0.03 — 0.2		gm.
Nicotine	1/60 — 1/20	gr.	0.001 — 0.003		gm.
Nitro-glucose (1% sol.)	1/4 — 1	m.	0.015 — 0.06		c. c.
Nitroglycerin	1/100 — 1/30	gr.	0.0006 — 0.002		gm.
Nungall	5—15	grs.	0.3 — 1.0		gm.
Oil amber	5—10	m.	0.3 — 0.6		c. c.
animal (Dippel's)	5—20	m.	0.3 — 1.3		c. c.
anise	1— 5	m.	0.06 — 0.3		c. c.
betula volatile	5—15	m.	0.3 — 1.0		c. c.
bitter almond	1/4 — 1	m.	0.015 — 0.06		c. c.
cade	3— 5	m.	0.2 — 0.3		c. c.
cajuput	1— 5	m.	0.06 — 0.3		c. c.
camphor	2— 3	m.	0.12 — 0.2		c. c.
caraway	1— 5	m.	0.06 — 0.3		c. c.
castor	1— 8	fl. drs.	4.0 — 30.0		c. c.
celery seed	1— 2	m.	0.06 — 0.12		c. c.
chamomile	1— 5	m.	0.06 — 0.3		c. c.
chaulmoogra	5—10	m.	0.3 — 0.6		c. c.
chenopodium	5—15	m.	0.3 — 1.0		c. c.
cherry-laurel	1/4 — 1/2	m.	0.01 — 0.03		c. c.

REMEDIES.	DOSES. Apothecaries'.		Metric.			
Oil cinnamon	1— 5	m.	0.06	—	0.3	c. c.
cloves	1— 4	m.	0.06	—	0.25	c. c.
cod liver	1— 2	fl. drs.	4.0	—	8.0	c. c.
cod liver, ferrated	1— 2	fl. drs.	4.0	—	8.0	c. c.
copaiba	10—15	m.	0.6	—	1.0	c. c.
corriander	2— 5	m.	0.12	—	0.3	c. c.
croton	⅓— 2	m.	0.02	—	0.12	c. c.
cubebs	5—20	m.	0.3	—	1.3	c. c.
cumin	1— 3	m.	0.06	—	0.2	c. c.
dill	2— 5	m.	0.12	—	0.3	c. c.
erigeron	10—30	m.	0.6	—	2.0	c. c.
eucalyptus	5—30	m.	0.3	—	2.0	c. c.
fennel	2— 5	m.	0.12	—	0.3	c. c.
fireweed	2— 6	m.	0.12	—	0.4	c. c.
garlic	1— 2	drops.	0.05	—	0.1	c. c.
gaultheria	3—10	m.	0.2	—	0.6	c. c.
ginger	1— 3	m.	0.06	—	0.2	c. c.
hedeoma (pennyroyal)	2—10	m.	0.12	—	0.6	c. c.
henbane (macerated)	1— 5	m.	0.06	—	0.3	c. c.
hops	1— 5	m.	0.06	—	0.3	c. c.
horsemint	1— 3	m.	0.06	—	0.2	c. c.
juniper	5—15	m.	0.3	—	1.0	c. c.
lavender flos	1— 5	m.	0.06	—	0.3	c. c.
lemon	1— 5	m.	0.06	—	0.3	c. c.
linseed	½— 2	fl. ozs.	15.0	—	60.0	c. c.
male fern	12—25	m.	0.8	—	1.5	c. c.
melissa	1— 2	m.	0.06	—	0.12	c. c.
mountain pine	5—10	m.	0.3	—	0.6	c. c.
mustard, volatile	⅛— ¼	m.	0.008	—	0.015	c. c.
nutmeg	1— 5	m.	0.06	—	0.3	c. c.
nutmeg (butter)	2— 5	grs.	0.12	—	0.3	gm.
olive	4— 8	fl. drs.	15.0	—	30.0	c. c.
orange peel	1— 5	m.	0.06	—	0.3	c. c.
peppermint	1— 5	m.	0.06	—	0.3	c. c.
phosphorated	1— 5	m.	0.06	—	0.3	c. c.
pimenta	2— 6	m.	0.12	—	0.4	c. c.
rosemary	1— 2	m.	0.06	—	0.12	c. c.
rue	1— 5	m.	0.06	—	0.3	c. c.
santal (sandalwood)	10—30	m.	0.6	—	2.0	c. c.
sassafras	1— 4	m.	0.06	—	0.25	c. c.
savine	1— 5	m.	0.06	—	0.3	c. c.
spearmint	2— 5	m.	0.12	—	0.3	c. c.
tansy	1— 2	m.	0.06	—	0.12	c. c.
thuja	1— 5	m.	0.06	—	0.3	c. c.
thyme	1— 5	m.	0.06	—	0.3	c. c.
turpentine	5—15	m.	0.3	—	1.0	c. c.
valerian	2— 5	m.	0.12	—	0.3	c. c.
wormwood	1— 2	m.	0.06	—	0.12	c. c.
yarrow	1— 5	m.	0.06	—	0.3	c. c.
Oleo-creosote	5—30	m.	0.3	—	2.0	c. c.
Oleo-guaiacol	5—10	m.	0.3	—	0.6	c. c.
Oleoresin aspidium	30—60	m.	2.0	—	4.0	c. c.
capsicum	1— 5	m.	0.06	—	0.3	c. c.
cubeb	5—30	m.	0.3	—	2.0	c. c.
ginger	½— 1	m.	0.03	—	0.06	c. c.
lupulin	2— 5	grs.	0.12	—	0.3	gm.
matico	3—15	grs.	0.2	—	1.0	gm.
mezereon	½— 1	m.	0.03	—	0.06	c. c.
pepper	¼— 1	m.	0.015	—	0.06	c. c.
Olibanum	10—30	grs.	0.6	—	2.0	gm.
Opium	¼— 2	grs.	0.015	—	0.12	gm.
Orexine	2— 4	grs.	0.12	—	0.25	gm.
Orthine hydrochlor	3— 7	grs.	0.2	—	0.45	gm.
Ouabain (to children)	1/1000	gr.			0.00006	gm.
Ox gall, purified	5—15	grs.	0.3	—	1.0	gm.
Oxy-sparteine	½—1½	grs.	0.03	—	0.1	gm.
hydrochlor.	¾—1½	grs.	0.05	—	0.1	gm.
Pancreatin	1—10	grs.	0.06	—	0.6	gm.
Papain	1— 3	grs.	0.06	—	0.2	gm.
Papaverine (to children)	1/12— ⅓	gr.	0.005	—	0.02	gm.
Papayotin	2— 5	grs.	0.12	—	0.3	gm.
Paracotoin	3— 8	grs.	0.2	—	0.5	gm.
Paraformaldehyde	8—15	grs.	0.5	—	1.0	gm.
Paraldehyde	30—150	m.	2.0	—	10.0	c. c.

REMEDIES.	Doses.					
	Apothecaries'.		*Metric.*			
Parthenicine	¾—2	grs.	0.05	— 0.12		gm.
Pelletierine tannate	5—20	grs.	0.3	— 1.3		gm.
Pental (by inhalation)	180—300	m.	12.0	— 20.0		c. c.
Pepsin	1—5	grs.	0.06	— 0.3		gm.
Pereirine	8—30	grs.	0.5	— 2.0		gm.
Petroleum, crude	3—5	grs.	0.2	— 0.3		gm.
Phenacetine	2—10	grs.	0.12	— 0.6		gm.
Phenocoll hydrochlorate	5—30	grs.	0.3	— 2.0		gm.
salicylate	10—15	grs.	0.6	— 1.0		gm.
Phenoxy-caffeine	4	grs.		0.25		gm.
Phloridzin	10—15	grs.	0.6	— 1.0		gm.
Phosphorus	1/200—1/12	gr.	0.0003	— 0.005		gm.
Physostigmine	1/240—1/32	gr.	0.0003	— 0.002		gm.
sulphate	1/100—1/50	gr.	0.0006	— 0.0012		gm.
Phytolaccin	½—2	grs.	0.03	— 0.12		gm.
Picrotoxin	1/60—1/30	gr.	0.001	— 0.002		gm.
Piliganine	⅙—⅓	gr.	0.01	— 0.02		gm.
Pilocarpine borate	⅛—⅓	gr.	0.008	— 0.02		gm.
hydrochlorate	⅛—¼	gr.	0.008	— 0.015		gm.
Piperazin hydrochlorate	5—10	grs.	0.3	— 0.6		gm.
Piperin	1—10	grs.	0.06	— 0.6		gm.
Podophyllotoxin	1/12—⅛	gr.	0.005	— 0.008		gm.
Potassa, sulphurated	2—10	grs.	0.12	— 0.6		gm.
Potassium acetate	5—60	grs.	0.3	— 4.0		gm.
and sod. borotartrate	1—4	drs.	4.0	— 15.0		gm.
and sod. tartrate	½—1	oz.	15.0	— 30.0		gm.
antimonate	8—24	grs.	0.5	— 1.5		gm.
arsenate	1/20—1/10	gr.	0.003	— 0.006		gm.
arsenite	1/30—1/15	gr.	0.002	— 0.004		gm.
benzoate	5—20	grs.	0.3	— 1.3		gm.
bicarbonate	5—30	grs.	0.3	— 2.0		gm.
bichromate	1/16—⅓	gr.	0.004	— 0.02		gm.
binoxalate	⅛—1½	grs.	0.008	— 0.1		gm.
bisulphate	60—120	grs.	4.0	— 8.0		gm.
bisulphite	5—30	grs.	0.3	— 2.0		gm.
bitartrate	20—240	grs.	1.3	— 15.0		gm.
bromide	5—60	grs.	0.3	— 4.0		gm.
camphorate	10—30	grs.	0.6	— 2.0		gm.
carbolate	1—5	grs.	0.06	— 0.3		gm.
carbonate	2—20	grs.	0.12	— 1.3		gm.
chlorate	5—20	grs.	0.3	— 1.3		gm.
citrate	10—30	grs.	0.6	— 2.0		gm.
citrate effervescent	60—120	grs.	4.0	— 8.0		gm.
cyanide	1/20—½	gr.	0.003	— 0.03		gm.
ferrocyanide	5—15	grs.	0.3	— 1.0		gm.
glycero-phosphate (by injec.)	½—1	gr.	0.03	— 0.06		gm.
hypophosphate	5—10	grs.	0.3	— 0.6		gm.
iodate	4—8	grs.	0.25	— 0.5		gm.
iodide	2—10	grs.	0.12	— 0.6		gm.
nitrate	10—30	grs.	0.6	— 2.0		gm.
nitrite	¼—2	grs.	0.015	— 0.12		gm.
osmate	1/60—1/50	gr.	0.001	— 0.0012		gm.
perchlorate	5—15	grs.	0.3	— 1.0		gm.
permanganate	½—3	grs.	0.03	— 0.2		gm.
phosphate	10—30	grs.	0.6	— 2.0		gm.
salicylate	6—15	grs.	0.4	— 1.0		gm.
salicylite	3—15	grs.	0.2	— 1.0		gm.
succinate	5—10	grs.	0.3	— 0.6		gm.
sulphate	20—240	grs.	1.3	— 15.0		gm.
sulphite	2—4	drs.	8.0	— 15.0		gm.
sulphocyanate	¾—3	grs.	0.05	— 0.2		gm.
tartraborate	10—20	grs.	0.6	— 1.3		gm.
tartrate	4—8	drs.	15.0	— 30.0		gm.
tellurate	½—¾	gr.	0.03	— 0.05		gm.
valerianate	2—5	grs.	0.12	— 0.3		gm.
Powder, antimonial	3—8	grs.	0.2	— 0.5		gm.
aromatic	10—30	grs.	0.6	— 2.0		gm.
compound chalk	5—60	grs.	0.3	— 4.0		gm.
glycyrrhiza comp	30—60	grs.	2.0	— 4.0		gm.
ipecac and opium	2—15	grs.	0.12	— 1.0		gm.
jalap comp	10—60	grs.	0.6	— 4.0		gm.
morphine, comp	5—15	grs.	0.3	— 1.0		gm.
propylamine	30—60	grs.	2.0	— 4.0		gm.
ptyalin	10—30	grs.	0.6	— 2.0		gm.

REMEDIES.	DOSES. Apothecaries'.		DOSES. Metric.		
Pyoktanin, blue	1—5	grs.	0.06	— 0.3	gm.
yellow	1—8	grs.	0.06	— 0.5	gm.
Pyridine	2—3	grs.	0.12	— 0.2	gm.
Pyrogallol	1—2	grs.	0.06	— 0.12	gm.
Quassin (cryst.)	1/30—1/3	gr.	0.002	— 0.02	gm.
Quassin (french)	2/5—2½	grs.	0.025	— 0.15	gm.
Quebrachine	1—2	grs.	0.06	— 0.12	gm.
hydrochlorate	¾—1½	grs.	0.05	— 0.1	gm.
Quinaigen	8—15	grs.	0.5	— 1.0	gm.
Quinetum	1—8	grs.	0.06	— 0.5	gm.
Quinidine and salts	3—30	grs.	0.2	— 2.0	gm.
Quinine acetate	1—15	grs.	0.06	— 1.0	gm.
albuminate	1—15	grs.	0.06	— 1.0	gm.
and iron tannate	2—10	grs.	0.12	— 0.6	gm.
and urea hydrochlor.	1—5	grs.	0.06	— 0.3	gm.
arsenate	1/16—⅛	gr.	0.004	— 0.008	gm.
benzoate	2—20	grs.	0.12	— 1.3	gm.
bisulphate	½—10	grs.	0.03	— 0.6	gm.
citrate	2—20	grs.	0.12	— 1.3	gm.
dihydrobromate	2—20	grs.	0.12	— 1.3	gm.
ethyl-sulphate	3—8	grs.	0.2	— 0.5	gm.
ferrocyanide	5—10	grs.	0.3	— 0.6	gm.
hydrobromate	½—20	grs.	0.03	— 1.3	gm.
iodo-hydro-iodate	1—5	grs.	0.06	— 0.3	gm.
peptonate	5—60	grs.	0.3	— 4.0	gm.
salicylate	2—20	grs.	0.12	— 1.0	gm.
sulphate	½—10	grs.	0.03	— 0.6	gm.
sulpho-carbolate	1—8	grs.	0.06	— 0.5	gm.
tannate	2—10	grs.	0.12	— 0.6	gm.
valerianate	2—6	grs.	0.12	— 0.4	gm.
Quinoidine (Chinoidine)	2—15	grs.	0.12	— 1.0	gm.
borate	8—15	grs.	0.5	— 1.0	gm.
citrate	5—25	grs.	0.3	— 1.6	gm.
tannate	2—12	grs.	0.12	— 0.8	gm.
Quinoline	15—30	m.	1.0	— 2.0	c. c.
salicylate	8—15	grs.	0.5	— 1.0	gm.
tartrate	5—15	grs.	0.3	— 1.0	gm.
Rennet powder	10—30	grs.	0.6	— 2.0	gm.
Resin copaiba	1—5	grs.	0.06	— 0.3	gm.
guaiac	5—30	grs.	0.3	— 2.0	gm.
jalap	2—10	grs.	0.12	— 0.6	gm.
podophyllum	1/40—1	gr.	0.0015	— 0.01	gm.
scammony	3—8	grs.	0.2	— 0.5	gm.
Resopyrin	5—10	grs.	0.3	— 0.6	gm.
Resorcin	5—30	grs.	0.3	— 2.0	gm.
Resorcin-salol	3—9	grs.	0.2	— 0.6	gm.
Rubid. and ammon. bromide	10—20	grs.	0.6	— 1.3	gm.
Rubidium bromide	5—10	grs.	0.3	— 0.6	gm.
iodide	5—30	grs.	0.3	— 2.0	gm.
tartrate	3—5	grs.	0.2	— 0.3	gm.
Saccharin	2—5	grs.	0.12	— 0.3	gm.
Safrol	1—2	m.	0.06	— 0.12	c. c.
Salacetol	15—45	grs.	1.0	— 3.0	gm.
Salicin	2—15	grs.	0.12	— 1.0	gm.
Salicylamide	3—5	grs.	0.2	— 0.3	gm.
Salicyl-resorcin	5—15	grs.	0.3	— 1.0	gm.
Salipyrin	10—30	grs.	0.6	— 2.0	gm.
Salol	2—20	grs.	0.12	— 1.3	gm.
camphorated	3—10	grs.	0.2	— 0.6	gm.
Salophen	5—15	grs.	0.3	— 1.0	gm.
Sanguinarine	1/12—⅛	gr.	0.005	— 0.008	gm.
Santonica	10—60	grs.	0.6	— 4.0	gm.
Santonin { children	¼—1	gr.	0.015	— 0.06	gm.
Santonin { adults	1—5	grs.	0.06	— 0.3	gm.
Santonin-oxim	1—3	grs.	0.06	— 0.2	gm.
Scammony	5—10	grs.	0.3	— 0.6	gm.
Scillipicrin (once daily)	⅓—1	gr.	0.02	— 0.06	gm.
Scillitin	⅙—½	gr.	0.01	— 0.03	gm.
Scillitoxin	1/60—1/30	gr.	0.001	— 0.002	gm.
Scoparin	8—15	grs.	0.5	— 1.0	gm.
Scopolamine salts (by inject.)	1/250—1/64	gr.	0.00025	— 0.001	gm.
Scutellarin	¾—4	grs.	0.05	— 0.25	gm.
Senegin	½—2	grs.	0.03	— 0.12	gm.
Silver arsenite	1/100—1/60	gr.	0.0006	— 0.001	gm.

Remedies.	Doses.			
	Apothecaries'.		Metric.	
Silver chloride....... ...	1/3— 1	gr.	0.02 — 0.06	gm.
iodide....	1/4— 1	gr.	0.015 — 0.06	gm.
nitrate.	1/8— 1/2	gr.	0.008 — 0.03	gm.
oxide.....	1/2— 2	grs.	0.03 — 0.12	gm.
Smilacin.	1— 3	grs.	0.06 — 0.2	gm.
Sodium acetate....	20—60	grs.	1.3 — 4.0	gm.
and mag. borocitrate.... ..	5—30	grs.	0.3 — 2.0	gm.
and mag. tartrate.....	2— 4	drs.	8.0 — 15.0	gm.
anisate.	5—15	grs.	0.3 — 1.0	gm.
arsenate (cryst.).........	1/16— 1/8	gr.	0.004 — 0.008	gm.
benzoate	5—60	grs.	0.3 — 4.0	gm.
bicarbonate........	10—60	grs.	1.3 — 4.0	gm.
bisulphite.	3—10	grs.	0.2 — 0.6	gm.
borate.	10—30	grs.	0.6 — 2.0	gm.
borobenzoate. ..	30 120	grs.	2.0 — 8.0	gm.
borocitrate.	15 20	grs.	1.0 — 1.3	gm.
borosalicylate.............	5—15	grs.	0.3 — 1.0	gm.
borotartrate..	30—120	grs.	2.0 — 8.0	gm.
bromide.	5—60	grs.	0.3 — 4.0	gm.
carbolate.	2—10	grs.	0.12 — 0.6	gm.
carbonate	5—30	grs.	0.3 — 2.0	gm.
cetrarate........	2 15	grs.	0.12 — 1.0	gm.
chlorate..	5—20	grs.	0.3 — 1.3	gm.
chloride........	5—20	grs.	0.3 — 1.3	gm.
choleate........	5 10	grs.	0.3 — 0.6	gm.
citrate, acid........	5—40	grs.	0.3 — 2.0	gm.
citrate, neutral........	10—60	grs.	0.6 — 4.0	gm.
copaivate	10 30	grs.	0.6 — 2.0	gm.
cyanide	1/20— 1/4	gr.	0.003 — 0.015	gm.
diiodosalicylate	5 15	grs.	0.3 — 1.0	gm.
dithiosalicylate..	5—15	grs.	0.3 — 1.0	gm.
ethylsulphate......	60—300	grs.	4.0 — 20.0	gm.
fluoride...	1/12— 1/6	gr.	0.005 — 0.01	gm.
formate............... .	1/5— 3	grs.	0.012 — 0.2	gm.
glycero-phosphate (by injec.)	1/4— 1	gr.	0.015 — 0.06	gm.
gyno-cardate	5—15	grs.	0.3 — 1.0	gm.
hypophosphite.......	5 10	grs.	0.3 — 0.6	gm.
hyposulphite.	5—20	grs.	0.3 — 1.3	gm.
iodide...	5 60	grs.	0.3 — 4.0	gm.
lactate.	2— 4	drs.	8.0 — 15.0	gm.
nitrate...	1— 4	drs.	4.0 — 15.0	gm.
nitrite	1/2— 5	grs.	0.03 — 0.3	gm.
paracresotate.	1—20	grs.	0.06 — 1.3	gm.
phosphate........	1— 8	drs.	4.0 — 30.0	gm.
pyrophosphate.	2—20	grs.	0.12 — 1.3	gm.
salicylate	5—20	grs.	0.3 — 1.3	gm.
santoninate................	1/4— 1	gr.	0.015 — 0.06	gm.
sozoiodolate..	5 30	grs.	0.3 — 2.0	gm.
sulphate . ..	1/2— 1	oz.	15.0 — 30.0	gm.
sulphite...................	5—20	grs.	0.3 — 1.3	gm.
sulpho-carbolate...........	10—30	grs.	0.6 — 2.0	gm.
sulpho-salicylate.	10—30	grs.	0.6 — 2.0	gm.
sulpho-vinate	2— 4	drs.	8.0 — 15.0	gm.
tartrate	4— 8	drs.	15.0 — 30.0	gm.
taurocholate.......... ..	2— 6	grs.	0.12 — 0.4	gm.
tellurate..	1/4 3/4	gr.	0.015 — 0.05	gm.
valerianate.	1— 5	grs.	0.06 — 0.3	gm.
Solanin..	1/6— 1	gr.	0.01 — 0.06	gm.
Solution of ammon. acetate	1 8	fl. drs.	4.0 — 30.0	c. c.
arsenic and merc. iodide....	2— 8	m.	0.12 — 0.5	c. c.
arsenous acid............	2— 8	m.	0.12 — 0.5	c. c.
chlorinated soda.	10 60	m.	0.6 — 4.0	c. c.
ferric acetate..............	2 10	m.	0.12 — 0.6	c. c.
ferric chloride..............	2—10	m.	0.12 — 0.6	c. c.
ferric citrate...	5—15	m.	0.3 — 1.0	c. c.
ferric nitrate...............	5—15	m.	0.3 — 1.0	c. c.
ferric subsulph.............	3—10	m.	0.2 — 0.6	c. c.
hydrogen dioxide...........	1— 3	fl. drs.	4.0 — 12.0	c. c.
iodine comp...............	1—10	m.	0.06 — 0.6	c. c.
iron and ammon. acetate....	2— 5	fl. drs.	8.0 — 20.0	c. c.
lime.......	1/2— 2	fl. ozs.	15.0 — 60.0	c. c.
magnesium citrate..........	4— 6	fl. ozs.	120.0 —180.0	c. c.
morph. sulph. (Magendie's)..	2— 8	m.	0.12 — 0.5	c. c.
potassa.	5—30	m.	0.3 — 2.0	c. c.

REMEDIES.	Apothecaries'.		Metric.	
Solution of potassium arsenite	2 – 8	m.	0.12 – 0.5	c.c.
potassium citrate	4 – 8	fl.drs.	15.0 – 30.0	c.c.
soda	5–30	m.	0.3 – 2.0	c.c.
sodium arsenate	2–15	m.	0.12 – 1.0	c.c.
Somnal	20–30	m.	1.3 – 2.0	c.c.
sparteine sulphate	⅛ – ½	gr.	0.03 – 0.03	gm.
Spermine hydrochlor. (2% sol.)	3–10	m.	0.2 – 0.6	c.c.
Sphacelotoxin	¼–1½	grs.	0.03 – 0.1	gm.
Spirit of ammonia	10 – 60	m.	0.6 – 4.0	c.c.
ammonia aromatic	½ – 2	fl.drs.	2.0 – 8.0	c.c.
anise	1 – 2	fl.drs.	4.0 – 8.0	c.c.
camphor	5 – 30	m.	0.3 – 2.0	c.c.
chloroform	10–60	m.	0.6 – 4.0	c.c.
cinnamon	5–30	m.	0.3 – 2.0	c.c.
ether	10 – 60	m.	0.6 – 4.0	c.c.
ether comp.	5 – 60	m.	0.3 – 4.0	c.c.
gaultheria	30 – 120	m.	2.0 – 8.0	c.c.
glonoin (nitro-glycerin)	½–10	m.	0.03 – 0.6	c.c.
juniper	1 – 4	fl.drs.	4.0 – 15.0	c.c.
juniper comp	1 – 4	fl.drs.	4.0 – 15.0	c.c.
lavender	30 – 60	m.	2.0 – 4.0	c.c.
nitrous ether	½ – 4	fl.drs.	2.0 – 15.0	c.c.
nutmeg	1 – 2	fl.drs.	4.0 – 8.0	c.c.
peppermint	10–30	m.	0.6 – 2.0	c.c.
phosphorus	5–60	m.	0.3 – 4.0	c.c.
spearmint	10 – 40	m.	0.6 – 2.5	c.c.
Storax	5 – 20	grs.	0.3 – 1.3	gm.
Strontium acetate	¼ – ¾	gr.	0.015 – 0.05	gm.
arsenite	1/30 – 1/15	gr.	0.002 – 0.004	gm.
bromide	5–30	grs.	0.3 – 2.0	gm.
iodide	5–30	grs.	0.3 – 2.0	gm.
lactate	5–30	grs.	0.3 – 2.0	gm.
phosphate	10–30	grs.	0.6 – 2.0	gm.
salicylate	10–40	grs.	0.6 – 2.6	gm.
Strophanthin	1/300 – 1/100	gr.	0.0002 – 0.0005	gm.
tannate	1/120 – 1/60	gr.	0.0005 – 0.001	gm.
Strophanthus	1/30 – ¼	gr.	0.003 – 0.015	gm.
Strychnine	1/200 – 1/16	gr.	0.0003 – 0.004	gm.
arsenate	1/64 – 1/16	gr.	0.001 – 0.004	gm.
arsenite	1/36 – 1/15	gr.	0.001 – 0.004	gm.
hydrobromate	1/30 – 1/12	gr.	0.002 – 0.005	gm.
hypophosphite	1/32 – 1/12	gr.	0.002 – 0.005	gm.
nitrate	1/60 – 1/20	gr.	0.001 – 0.003	gm.
sulphate	1/120 – 1/16	gr.	0.0003 – 0.004	gm.
Stypticin	½ – 1	gr.	0.025 – 0.06	gm.
Sulphaminol	3 – 4	grs.	0.2 – 0.25	gm.
salicylate	3 – 6	grs.	0.2 – 0.4	gm.
Sulphonal	15–40	grs.	1.0 – 2.5	gm.
Sulphur	10–60	grs.	0.6 – 4.0	gm.
iodide	1 – 4	grs.	0.06 – 0.25	gm.
Syrup of lime	½ – 2	fl.drs.	2.0 – 8.0	c.c.
Tar (pine)	5–10	grs.	0.3 – 0.6	gm.
Tartar emetic—see ant. and pot. tartrate.				
Terebene	5 –20	m.	0.3 – 1.3	c.c.
Terpene hydrochlorate	15–30	grs.	1.0 – 2.0	gm.
Terpin hydrate	2–10	grs.	0.12 – 0.6	gm.
Terpinol	2 – 5	grs.	0.12 – 0.3	gm.
Tetronal	15–30	grs.	1.0 – 2.0	gm.
Thalline and salts	2 – 15	grs.	0.12 – 1.0	gm.
Theobromine	5–15	grs.	0.3 – 1.0	gm.
and lith. benzoate	5–15	grs.	0.3 – 1.0	gm.
and sod. benzoate	10–20	grs.	0.6 – 1.3	gm.
and sod. iodosalicylate	4 – 8	grs.	0.25 – 0.5	gm.
and sod. salicylate	15	grs.	1.0	gm.
Thermingin	4	grs.	0.25	gm.
Thermodin	5 – 20	grs.	0.3 – 1.3	gm.
Thiol	5–30	grs.	0.3 – 2.0	gm.
Thiosinamine (hypoderm., daily)	4 – 8	grs.	0.25 – 0.5	gm.
Thymacetin	5–15	grs.	0.3 – 1.0	gm.
Thymol	½ – 2	grs.	0.03 – 0.12	gm.
Thyroidin	5	grs.	0.3	gm.
Tincture of ferric chloride	5–20	m.	0.3 – 1.3	c.c.
iodine	1 – 5	m.	0.06 – 0.3	c.c.
musk	1 – 2	fl.drs.	4.0 – 8.0	c.c.

Remedies.	Doses.			
	Apothecaries'.		*Metric.*	
Tincture of saffron	1— 2	fl. drs.	4.0 — 8.0	c. c.
Tolypyrine	5—15	grs.	0.3 — 1.0	gm.
Tolysal	5—45	grs.	0.3 — 3.0	gm.
Tribromophenol-bismuth	8	grs.	0.5	gm.
Trimethylamine hydrochlorate	2— 3	grs.	0.12 — 0.2	gm.
Trional	15—30	grs.	1.0 — 2.0	gm.
Trituration of elaterin	½— 1	gr.	0.03 — 0.06	gm.
Tuberculin...(initial dose hypo.)	1/200—1/125	gr.	0.0003 — 0.0005	gm.
Turpentine (oleoresin)	5—30	grs.	0.3 — 2.0	gm.
Chian	3— 5	grs.	0.2 — 0.3	gm.
Ulexine	1/20—1/10	gr.	0.003 — 0.006	gm.
Uranium nitrate	1/6—⅓	gr.	0.01 — 0.02	gm.
Urethan	15—60	grs.	1.0 — 4.0	gm.
Vallet's mass	2— 5	grs.	0.12 — 0.3	gm.
Vanillin	1/6—⅓	gr.	0.01 — 0.02	gm.
Veratrine	1/60—1/10	gr.	0.001 — 0.006	gm.
Vicrin	1— 4	grs.	0.06 — 0.25	gm.
Water, ammonia	5—30	m.	0.3 — 2.0	c. c.
camphor	1— 4	fl. drs.	4.0 — 15.0	c. c.
cherry laurel	5—30	m.	0.3 — 2.0	c. c.
chlorine	10—20	m.	0.6 — 1.3	c. c.
creosote	1— 4	fl. drs.	4.0 — 15.0	c. c.
lime	½— 2	fl. ozs.	15.0 — 60.0	c. c.
Wine of antimony	5—15	m.	0.3 — 1.0	c. c.
Xylene	5—15	m.	0.3 — 1.0	c. c.
Xylenol-salol	2— 6	grs.	0.12 — 0.4	gm.
Zinc acetate	½— 2	grs.	0.03 — 0.12	gm.
bromide	½— 2	grs.	0.03 — 0.12	gm.
chloride	½— 1	gr.	0.03 — 0.06	gm.
cyanide	1/10—¼	gr.	0.006 — 0.015	gm.
ferrocyanide	½— 4	grs.	0.03 — 0.25	gm.
hypophosphite	½—1½	grs.	0.03 — 0.1	gm.
iodide	½— 2	grs.	0.03 — 0.12	gm.
lactate	½— 1	gr.	0.03 — 0.06	gm.
oxide	1—10	grs.	0.06 — 0.6	gm.
phosphate	1½—4½	grs.	0.1 — 0.3	gm.
phosphide	1/10— 1	gr.	0.006 — 0.06	gm.
subgallate	½— 4	grs.	0.03 — 0.25	gm.
sulphate...... ton. and alt.	1/10— 2	grs.	0.006 — 0.12	gm.
sulphate...... emetic	10—30	grs.	0.6 — 2.0	gm.
sulphocarbolate	¼— 5	grs.	0.015 — 0.3	gm.
sulphydrate	½— 2	grs.	0.03 — 0.12	gm.
tannate	1½—4½	grs.	0.1 — 0.3	gm.
valerianate	½— 4	grs.	0.03 — 0.25	gm.

APPROXIMATE MEASURES.

A drop=usually about 1 m.
A teaspoonful=60 drops or 1 fluid dram.
A dessertspoonful=2 fluid drams.
A tablespoonful=4 fluid drams.
A wineglassful=2 fluid ounces.
A teacupful=4 fluid ounces.

TABLE TO ASSIST THE BEGINNER

IN PRESCRIBING LIQUIDS.

Having fixed upon the bulk of his liquid, he will remember that there are in—

1 fluid ounce, 8 teaspoonfuls each 1 fluid dram.
2 fluid ounces, 16 teaspoonfuls each 1 fluid dram.
4 fluid ounces, 32 teaspoonfuls each 1 fluid dram.
4 fluid ounces, 16 dessertspoonfuls each 2 fluid drams.
6 fluid ounces, 24 dessertspoonfuls each 2 fluid drams.
6 fluid ounces, 12 tablespoonfuls each ½ fluid ounce.
8 fluid ounces, 16 tablespoonfuls each ½ fluid ounce.
1 pint, 32 tablespoonfuls each ½ fluid ounce.
1 pint, 8 wineglassfuls each 2 fluid ounces.

GENERAL PRINCIPLES
OF THE
INCOMPATIBILITY OF DRUGS.

Incompatibility may be defined as that relation between various substances which, upon their combination or admixture, produces an undesirable change either in their chemical nature, physical characters or the therapeutic value of the resulting compound. The following are the general principles underlying the great majority of incompatibilities:

1. In general, it may be stated that, whenever two soluble substances by direct combination or interchange of radicles are capable of producing an insoluble or less soluble compound, the mixing of their solutions will cause precipitation. Therefore, in combining soluble salts with each other or with infusions, be careful to see that an insoluble precipitate is not unintentionally formed. The precipitation of quinine acetate upon the addition of potassium acetate to an acid solution of quinine, and the precipitation glycyrrhizin when fluid extract of licorice is added to the same kind of solution, are examples of this class.

2. As a rule, a drug is incompatible with its antidotes and its chemical tests, especially if the latter depend upon the forming of an insoluble precipitate.

3. Mineral acids, especially when concentrated, will displace from their combinations the weaker acids. They also form ethers with alcoholic preparations.

4. The alkalies and their carbonates decompose metallic salts, generally with the formation of a precipitate. The fixed alkalies also liberate ammonia from its combinations and decompose chloral hydrate with separation of chloroform.

5. Strong mineral acids, chlorine water, chlorate of potash, chlorinated lime and solution of chlorinated soda will liberate iodine from the soluble iodides, syrup iodide of iron and syrup of hydriodic acid.

6. Alkaloids are liberated from their combinations by the alkalies and their carbonates; they form insoluble compounds with tannic acid, iodine and iodides; they may be destroyed by chlorinous compounds.

7. The glucosides, such as salicin, santonin and colocynthin, are decomposed by free acids or emulsin.

8. Tannic acid is incompatible with alkaloidal solutions, metallic salts, gelatin and albumen.

9. Alkalies as a rule modify the action of the cathartic resins and of preparations of lactucarium.

10. A change in the solvent power of the menstruum contained in fluid extracts or tinctures will cause precipitation: (1) Of resinous or oily matter when the alcoholic strength is reduced by the addition of water; (2) of gum, mucilage and albuminous matter if the alcoholic strength is increased.

11. Pepsin is incompatible with alkalies and the metallic salts generally.

12. Gold and silver salts, corrosive sublimate and potassium permanganate are decomposed by contact with organic matter.

13. Carbonates added to acidulous mixtures or to a mixture of borax and glycerin evolve carbon dioxide which may cause an explosion when in a tightly closed container.

14. Mixtures of energetic oxidizing agents with substances readily oxidized are explosive more especially when in the dry state. Thus, strong nitric acid, chromic acid, oxide of silver, potassium bichromate, potassium permanganate and potassium chlorate may become explosive when mixed with dry organic substances as sugar, tannin, etc., glycerin, carbolic acid, alcohols, ethers, oils, sulphur, sulphides, phosphorus, hypophosphites, etc. Nitrate of silver with creosote has caused explosion and tincture of iodine with ammonia precipitates the highly explosive iodide of nitrogen.

Poisons and Antidotes.

The antidotes for poisonous vegetable drugs, and their constituents, are given under the heading of the corresponding fluid extracts and to avoid repetition, are so referred to in the following table.

POISONS.	ANTIDOTES.
Acids, Mineral	Chalk, magnesia (plaster of wall in emergency), solution carbonate of soda, emollient drinks, fixed oils.
Aconite	See Fl. Ext. Aconite Leaves, p. 6.
Alkalies, Caustic	Dilute acids, especially vegetable acids. Vinegar unites with them, producing innocuous acetates, albumen, milk, fixed oils.
Alkaloids	Emetics, stomach-pump. Tannin, animal charcoal, strong tea or coffee; solution of iodine (pot. iod., 60 grs.; tr. iodine, 15 m.; water, 5 fl. ozs.) in teaspoonful doses every 15 minutes.
Arsenic	Moist hydrated oxide of iron (obtained from perchloride of iron and calcined magnesia), dialyzed iron, charcoal, ammonia, artificial respiration, cold affusion.
Atropine	See Fl. Ext. Belladonna Leaves, p. 17.
Barium Salts	Sulphates of magnesium, sodium or potassium, diluted sulphuric acid.
Belladonna	See Fl. Ext. Belladonna Leaves, p. 17.
Calabar Bean	See Fl. Ext. Calabar Bean, p. 30.
Cantharides	See Fl. Ext. Cantharides, p. 32.
Carbolic Acid	Sulphates of magnesium or sodium, syr. of lime, soap, vegetable demulcents but no oils or glycerin. Locally solution of sodium carbonate.
Chloral Hydrate	Emetics, stomach-pump. Heat to body and limbs, frictions, amyl nitrite, strychnine, atropine, morphine,
Chlorine Water	Albumen, white of egg, milk, flour.
Chloroform	Fresh air, flagellation, coffee, electricity, artificial respiration (including head down, pulling tongue forward), galvanism to pneumogastric and through diaphragm, brandy and ammonia enemata. Tracheotomy was successfully performed in one case by Mr. Howse, Guy's Hospital. The hypodermic injection of 1/2 gr. digitalin, by Professor Larabee, Louisville, followed in four hours after by 1/5 gr. atropine, recovered a patient after galvanism had failed.
Cocaine	See Fl. Ext. Coca Leaves, p. 42.
Cocculus Indicus	See Fl. Ext. Cocculus Indicus, p. 42.
Colchicum	See Fl. Ext. Colchicum Root, p. 43.
Conium	See Fl. Ext. Conium Leaves, p. 45.
Copper Arsenite	See Arsenic.
Copper Salts	Albumen or white of egg, flour, milk, magnesia, potassium ferrocyanide.
Corrosive Sublimate	Albumen, white of egg (4 grs. sublimate require white of one egg), flour, milk, protochloride of tin or charcoal, followed by emesis or the stomach-pump.

POISONS.	ANTIDOTES.
Creosote	See Carbolic Acid.
Croton Oil	Emetic of sulphate of copper (gr. x) followed by mucilaginous fluids containing opium.
Cyanides	See Hydrocyanic Acid.
Digitalis	See Fluid Ext. Digitalis, p. 50.
Elaterium	Demulcent drinks and enemata, small doses of opium, and the warm bath.
Gelsemium	See Fl. Ext. Gelsemium, p. 59.
Gold Chloride	See Corrosive Sublimate.
Hydrocyanic Acid	Fresh air and artificial respiration, with cold affusion; freshly precipitated oxide of iron, with an alkaline carbonate, or with magnesia.
Hyoscyamus	See Fl. Ext. Henbane, p. 65.
Ignatia Bean	See Fl. Ext. Ignatia, p. 68.
Iodine	Emetics and demulcent drinks, starch or flour diffused in water.
Lead Salts	Sulphate or phosphate of soda, epsom salts, followed by emetics, and afterwards opium and milk.
Lobelia	See Fl. Ext. Lobelia Herb, p. 78.
Mercury Biniodide	See Corrosive Sublimate.
Morphine	See Fl. Ext. Opium, Aqueous, p. 88.
Nitrites	Ergot, belladonna, nux vomica, digitalis. Stimulants, artificial respiration, cold and hot douche alternately, cold to the head.
Nitroglycerin	See Nitrites.
Nux Vomica	See Fl. Ext. Nux Vomica, p. 87.
Opium	See Fl. Ext. Opium, Aqueous, p. 88.
Oxalic Acid	Chalk, whiting, lime water, syr. of lime, wall-plaster, emollient drinks. Avoid soluble carbonates.
Paris Green	See Arsenic.
Phosphorus	Copper sulphate or carbonate, magnesia, turpentine, emetics and purgatives.
Picrotoxin	See Fl. Ext. Cocculus Indicus, p. 42.
Pilocarpine	See Fl. Ext. Jaborandi, p. 69.
Pulsatilla	See Fl. Ext. Pulsatilla, p. 96.
Silver Nitrate	Solution of common salt in demulcent drinks.
Stramonium	See Fl. Ext. Stramonium Seed, p. 114.
Strophanthus	Emetics, stomach-pump. Stimulants, aconite, veratrum viride.
Strychnine	See Fl. Ext. Nux Vomica, p. 87.
Tartar Emetic	Vegetable astringents, such as tannic acid, catechu.
Tin Salts	Albumen, milk, ammonium or sodium carbonates.
Tobacco	Emetics, stimulants external and internal, strychnine.
Veratrum Viride	See Fl. Ext. Veratrum Viride, p. 120.
Water Hemlock	See Fl. Ext. Water Hemlock, p. 123.
White Precipitate	Emetics (zinc sulphate), milk, albumen. Compare also corrosive sublimate.
Zinc Salts	Carbonate of soda, emetics, warm demulcent drinks.

WHEN ORDERING OR PRESCRIBING.

The Examination of Urine.

A. TABLE SHOWING THE NORMAL CONSTITUENTS AND CHARACTERISTICS OF URINE AND THEIR USUAL VARIATIONS FROM DISEASE OR OTHER CAUSES.

		NORMAL.	ABNORMAL.
PHYSICAL CHARACTERISTICS.	Color.	Varies from straw-yellow to amber yellow according to amount and concentration. Rendered very pale by nervousness or excessive drinking.	Pale or almost colorless (hysteria, diabetes, hydruria, chlorosis and granular kidney); highly colored (febrile conditions); blood-red, brown or nearly black (presence of blood or biliary coloring matter); green (biliverdin) or dirty-blue (cholera and typhus).
	Odor	Characteristic; aromatic when fresh, ammoniacal on standing, also changed by certain foods and medicines.	Rendered foul and repulsive in destructive disease of the kidney or bladder and by the presence of sulphuretted hydrogen.
	Transparency	Should be clear, showing on standing only a mucous cloud containing usually a small amount of epithelium.	May be clouded by suspended acid urates (disappear on heating), calcium carb., earthy phosphates, pus, blood, (increases on heating, the first two soluble on adding acetic acid); also mucus, bacteria and fatty matter.
	Consistence	Thin fluid, easily separating into drops.	Viscid or glairy (pus in alkaline urine) or coagulable on standing (fibrin).
	Amount.	Averages 1500 c.c. (50 fl. ozs.) in 24 hours. Varies with food and habits.	Much increased in hydruria and diabetes, diminished in fevers and kidney affections to entire suppression in uremia.
	Reaction	Normally acid, may be alkaline directly after a meal.	Strongly acid in articular rheumatism and gouty affections. Strongly alkaline in diseases of the bladder. May be alkaline after taking alkalies or alkaline mineral water.
	Spec. gravity	1.015 to 1.021.	1.003 to 1.040.
	Solids.	4.3 to 4.3% or 60 to 70 gm. in 24 hours urine. Reduced by fasting and dieting.	Increased in diabetes (200 gm.), decreased in hydruria (20 gm.). In urina potus the % is decreased but the amount for 24 hours is normal.
ORGANIC CONSTITUENTS.	Urea	2.5 to 3.2% or 30 to 40 gm. in 24 hours.	Decreased by a vegetable diet and in chronic disease and uremia. Increased in acute febrile processes and diabetes, also by animal diet.
	Uric acid	.03 to .05% or .4 to .8 gm. excreted in 24 hours mostly as neutral urates.	A yellowish red or brick-dust precipitate of uric acid or acid urates in fresh urine indicates stone or gravel. Generally uric acid increases or decreases as the excretion of urea.
	Coloring matters	Most important of these are urobilin and indican.	An excess of urobilin develops a green fluorescence on addition of ammonia and sol. zinc chloride. An increase of indican develops a violet or blue color on stirring 10 or 12 drops of urine into 4 c.c. of HCl.

<table>
<tr><td></td><td>NORMAL.</td><td>ABNORMAL.</td></tr>
</table>

	NORMAL.	ABNORMAL.
Creatinine...	.04 to .06% or ½ to 1 gm. in 24 hours.	Increased in pneumonia, intermittent and typhus fevers; decreased in advanced kidney disease and inanition.
Hippuric acid.......	.02 to .06% or .3 to 1 gm. in 24 hours. Characteristic of the urine of herbivora.	Increased by a vegetable diet, the administration of benzoic acid and in diabetes and fevers. Diminished by a strict animal diet.
Chlorides....	.7 to .8% or 10 to 15 gm. in 24 hours. Less during sleep or repose.	Increased in the paroxysms of intermittent fever, in diabetes insipidus, dropsy and by exercise or salty diet. Decreased in all acute febrile processes.
Phosphoric acid.	.19 to .22% or 2.5 to 3.5 gm. in 24 hours. Two thirds of this amount is combined with sodium and potassium as alkali phosphates, the remainder with calcium and magnesium as earthy phosphates. Of the latter there is usually present .07 to .08% or .9 to 1.3 gm. in 24 hours, ⅓ of which is calcium phosphate.	Total phosphates are usually increased in wasting diseases, decreased in acute diseases and during pregnancy. Continued elimination of an excess of phosphates constitutes what has been termed phosphatic diabetes. The earthy phosphates are increased in bone-diseases and certain rheumatic processes, also by the use of some mineral waters, medicines and a flesh diet; decreased in kidney affections. When the urine becomes alkaline the earthy phosphates are precipitated.
Sulphuric acid	.16 to .17% or 1.5 to 2.5 gm. in 24 hours as neutral sulphates.	Increased after the exhibition of sulphur or its combinations, by an exclusive flesh diet, also in meningitis, encephalitis, rheumatism and affections of the muscular system.

(Left margin, vertical: INORGANIC CONSTITUENTS.)

B. Abnormal Constituents.

Most important of these are albumen and sugar. Among the others are leucin, tyrosin, certain coloring matters, the bile acids, ammonium carbonate and sulphuretted hydrogen.

Albumen occurs in all disturbed conditions of the circulation, in such diseases as parenchymatous nephritis and Bright's disease, with functional disorders, sometimes with hydraemia and in urine containing blood or pus. In strongly acid or alkaline urine it may be present as non-coagulable acid or alkali albumen which can be reconverted to the ordinary variety by the careful addition respectively of alkali or acid.

Sugar in small amount may appear temporarily after certain diseases such as lesions of the brain, pneumonia, typhus, rheumatism, affections of the spinal cord and after the use of certain medicines, as turpentine, nitrite of amyl, nitrobenzole, etc. It is present persistently and in large amount only in glycosuria (diabetes).

Leucin and Tyrosin have been found in the urine in large amount only in acute atrophy of the liver and a few cases of phosphorus-poisoning. In such cases crystals of tyrosin are found in the sediment, or separate together with leucin from urine evaporated to a small bulk.

Abnormal coloring matters. The dark reddish-yellow color of fever urine is due in part to the presence of uroerythrin. A deposit of urates occurring in such urine is rose-colored to dark red. Many drugs when administered impart color to the urine; thus rhubarb and senna color it red when alkaline, becoming yellow on acidulation; santonin produces a bright-yellow color in acid urine; and madder, indigo, gamboge, logwood, etc. give to urine more or less of their peculiar color. Coloring matters of the blood when present are carried down with the phosphates when they are precipitated and color the precipitate correspondingly. Biliary coloring matters color such precipitate brown; they occur in phosphorus-poisoning and various pathologic processes of the liver.

Bile Acids are seldom found in the urine and then only in extremely small amounts.

Ammonium Carbonate arises from a transformation of urea accompanied by the assimilation of the elements of water. This occurs especially in catarrh of the bladder and hence the alkalinity of urine in bladder troubles.

Sulphuretted hydrogen occurs sometimes in albuminous urine and arises from the decomposition of albuminous bodies within the bladder.

C. Examination.

I. Of clear urine.

1. Note the appearance, odor and reaction (see A.).
2. Determine the specific gravity. Calculate the amount of solids by subtracting from the specific gravity 1.000 and multiplying the remainder by 2.33, the result = grams of solids in 1000 c.c.
3. Upon a quantity of nitric acid in a test-tube place a layer of urine by means of a pipette, being careful not to allow the two liquids to mix, or beneath a quantity of urine in a test-glass, place a layer of nitric acid by carefully pouring it along the side of the glass. If albumen is present a white zone, or flocculent, or even curdy precipitate appears in the zone of contact of the two liquids according to the quantity, whether small, considerable or large. Urates may give rise to a white cloud extending upward into the urine layer, giving place after a time to a crystalline precipitate of uric acid. If this occur in the presence of albumen the cloud of urates floats above the albumen precipitate. If neither albumen nor excess of urates is present there appears simply a brown ring. When biliary coloring matters are present a green zone is produced. With excess of indican a violet or blue zone. An excess of urea will give, after mixing and cooling, a crystalline precipitate.
4. Acidulate slightly with acetic acid (avoiding excess) and heat in a test-tube. A precipitate indicates albumen. If urine is not acid, phosphates may be precipitated, soluble on addition of a little acetic acid. Now add half as much sol. of potassa as there is urine, the albumen is dissolved, earthy phosphates are precipitated—white if no foreign coloring matters are present, blood red or dichroic in presence of blood, rose-red (albumen being absent) from plant-coloring matters, grayish from uroerythrin or brown from biliary coloring matter. Set aside and note the amount of precipitate; if occupying ⅓ or ⅙ of the space occupied by the entire liquid it is normal; if as much as ⅓, the quantity of earthy phosphates is increased; if there are only a few scattered flakes, they are diminished. Now heat the mixture, if it turns brown sugar in indicated.
5. Into a test-tube pour about 5 c.c. of Fehling's solution and heat it to boiling; if in good condition it will remain unaltered. Now add a little urine and boil, if sugar is present in considerable amount a yellow or red precipitate is produced. Should this not occur add more urine never adding a larger quantity, however, than the amount of test-solution used and boil again. If a small quantity of sugar is present a yellow precipitate appears. If the urine is free from sugar only a green color, or greenish flocculent precipitate of phosphates is produced.

6. Into a quantity of sulphuric acid in a test-glass pour, slowly and from a height of about four inches, double the amount of urine. With normal urine a deep garnet-red is produced; if there is present excess of coloring matter or altered bile pigments the mixture turns dark or nearly black; if a deficiency, the color is correspondingly light.

7. Into 5 or 6 c.c. of hydrochloric acid in a test-glass drop sufficient urine to distinctly color it and mix. Beneath this carefully pour a sub-layer of nitric acid. In the presence of bile pigments a play of colors (green being the most characteristic) is observed at the the zone of contact. If stirred it is repeated throughout the entire mixture. Urine containing bile also stains linen and paper permanently yellow. Decomposed bile pigments produce a brown stain.

8. If blood is suspected mix equal parts of fresh tinct. of guaiac and ozonized (by long exposure to air) oil of turpentine; pour carefully upon the surface of some urine in a test-tube. At the line of contact appears a grayish precipitate of resin and immediately above if blood is present an indigo-blue ring. Upon shaking a blue emulsion results.

9. Acidulate a portion of urine with nitric acid. Add one or two drops of sol. nitrate of silver. If a curdy precipitate falls chlorides are undiminished. If a milky cloudiness ensues chlorides are diminished; if no cloudiness they are wanting. If albumen is present it should be first removed by boiling with a few drops of acetic acid.

10. If there is an excess of earthy phosphates (see 4) remove by precipitating with an alkali and filter, if not add to 10 c.c. of raw urine 3 c.c. of magnesia mixture. A milky turbidity indicates alkaline phosphates in normal amount; a copious precipitate, giving a creamy appearance, signifies great increase and a slight turbidity only, a decrease.

11. Proceed as in No. 9 using sol. of barium chloride instead of silver nitrate. An opaque milky cloudiness results when sulphates are normal; greater or less turbidity indicates a corresponding increase or decrease in sulphates. If solutions of sulphate, chloride and phosphate of sodium, corresponding in strength to normal urine be kept on hand the last three tests can be made comparative.

II. Of urinary deposits.

Should the urine contain a sediment, allow to subside in a conical glass when it can be removed for examination with a pipette.

(a). Unorganized sedimentary matter.

1. Urates—Yellowish to reddish-yellow, soluble on heating.
2. Uric acid—Brick-red, crystalline, soluble on heating with an alkali.
3. Fat—Rises to the surface, dissolved on shaking with ether.
4. Phosphates—Amorphous or crystalline, soluble in acetic acid.
5. Calcium carbonate—Amorphous, soluble in acetic acid with effervescence.
6. Calcium oxalate—Crystalline, insoluble in acetic, soluble in hydrochloric acid.
7. Cystin—Crystalline, soluble in ammonia without heating, insoluble in acetic acid.

(b) Organized sedimentary matter.

1. Mucus—Ropy, tenacious and transparent; coagulated by acetic acid.
2. Pus—On the addition of a small piece of caustic soda or potash becomes greenish, stringy, and gelatinous, is always accompanied by albumen.
3. Blood corpuscles, epithelium, cylinders, etc. as well as all crystalline deposits should be identified by aid of the microscope.

The Treatment of Asphyxia.

The points to be aimed at are:

1—The restoration of breathing;

2—The promotion of warmth and circulation.

Treatment should be applied instantly, in the open air, if possible, freely exposing the face, neck and chest to the breeze except in severe weather. No time should be lost in trying to remove the patient. The use of bellows or any forcing instrument, also, the warm bath and all rough treatment, should be avoided.

I. THE RESTORATION OF BREATHING.

Dr. Marshall Hall's Method.

1. In order to clear the throat, place the patient gently on the face, with one wrist under the forehead, that all fluid, and the tongue itself, may fall forward, and leave the entrance into the windpipe free.

2. To excite respiration, turn the patient slightly on his side and apply some irritating or stimulating agent to the nostrils, as veratrine, dilute ammonia, etc.

3. Make the face warm by brisk friction; then dash cold water upon it.

4. If not successful, lose no time; but, to imitate respiration, place the patient on his face and turn the body gently, but completely, on the side and a little beyond; then again on the face, and so on alternately. Repeat these movements deliberately and perseveringly fifteen times only in a minute. (When the patient lies on the thorax, the cavity is compressed by the weight of the body, and expiration takes place. When he is turned on the side, this pressure is removed, and inspiration occurs.)

5. When the prone position is resumed, make a uniform and efficient pressure along the spine, removing the pressure immediately, before rotation on the side. (The pressure augments the expiration; the rotation commences inspiration). Should these measures not prove successful in the course of five minutes employ the following:

Dr. Silvester's Method.

1. Place the patient on the back upon a flat surface slightly elevated towards the head. Place under the shoulder-blades a small firm cushion or a pad made from articles of clothing.

2. Cleanse the mouth and nostrils. Draw forwards the patient's tongue and keep it projecting beyond the lips by an elastic band or string passed under the chin and over the tongue or, by raising the lower jaw until the tongue is held between the teeth.

3. Remove all tight clothing from the neck and chest.

4. To induce inspiration stand at the patient's head, grasp the arms just above the elbows and gently and steadily raise them until extended full length above the head. Keep them in this position two seconds.

5. To induce expiration turn down the patient's arms and press them gently but firmly against the sides of the chest for two seconds.

6. Repeat these measures about fifteen times a minute until spontaneous efforts to respire are perceived.

Dr. Howard's Method.

1. Instantly place the patient face downward with one of his arms under his forehead and a large firm roll of clothing under his stomach and chest.

2. Press upon patient's back with all your weight for four or five seconds and repeat two or three times so that the lungs and stomach may be relieved of the water present.

3. Quickly turn the patient on his back with the roll of clothing under his shoulder-blades, leaving the head hang back as low as possible; place the hands above his head.

4. Kneel with the patient's hips between your knees and firmly fixing your elbows against your hips, grasp the lower part of the patient's naked chest, squeezing his sides together and press gradually forward with all your weight for about three seconds, until your mouth is nearly over that of the patient, then with a push suddenly jerk yourself back.

5. Rest about three seconds then repeat. These movements should be continued about eight or ten times a minute, for at least an hour, or, until natural respiration is established.

II. THE RESTORATION OF WARMTH AND CIRCULATION.

1. Substitute for the patient's wet clothing such dry covering as can be instantly procured; each bystander supplying a coat or cloak, etc.

2. Rub the body briskly until it is dry and warm, then dash cold water upon it and repeat the rubbing.

3. Rub the limbs upward with firm pressure and with energy. (The object being to aid the return of venous blood to the heart).

4. Make dry hot applications (hot flannels etc.) to the pit of the stomach, armpits, between the thighs, to the soles of the feet.

5. When the patient has recovered the power of swallowing give a small quantity of some stimulant (wine, brandy and water, coffee, etc).

Eruption of the Teeth.

DECIDUOUS TEETH.	PERMANENT TEETH.
(The lower generally precede the upper by two or three months.)	First molars........ ... 5 to 6 yrs.
	Central incisors....... 6 to 8 yrs.
	Lateral incisors....... 7 to 9 yrs.
Central incisors...... 5 to 8 mos.	First bicuspids........ 9 to 10 yrs.
Lateral incisors...... 7 to 10 mos.	Second bicuspids....10 to 11 yrs.
First molars.........12 to 16 mos.	Canines..............11 to 12 yrs.
Canines............15 to 20 mos.	Second molars........12 to 14 yrs.
Second molars.......20 to 36 mos.	Third molars.....17 to 21 yrs.

Temperature of the Body.

The average normal temperature of adults is 98.6° F.; of the aged, 98.8°; of children, 99°. The daily variation is from 1° to 1.5°, the maximum temperature being reached between 9 a. m. and 2 p. m.

Relation of Pulse and Temperature.

A variation of one degree in temperature, above 98° F., is approximately equivalent to a difference of 10 beats in the pulse, thus:

A temperature of 98° F. corresponds with a pulse of 60.
"   99°   "   "   "   70.
"   100°   "   "   "   80.
"   101°   "   "   "   90.
"   102°   "   "   "   100.
"   103°   "   "   "   110.
"   104°   "   "   "   120.
"   105°   "   "   "   130.
"   106°   "   "   "   140.

The Pulse.

AVERAGE FREQUENCY AT DIFFERENT AGES, IN HEALTH.

AGE.	BEATS PER MINUTE. (CARPENTER.)	BY OTHER AUTHORITIES.
In the fœtus *in utero*.....	between.. 150 and 140..	
New-born infants.........	between.. 140 and 130..	
During first year...	from..... 130 down to 115..	130 108
During second year.......	from..... 115 down to 100.	108- 90
During third year........	from..... 105 down to 95	90- 80
From 7th to 14th year....	from.... 90 down to 80	80- 72
From 14th to 21st year ..	from .... 85 down to 75.	85- 80
From 21st to 60th year..	from..... 75 down to 70.	70- 60
In old age	between.. 75 and 80	

The pulse is generally more frequent in females, by 10-14 beats per minute; during and after exertion, unless long continued; during digestion or mental excitement; generally more frequent in the morning; and less frequent, in health, in the nervous as well as in the phlegmatic temperament.

THE PULSE MAY BE:

1. In regard to force—deficient, depressed, feeble or weak, full, hard, languid, large, low, natural, resisting, sharp, jerking, small, soft, strong, tense.

2. In regard to frequency and succession—developed, equal, febrile, frequent, hectic, intercurrent, intermittent, intricate, irregular, irritative, quick, regular, slow, unequal, and the PULSUS SERRINUS (saw-like, alternately strong and feeble).

3. In regard to form or manner of striking (force included)—ardent, caprizant (double blow, the latter part stronger), contracted, convulsive, critical, deep, dicrotic, (double), formicant, hemorrhoidal, long, simple, supple, sudoral, thread-like, tremulous, undulating, uterine, vermicular, vibrating; also, the PULSUS STRIATUS (striking in a narrow line), P. VACUUS (empty). Other forms not so readily observed, or of doubtful value, are named.

Respiration at Various Ages.

AGE.	NO. OF RESPIRATIONS PER MINUTE.
First year..........................	35
At puberty..........................	20
Adult age	18

Indications of the Tongue.

A white tongue indicates febrile disturbance; a brown moist tongue, indigestion; a brown dry tongue, depression, blood-poisoning, typhoid fever; a red moist tongue, inflammatory fever; a red glazed tongue, general fever, loss of digestion; a tremulous, moist and flabby tongue, feebleness, nervousness; a glazed tongue with blue appearance, tertiary syphilis.

TABLE OF ERUPTIVE FEVERS.

NAME.	PERIODS OF INCUBATION.	OCCURRENCE OF RASH.	CHARACTER OF RASH.	DISAPPEARANCE OF RASH.	DURATION OF ILLNESS.
Chicken pox..	4 days.	2d day of fever, or after 24 hours illness.	Small rose blisters, becoming vesicles.	Slight scabs form about the 4th day of fever.	6 to 7 days....
Erysipelas...	3 to 7 days.	2d or 3d day.	diffused redness and swelling.	Uncertain.	Uncertain.......
Measles	10 to 14 days.	4th day of fever, or after 72 hours illness.	Small red dots like flea bites, crescentic.	On the 7th day of fever.	6 to 10 days....
Rotheln	7 to 14 days.	4th to 6th day.	Like measles but less distinct, patches are brighter near center.	Often desquamation on 4th day. Uncertain.	8 to 10 days....
Scarlet fever..	4 to 10 days.	2d day of fever, or after 24 hours illness.	Bright scarlet, diffused.	On the 5th day of fever.	8 to 15 days....
Small pox.....	12 days.	3d day of fever, or after 48 hours illness.	Small red pimples, becoming vesicles, then pustules.	Scabs form on 9th or 10th day of fever and fall on about the 14th.	14 to 21 days...
Typhoid fever	10 to 14 days, or suddenly.	7th to 10th day.	Rose colored spots, few in number.	Uncertain.	20 to 30 days...
Typhus fever..	1 to 12 days.	4th to 7th day.	Mulberry color, generally over abdomen.	Uncertain.	14 to 21 days...

PERIODS OF ISOLATION OF PATIENTS.

Diphtheria, measles, scarlet fever and small-pox, 40 days; chicken-pox and mumps, 25 days, counting in all cases from the inception of the disease.

Table for Calculating the Period of Utero-Gestation.

Confinement (expected)	Last menses ceased (month)	1	2	3	4	5	6	7	8	9	10	11	12	13	14	15	16	17	18	19	20	21	22	23	24	25	26	27	28	29	30	31
Oct.	Jan.	25	26	27	28	29	30	31	1	2	3	4	5	6	7	8	9	10	11	12	13	14	15	16	17	18	19	20	21	22	23	24
Nov.	Feb.	25	26	27	28	29	30	31	1	2	3	4	5	6	7	8	9	10	11	12	13	14	15	16	17	18	19	20	21	22	23	
Dec.	Mar.	24	25	26	27	28	1	2	3	4	5	6	7	8	9	10	11	12	13	14	15	16	17	18	19	20	21	22	23	24	25	26
Jan.	April	27	28	29	30	31	1	2	3	4	5	6	7	8	9	10	11	12	13	14	15	16	17	18	19	20	21	22	23	24	25	26
Feb.	May	27	28	29	30	1	2	3	4	5	6	7	8	9	10	11	12	13	14	15	16	17	18	19	20	21	22	23	24			
Mar.	June	25	26	27	28	29	30	31	1	2	3	4	5	6	7	8	9	10	11	12	13	14	15	16	17	18	19	20	21	22	23	24
April	July	25	26	27	28	29	30	1	2	3	4	5	6	7	8	9	10	11	12	13	14	15	16	17	18	19	20	21	22	23	24	
May	Aug.	25	26	27	28	29	30	31	1	2	3	4	5	6	7	8	9	10	11	12	13	14	15	16	17	18	19	20	21	22	23	24
June	Sept.	25	26	27	28	29	30	31	1	2	3	4	5	6	7	8	9	10	11	12	13	14	15	16	17	18	19	20	21	22	23	
July	Oct.	24	25	26	27	28	29	30	1	2	3	4	5	6	7	8	9	10	11	12	13	14	15	16	17	18	19	20	21	22	23	24
Aug.	Nov.	25	26	27	28	29	30	31	1	2	3	4	5	6	7	8	9	10	11	12	13	14	15	16	17	18	19	20	21	22	23	24
Sept.	Dec.	25	26	27	28	29	30	1	2	3	4	5	6	7	8	9	10	11	12	13	14	15	16	17	18	19	20	21	22	23	24	

Normal labor occurs about 280 days after the last menstrual period and the above table is designed to show at a glance the probable date of confinement. In the body of the table (within the double rules) find the date of cessation of the last menstrual period, at the head of the column will be found the day, and at the extreme left (on the same line as date of last menses) will be found the month when confinement may be expected. For instance, the menses having ceased July 21, confinement may be expected about April 27; or if July 25, confinement will occur about May 1, etc.

DEFINITIONS

OF

Therapeutic Terms.

Abortifacient— Producing abortion.
Absorbent— A medicine or dressing which acts by absorbing gases or liquids.
Abstergent— A cleansing application.
Acro-narcotic— Having both acrid and narcotic properties.
Adjuvant—Any substance designed to assist the action of the principal means.
Alexipharmic— Acting as a prophylactic or as an antidote.
Alexipyretic— Preventing or curing fever.
Aliment— A food, a nutrient.
Alkaluretic— Promoting the secretion of alkaline urine.
Alterant }
Alterative } Promoting healthy changes in the system.
Amblotic }
Ambolic } Producing abortion.
Anabrotic— Corrosive, caustic.
Anacathartic— Promoting expectoration or vomiting.
Analeptic— Supporting, restorative.
Analgesic—Relieving pain.
Anaphrodisiac— Subduing sexual desire.
Anaplerotic— Promoting granulation of wounds.
Anastaltic— Arresting hemorrhages.
Anesthetic— Having the power of producing insensibility to pain.
Anodyne—Allaying pain.
Antacid—Counteracting acidity.
Antalgic—Relieving pain.
Antatrophic— Repairing diseased tissues.
Antemetic— Allaying vomiting.
Antephialtic—Efficacious against nightmare.
Anterethic— Relieving irritation.
Anterotic—Diminishing sexual appetite.
Anthelmintic—Destroying or expelling worms.
Antiarthritic—A remedy for gout.
Antiasthenic— Relieving debility, strengthening.
Antiblenorrhagic—Reducing or curing mucus discharges, anti-gonorrheal.
Antibromic—Deodorizing.
Anticausodic— Antipyretic.
Anticaustic—Preventing or mitigating the action of caustics.
Antidrotic—Diminishing perspiration.
Anticephalalgic—Efficacious against headache.
Antichlorotic—Efficacious against chlorosis.
Antichoradic— Efficacious against scrofulous glandular swelling.
Anticholeric—Efficacious against cholera or the disturbances of a choleric temperament.
Anticteric—A remedy for jaundice.
Antidinic—Efficacious against vertigo.
Antidote—A remedy destroying, or counteracting the effects of a poison.
Antidysuric—Efficacious against strangury.
Antiemetic—Efficacious against vomiting.
Antiepileptic—Efficacious against epilepsy.
Antifermentative—Preventing or stopping fermentation.
Antigalactic—Preventing or diminishing the secretion of milk.
Antihectic—Efficacious against consumption.
Antiherpetic—A remedy for tetter.
Antihidrotic—Diminishing perspiration.
Antihydropic—Efficacious against dropsy.
Antihypnotic—A remedy preventing sleep.
Antihysteric—A remedy for hysteria.
Antilithic—Tending to cure stone and gravel.
Antiloimic—Efficacious against the plague.
Antimiasmatic—Efficacious against miasmatic affections.
Antimycetic—Destroying fungi.
Antinephritic—A remedy for kidney diseases.
Antineuralgic—Relieving neuralgia.
Antineurotic—Nervine.
Antiparasitic—Destructive to parasites.

Antiperiodic—Preventing the recurrence of periodic diseases.
Antiphlogistic—Diminishing fever and inflammation.
Antiphthisic—A remedy for consumption.
Antiphysetic—Carminative.
Antipodagric—A remedy for gout.
Antipruritic—Relieving itching.
Antipsoric—Efficacious against the itch.
Antipurulent—Preventing or checking suppuration.
Antiputrescent—Preventing or arresting putrefaction.
Antipyic—Preventing or checking suppuration.
Antipyretic—Febrifuge; efficacious against fever, reducing the temperature of the body.
Antipyrotic—Relieving burns or pyrosis.
Antirachitic—Efficacious against rickets.
Antirheumatic—Relieving or curing rheumatism.
Antiscorbutic—Curing scurvy.
Antiscrofulic—Tending to prevent and cure scrofula.
Antiseptic—Preventing or arresting putrefaction.
Antispasmodic—Allaying spasms.
Antispastic—Revulsive, counter-irritant or antispasmodic.
Antisplenetic—Relieving hypochondriasis.
Antisquamic—Curing skin disease.
Antistrumous—Antiscrofulous.
Antisudorific—Diminishing perspiration.
Antisyphilitic—Overcoming venereal disease.
Antithermic—Antipyretic.
Antitoxic—Antidoting poison.
Antivenereal—Efficacious in the treatment of venereal diseases; preventing venereal infection.
Antizootic—Destroying animal life, preventing contagion.
Antizymic—Preventing or retarding fermentation.
Antizymotic—Preventing zymotic diseases.
Antodontalgic—Relieving tooth-ache.
Antophthalmic—A remedy for ophthalmia.
Antorgastic—Calming venereal excitement.
Aperient—Gently laxative.
Aphrodisiac—Stimulating venereal desire.
Apulotic—Healing, causing cicatrization.
Astringent—Contracting organic texture.

Bacillicide—A substance that destroys bacilli.
Bactericide—A substance that destroys bacteria.
Blennostatic—Checking mucous secretion.

Caccagogue—Purgative.
Calmative—Quieting.
Calorifacient—Heat-producing.
Cardiac—A heart stimulant or tonic.
Carminative—Correcting flatulency.
Carotic—Producing sleep or stupor.
Catarrhectic—Purgative.
Catastaltic—Checking evacuations, secretions or hemorrhage; also calming, soothing.
Cathartic / **Cathartic**—Producing evacuation.
Catheretic—Feebly caustic.
Catoteric—Causing a downward flow, cathartic.
Catulotic—Tending to promote cicatrization.
Caustic / **Cauterant** / **Cauteretic**—Destroying tissue as if by burning.
Cenotic—Producing painful purging.
Cerebrospinant—A remedy acting upon both the brain and spinal chord.
Chalybeate—Containing iron.
Cholagogue—Increasing the flow of bile.
Cicatrizant—Promoting cicatrization or healing of wounds.
Coagulant—A remedy supposed to thicken the blood and other fluids of the body.
Convulsivant—Causing convulsions.
Copragogue—A cathartic.
Corrective / **Corrigent**—Modifying so as to prevent severe or unpleasant effects.
Corroborant—Strengthening.
Corrodent / **Corrosive**—Destroying organic or inorganic matter more or less rapidly.
Counterirritant—An irritant applied to one part to relieve pain in another.

Decalvant—Causing baldness.
Deliriant
Delirifacient} Causing delirium.
Demulcent—Soothing.
Deobstruent—Removing obstructions.
Deodorant
Deodorizant} Removing or correcting foul odors.
Depilatory—An agent used to remove hair.
Depletive
Depletory} Reducing the quantity of any liquid in the body.
Depressant—Causing melancholy or nervous debility.
Depurative—Removing impurities from the fluids of the body; cleansing.
Derivative—Diverting from one part to another; revulsive.
Desiccant—An agent removing moisture; drying.
Detergent—Cleansing.
Diabrotic—Corroding the flesh or skin.
Dialytic—Relaxing.
Diaphoretic—Tending to produce or increase perspiration.
Diapnoic—Promoting perspiration.
Diapyetic—Promoting suppuration.
Diarrhetic—Producing profuse stools.
Dietetic—Pertaining to diet or the regulation of the diet.
Digestant—Aiding digestion.
Diluent—A drink serving the purpose of diluting the various fluids of the body.
Dipsetic—Causing thirst.
Discutient—Dispersing or repelling morbid swellings; resolvent.
Disinfectant—Destroying the cause of infection.
Dissolvent—Disintegrating and dissolving concretions, such as calculi, etc.
Diuretic—Increasing the secretion of urine.
Drastic—Acting quickly and violently; said of cathartics.

Ecbolic—Inducing abortion.
Eccoprotic—A mild purgative; gently cathartic.
Eccorthatic—Causing copious discharges of feces.
Ectrotic—Causing abortion.
Ectylotic—Tending to remove warts, callosities and indurations of the skin.
Emetic—Causing vomiting.
Emetocathartic—Producing both vomiting and catharsis.
Emmenagogue—Promoting menstruation.
Emollient—Softening, soothing.
Emulgent—Exciting the flow of bile.
Emundant—Cleansing, detergent.
Epechontocic—Moderating uterine contraction.
Epispastic—Irritating, blistering.
Epizoicide—Destroying epizoa, parasiticide.
Epulotic—Promoting cicatrization.
Erodent—Caustic, corrosive.
Errhine—Exciting nasal discharges; sternutatory.
Escharotic—Searing or destroying flesh; caustic.
Eutrophic—Nutritious.
Evacuant—Producing a discharge from a particular organ; a purgative and cathartic.
Excitant—Stimulating the action of any of the organs, especially the nervous system.
Exhilarant—An agent that exhilarates or enlivens.
Expectorant—Promoting mucus discharges from the air passages.
Exsiccative—Drying, desiccant.
Extergent—Detergent, cleansing.

Febrifacient—Producing fever.
Febrifuge—Allaying fever.
Frigefacient—Refrigerant, cooling.

Galactagogue
Galactophorous} Promoting the secretion of milk.
Galactophygous—Preventing or checking the secretion of milk.
Galactopoietic—Promoting the secretion of milk.
Germicide—A substance or agent that destroys germs.

Helminthagogue—Destroying or expelling worms.
Hemagogue—Promoting menstrual discharges.
Hematic—Acting on or through the blood.
Hematinic—Increasing the coloring matter of the blood.
Hemostatic—Arresting the flow of blood.
Hepatic—Promoting the healthful action of the liver.
Herpetic—Curing diseases of the skin.

Hidroteric }
Hidrotic } Causing perspiration.
Hydragogue }
Hydrotic } Causing copious watery stools.
Hygiastic—Curative.
Hygienic—Tending to preserve health.
Hypnetic }
Hypagogue } Slightly purgative.
Hypercathartic—Causing excessive purging.
Hyperorexic—Increasing the appetite.
Hypnotic—Inducing sleep or stupor.
Hypochoretic—Purgative.

Icteric—A remedy for jaundice.
Insecticide—A substance that destroys insects.
Irritant—Exciting soreness and inflammation.

Lactagogue—Promoting the secretion of milk.
Lactifuge—Decreasing or arresting the secretion of milk.
Laxative—Producing gentle action of the bowels.
Lenitive—Assuaging, palliating, demulcent.
Lithagogue—Expelling calculi.
Litholytic }
Lithontriptic } Capable of dissolving vesical calculi.

Menagogue—Promoting the menstrual flow.
Methystic—Intoxicating.
Microbicide—A substance that destroys microbes.
Mydriatic—Dilating the pupil of the eye.
Myositic }
Myotic } Contracting the pupil of the eye.

Narcotic—Inducing sleep or stupor.
Nauseant—Causing vomiting, or inclination to vomit.
Nephritic—Efficacious in kidney complaints.
Nervine—Nervous sedative.
Nutrient }
Nutritive } Nourishing or sustaining life.

Obtundent—Serving to reduce irritability or deaden the sensibility of a part.
Odinagogue—Hastening labor.
Orectic—Exciting an appetite.
Oxytocic—Hastening labor.

Palliative—Relieving morbid conditions without curing.
Paralyzant—A drug suspending or abolishing functional power.
Parasiticide—A drug which destroys parasites, an insecticide; a vermifuge.
Parturient }
Parturifacient } Hastening labor.
Pectoral—Relieving diseases of the lungs.
Phlegmagogue—Expelling mucus.
Phlogogenic—Producing inflammation.
Prophylactic—Preventing disease.
Pustulant—Producing pustules.
Pyogenic—Causing the formation of pus—said of microbes.
Pyrogenic—Producing heat or fever.
Pyrotic—Caustic, burning.
Refrigerant—Cooling, mitigating heat.
Relaxant—Relieving tension, relaxing; also a laxative.
Resolvent—Allaying inflammation and dispersing morbid swelling.
Restorative—Bringing back the natural functions.
Revulsive—Acting by producing irritation in one part to divert diseased actions from another.
Rhophetic—An absorbent medicine.
Roborant—Strengthening, tonic.
Rubefacient—Producing superficial irritation or redness.

Salivant—Promoting the production of saliva.
Sarcotic—Flesh-producing.
Sedative—Diminishing vital actions.
Sialagogue—Stimulating the secretion of saliva.
Siccative—Desiccant, drying.
Somnifacient }
Sopient } Inducing sleep.
Sorbefacient—Causing abortion.
Spastic—Producing involuntary muscular contraction.
Spinant—Acting upon the spinal marrow.

Sternutatory—Exciting sneezing.
Stimulant—Exciting or increasing vital action.
Stomachic—Inducing a healthy action of the stomach.
Styptic—Arresting hemorrhage.
Sudorific—Causing perspiration.
Suppurant—Producing suppuration.

Tenifuge—A medicine which expels tape worm from the intestines.
Tonic—Producing a permanent increase in the tone of the system.
Toxic—Poisonous.

Ulotic—Promoting the healing of wounds.
Uretic ⎱
Uropoietic ⎰ Promoting the secretion of urine.

Vermifuge—Destroying or expelling worms.
Vesicant ⎱
Vesicatory ⎰ Producing blisters.
Vulnerary—Favoring the healing of wounds.

Zymogenic—Producing fermentation.

Phrases and Abbreviations

USED IN PRESCRIPTIONS.

WORD OR PHRASE.	ABBREVIATION.	TRANSLATION.
Absente febre	Abs. feb.	In the absence of fever.
Ad		To, up to.
Adde or addantur	Add. or ad.	Let it or them be added.
Ad defectionem animi	Ad def. animo.	To fainting.
Ad duas vices	Ad 2 vic.	At twice taking (second time).
Ad gratam aciditatem	Ad grat. acid.	To an agreeable sourness.
Adhibendus		To be administered.
Adjacens	Adjac.	Adjacent.
Ad libitum	Ad lib.	At pleasure.
Admove, or admoveatur	Admov.	Apply, or let it be applied.
Ad secundum vicem	Ad sec. vic.	To the second time.
Adstante febre	Adst. feb.	When the fever is on.
Ad tertiam vicem	Ad ter. vic.	For three times.
Adversum	Adv.	Against.
Aggrediente febre	Aggred. feb.	While the fever is coming on.
Agitato vase		The vial being shaken.
Aliquot		Some.
Alter		The other.
Alternis horis		Every other hour.
Aluta		Leather.
Alvo adstricta	Alv. adst.	The bowels being confined.
Alvus		The belly.
Amplus		Large.
Ampulla		A large bottle.
Ana	A. or aa.	Of each.
Aqua	Aq.	Water.
Aqua astricta	Aq. astr.	Frozen water.
Aqua bulliens	Aq. bull.	Boiling water.
Aqua communis	Aq. comm.	Ordinary water.
Aqua fervens	Aq. ferv.	Hot water.
Aqua fluviatilis	Aq. fluv.	River water.
Aqua fontana	Aq. font.	Spring or well water.
Aqua marina	Aq. mar.	Sea water.
Aqua nivalis	Aq. niv.	Snow water.
Aqua pluvialis	Aq. pluv.	Rain water.
Aut		Or.
Balneum arenæ	B. A.	A sand bath.
Balneum maris	B. M.	A salt water bath.
Balneum vaporis	B. V.	A vapor bath.
Barbadensis	B. B., or B. B. S.	Barbadoes.
Bene		Well.
Bibe	Bib.	Drink.
Biduum		Two days.
Bis		Twice.

WORD OR PHRASE.	ABBREVIATION.	TRANSLATION.
Bis in dies.	Bis. in d.	Twice daily.
Bulliat, bulliant.	Bull.	Let boil.
Caeruleus.	Caerul.	Blue.
Calefactus.		Warmed.
Calomelas.		Calomel.
Cape; capiat.	Cap.	Take; let him (or her) take.
Capsula.	Caps.	A capsule.
Cataplasma.		A poultice.
Caute.		Cautiously.
Charta.	Chart.	A paper (medicated).
Chartula.	Chart.	A little paper for a powder.
Cibus.	Cib.	Food.
Cochleare amplum.	Coch. amp.	A tablespoonful.
Cochleare magnum.	Coch. mag.	A tablespoonful.
Cochleare modicum.	Coch. mod.	A dessertspoonful.
Cochleare parvum.	Coch. parv.	A teaspoonful.
Cochleatin.	Cochleat.	By spoonfuls.
Coctio.	Coct.	Boiling.
Cola; colatus.	Col.	Strain; strained.
Colatura.	Colatur.	To, or of, the strained liquid.
Coletur; colentur.	Colet. colent.	Let it, or them, be strained.
Collutorium.	Collut.	A mouth wash.
Collyrium.	Collyr.	An eye wash.
Coloretur.		Let it be colored.
Compositus.	Co. comp.	Compound.
Concisus.		Cut.
Confectio.	Conf.	A confection.
Congius.	Cong.	A gallon.
Conserva.	Cons.	A conserve; also, keep (thou).
Continuantur remedia.	Cont. rem.	Let the medicine be continued.
Contusus.		Bruised.
Coque; coquantur.	Coq.	Boil; let them be boiled.
Coque ad medietatis consumptionem.	Coq. ad med. consump.	Boil until reduced (consumed) to one-half.
Coque in sufficiente quantitate aquae.		Boil in a sufficient quantity of water.
Cor, cordis.		The heart.
Cortex.	Cort.	The bark.
Coxa.		The hip.
Cras, crastinus.	Crast.	To-morrow.
Cras mane sumendus.		To be taken tomorrow morning
Cras nocte.		To-morrow night.
Cras vespere.		To-morrow evening.
Cujus; cujuslibet.	Cuj.	Of which; of any.
Cum.	C.	With.
Cyatho theæ.		In a cup of tea.
Cyathus; cyathus vinarius	Cyath., c. vinar.	A wineglass.
Da; detur.	D.; det.	Give; let be given.
De.		Of or from.
Deaurentur pilulæ.	Deaur. pil.	Let the pills be gilt.
Debita spissitudo.	Deb. spiss.	A proper consistence.
Debitus.		Due, proper.
Decanta.	Dec.	Decant.
Decem; decimus.		Ten; the tenth.
Decoctum.	Decoc.	A decoction.
Decubitus.	Decub.	Lying down.
De die in diem.	De d. in d.	From day to day.
Dein.		Thereupon.
Deglutiatur.	Deglut.	May, or let, be swallowed.
Dentur tales doses.	D. t. d.	Let of such doses be given.
Detur in duplo.		Let twice as much be given.
Dexter, dextra.		The right.
Diebus alternis.	Dieb. alt.	Every other day.
Diluculo.	Diluc.	At break of day.
Dilue, dilutus.	Dil.	Dilute; diluted.
Dimidius.	Dim.	One-half.
Directione propria.	D. P. or direc. prop.	With a proper direction.
Dividatur in partes æquales	D. in p. æq.	Let it be divided into equal parts.
Divide.	D., Div.	Divide (thou).
Dividendus.	Dividend.	To be divided.
Donec alvus bis dejiciatur		Until the bowels have twice moved.
Donec alvus soluta fuerit		Until the bowels shall be moved (opened).
Lotio.		A lotion.

WORD OR PHRASE.	ABBREVIATION.	TRANSLATION.
Donec dolor exulaverit....		Until the pain is removed.
Durante dolore.		While the pain lasts.
Eadem...............		The same.
Ejusdem.............	Ejusd.........	The same.
Electuarium............	Elect.......	An electuary.
Emesis.		Vomiting.
Emplastrum............	Emp........	A plaster.
Enema.	Enem......	An enema, a clyster.
Et..............		And.
Evanuerit.............		Shall have disappeared.
Exhibeatur.............	Exhib.......	Let it be exhibited.
Extende supra...........	Ext. sup.	Spread upon.
Extende super alutam mollem.	Ex. sup. alut. moll........	Spread upon soft leather.
Extractum.	Ext	An extract.
Fac; fiat; fiant........	F.; Ft.......	Make; let it be made; let them be made.
Fasciculus...........		A bundle.
Febre durante	Feb. dur.......	During the fever.
Fiat lege artis............	F. L. A..	Let it be made according to art.
Fiat solutio........	Ft. sol........	Make a solution.
Fiat venæsectio		Bleed.
Fictilis		Earthen.
Filtra.............		Filter.
Filtram, filtrum.....		A filter.
Fistula armata. ...		A syringe fitted for use.
Fluidus......	Fl..........	Fluid.
Frustillatim..	Frust........	In little pieces.
Fuerit.........		Shall have been.
Gargarisma.....	Garg........	A gargle.
Gradatim.....		Gradually, by degrees.
Grana sex pondere....		Weighing six grains.
Granum; grana........	Gr........	Grain; grains.
Gratus.....		Pleasant.
Gutta; guttæ......	Gtt.......	A drop; drops.
Guttatim....	Guttat........	Drop by drop.
Guttis quibusdam......	Gutt. quibus....	With a few drops.
Harum pilularum sumantur tres...........	Har. pil. sum. 3	Let three of these pills be taken.
Haustus.........	Haust........	A draught.
Haustus purgans noster.....	H. p. n	A purging draught made by the prescriber's own formula.
Hebdomada............		A week.
Heri.............		Yesterday.
Hic, hæc, hoc.........		This.
Hirudo		A leech.
Hora...........	H.........	An hour
Hora somni..	H. S.	Just before retiring.
Hora undecima matutina...		At the eleventh hour of the morning.
Hora decubitus...........	H. D........	At the hour of retiring.
Horæ unius spatio.	Hor. un. spat..	At the expiration of an hour.
Horis intermediis..........	Hor. intermed...	In the intermediate hours.
Idem		The same.
Idoneus................		Proper.
Imprimis..............		First.
Incide; incisus		Cut; being cut.
In dies...............	In d........	Daily.
Infunde..	Inf........	Pour in.
Infusum.............	Inf........	An infusion.
Injectio....	Inj	An injection.
Injiciatur enema..........		Let a clyster be given.
In pulmento...........		In gruel.
Instar.............	Inst........	Like, as large as.
Inter...............		Between.
Jam.............		Now.
Jusculum....		A broth.
Juxta		Near to.
Lac..............		Milk.
Lana..		Flannel.
Languor............		Faintness.
Lateris dolenti.	Lat. dol........	To the side that is painful.
Lectus................		A bed.
Libra............•........	Lib. lb..........	A pound.
Linteum.		Lint.
Liquor..............	Liq.........	A solution.

WHEN ORDERING OR PRESCRIBING.

WORD OR PHRASE.	ABBREVIATION.	TRANSLATION.
Macera.	Mac.	Macerate.
Magnus.	Mag.	Large.
Mane primo.	Mane pr.	Very early in the morning.
Manspulus.	M. or Man.	A handful.
Manus		The hand.
Massa pilularis.	Mass. pil.	A pill mass.
Matutinus.		In the morning.
Medius.		Middle.
Mensura		By measure.
Mica panis.	Mic. pan.	Crumb of bread.
Minimum.	M. or Min.	A minim.
Minutum.		A minute.
Misce	M.	Mix.
Mistura.	Mist.	A mixture.
Misce; mittatur		Send; let it be sent.
Modicus.		Middle-sized.
Modo præscripto.	Mod. præsc.	In the manner prescribed.
Mora.		Delay.
More dictu.	More dict.	In the manner directed.
More solito.	More sol.	In the usual manner.
Mortarium.		A mortar.
Ne tradas sine nummo.	Ne tr. s. num.	Do not deliver unless paid for
Necnon.		Also.
Nisi.		Unless.
Non		Not.
Nox; Noctis.		Night.
Nocte maneque.		At night and in the morning
Nucha.		The nape of the neck.
Numerus; numero.	No.	A number, in number.
Nux moschata.		A nutmeg.
Octarius.	O.	A pint.
Octavus; octo		The eighth, eight.
Oleum lini sine igne.		Cold-drawn linseed oil.
Omni hora.	Omn. hor.	Every hour.
Omni bihori	Omn. bih.	Every two hours.
Omni quadrante horæ.	Omn. quad. hor.	Every quarter of an hour.
Omni mane.		Every morning.
Omni nocte.		Every night.
Optimus.	Opt.	Best.
Opus.		Need, occasion.
Ovum.	Ov.	An egg.
Pannus.		A rag.
Pars, partis.	Par.	A part.
Partes æquales.	P. æ.	Equal parts.
Partitis vicibus	Part. vic.	In divided doses.
Parvulus.		An infant.
Parvus.	Parv.	Small.
Pediluvium.		A foot bath.
Penicilium Camelinum.	Penicil. Cam.	A camel's-hair pencil or brush.
Per.		Through, by.
Peracta operatio emetici.		When the operation of the emetic is finished.
Per deliquium.		By deliquescence.
Pergo, pergere.		To go on with.
Per fistulam vitream.		Through a glass tube.
Phiala.	Phil.	A vial, a small bottle.
Phiala prius agitata	P. P. A.	The bottle having first been shaken.
Pilula.	Pil.	A pill.
Poculum; pocillum.	Pocul; pocill.	A cup, a little cup.
Pondere.	P.	By weight.
Pondus civile.		Civil (commercial or avoirdupois) weight.
Pondus medicinale.		Medicinal (Apothecaries') weight.
Pone aurem.		Behind the ear.
Post singulas sedes liquidas		After each loose stool.
Potus.		Drink.
Primo mane.		Very early in the morning.
Primus.		The first.
Pro.		For.
Pro ratione ætatis.		According to age.
Pro re nata.	P. r. n.	According to circumstances, occasionally.
Pugillus.	Pug.	A pinch.
Pulvis.	Pulv.	A powder.

WORD OR PHRASE.	ABBREVIATION.	TRANSLATION.
Pyxis ..		A pill-box.
Quantum libet, or q. placet, or q. vis, or q. volueris....	Q. l., Q. p., Q. v.	As much as you please.
Quantum sufficiat or q. satis.	Q. S	As much as is sufficient.
Quaqua hora..	Q. h	Every hour.
Quaque.......	Q. Q.	Each or every.
Quartus; quatuor.		The fourth; four.
Quater...		Four times.
Quibus.		From which.
Quinque; quintus.		Five; the fifth.
Quoque......	Q. Q	Also.
Quorum.	Quor.	Of which.
Quofi die......		Daily.
Recens..........		Fresh.
Recipe......	R......	Take.
Redigatur in pulverem	Redig. in pulv.	Let it be reduced to powder.
Reliquus.		Remaining.
Repetatur; repetantur.....	Rept........	Let it (them) be repeated.
Respondere...		To answer.
Retinere		To keep.
Saltem.....		At least.
Saturatus.	Sat	Saturated.
Scatula........	Scat	A box.
Scilicet...............		Namely.
Secundum artem......		According to art.
Secundum artis regulas...		According to the rules of art.
Secundum naturam..		According to nature.
Secundus.		The second.
Sedes........		The alvine evacuation.
Semel.		Once.
Semissis or semis.	Ss..	A half.
Semidrachma.	Semidr	A half dram.
Semihora..	Semih.	A half hour.
Septem...		Seven.
Septimana.		A week.
Sesuncia.	Sesunc..	An ounce an a half.
Sesquihora....... ...		An hour and a half.
Sex; sextus.		Six; the sixth.
Si............		If.
Sic; sic?...		So; is it so?
Signa............	S, or Sig	Sign, or mark (thou).
Signetur nomine proprio...		Let it be labeled with its proper name.
Simul...		Together.
Sine		Without.
Singulorum	Sing.	Of each.
Si non valeat.............	Si, n. val......	If it does not answer
Si opus sit...		If necessary.
Si vires permittant....	Si vir. perm...	If the strength will permit.
Sit.		Let it be.
Solus		Alone.
Solve; solutus.... ..		Dissolve; dissolved.
Solutio..	Sol.	A solution.
Spiritus vini tenuis........		Proof spirit.
Statim	Stat.	Immediately.
Stet; stent..		Let it (them) stand.
Stratum super stratum......	S. S. S.	Layer upon layer.
Subactus.		Subdued.
Subfinem coctionis........		When the boiling is nearly finished.
Subinde.....		Frequently.
Sumat talem		Let there be taken one like this
Sumat; sumatur...	Sum......	Let him take; let it be taken.
Sume; sumendus....	Sum	Take; to be taken.
Summitates........		The tops.
Superbibendo haustum.....		Afterwards drinking this draught.
Supra...		Above.
Tabella...............	Tabel....	A tablet or lozenge.
Talis...........	Tal...	Such as or like this.
Ter die, or ter in die........	T. d., or t. i. d.	Three times a day.
Tere; tero.	Ter.	Rub; I rub.
Tere simul...............	Ter Sim...	Rub together.
Tertius......		The third.
Tres.............		Three.
Triduum...........		Three days.
Tritura...	Trit.	Triturate.
Trochischus.	Troch.	A troche.

WORD OR PHRASE.	ABBREVIATION.	TRANSLATION.
Tussis..............	....	A cough.
Ultimo præscriptus.........	Ult. præsc.......	The last ordered.
Una........	....	Together.
Uncia......	....	An ounce.
Ut dictum....	Ut dict.	As directed.
Utendum......	Utend...........	To be used.
Uto, uti.........	....	To make use of.
Vas vitreum......	....	A glass vessel.
Vehiculum	....	A vehicle.
Vel...........	....	Or.
Vesper, vesperis.	Vesp.............	The evening.
Vices..................	....	Turns, times or changes.
Vires..................	....	Strength.
Vitellus...............	Vit.............	The yolk (of an egg).
Vitello ovi solutus.........	V. O. S.........	Dissolved in the yolk of an egg.
Vitreum, vitrum.	....	Glass.
Vomitione urgente.........	Vom. urg.......	The vomiting being troublesome.

Latin Genitive Case Endings.

NOM.	GEN.	EXCEPTIONS.
-a........	æ	Cataplasma, enema, physostigma, aspidosperma, and gargarisma end in -atis; folia (pl.)=foliorum; coca is unchanged though cocæ is used by some.
-us -um -os -on ..	-i	Rhus, rhois; flos, floris; bos, bovis; limon, limonis; erigeron, erigerontis. Quercus, cornus, fructus, spiritus, haustus and potus remain unchanged.
-as.........	-atis.....	Asclepias, -adis; mas, maris. Sassafras does not change.
-is	-idis	Pulvis, -eris; arsenis, phospis, sulphis and all salts ending in -is take the ending -itis. Berberis, cannabis, digitalis, hydrastis and sinapis remain unchanged.
-o.........	onis	Mucilago, ustilago and solidago end in -inis. Condurango, kino, sago and matico do not change.
-l	lis.	Fel, fellis; mel, mellis; sumbul, sumbuli.
-en...... -ps......... -rs......... -r. .... -x.........	inis.... pis......... rtis....... ris ...... cis	Azedarach, buchu, catechu, curare, jaborandi and amyl also remain unchanged though amylis is sometimes used.

Symbols or Signs Used in Prescriptions.

M. Minim, ᵍᵇ part of a fluidrachm.

Gtt. Gutta, a drop; guttæ, drops.

℈. Scrupulus vel scrupulum, a scruple = 20 grains.

℥. Drachma, a dram = 60 grains.

f ℨ. Fluidrachma, a fluid or measured dram = 60 minims.

℥. Uncia, a troy ounce = 480 grains.

f ℥. Fluiduncia, a fluid ounce = 480 minims.

lb. Libra, a pound, understood in prescriptions to apply to a troy pound of 5,760 grains.

O. Octarius, a pint.

Gr. Granum, a grain, plural grana, grains.

Ss. Semis, one-half, affixed to signs as above.

Table for Making Solutions of Various Strengths with Water or Alcohol.

In the amount of solvent desired (see left-hand column), dissolve the quantity of material given on the same line and in the column headed by the strength of solution desired. Thus, 1 fl. oz. of distilled water + 10 grs. of material = a 4% solution. Where fractions are dropped or shortened the nearest figure is always given.

GRAINS OF SUBSTANCE REQUIRED FOR SOLUTIONS OF DIFFERENT STRENGTHS.

THE METRIC SYSTEM

OF

Weights and Measures.

The entire metric system is based upon the ten-millionth part of the distance from the equator to the pole. This distance as determined by careful measurements and calculations was taken as a unit of linear measure and called the *Meter*.

By taking the cube of $\frac{1}{10}$ meter or the thousandth part of 1 cubic meter the unit of volume measure was obtained. This is called the *Liter*.

The weight of one thousandth part of a liter, or one cubic centimeter of water at its greatest density was taken as the unit of weight and called the *Gram*.

There is then, in this system, a direct relation between measures of weight and capacity. As specific gravity is the weight of any substance as compared with the weight of an equal volume of water at the same temperature, then, the weight of one cubic centimeter of water being one gram, the weight in grams of one cubic centimeter of any substance, at the proper temperature, is its specific gravity. Consequently being given any two of the three terms—weight, volume or specific gravity—it is an easy matter to find the third. In no other system does this direct and simple relation exist and in no other system are computations made with equal ease and facility.

Multiples and sub-divisions of the above units increase and decrease by ten. The prefixes used are alike for all three of them, Greek being used for the multiples and Latin for the divisions, thus:

myria,	meaning.......................................	10,000.
kilo,	"	1,000.
hecto,	"	100.
deka,	"	10.
deci,	"	0.1
centi,	"	0.01
milli,	"	0.001

In prescription writing all of these may be dispensed with, and the gram (abbreviated gm.) and cubic centimeter (abbreviated c.c. which may be called fluigram, and written f. gm.) only, should be used. In fact, in the general use of the system, only a few of these prefixes are applied; each unit giving rise to larger and smaller units for denoting greater or lesser quantities. Thus, for long distances the kilometer is used much in the same way as we use the mile, though it is less; for ordinary distances the meter replaces the yard and foot, and for small distances the centi- and milli-meter are used. In capacity we have the *Ster* or kiloliter (1000 liters), the liter and the cubic centimeter (milliliter); in weight, the metric ton or millier (1000 kilos), the kilo or kilogram (1000 grams) and the gram. Quantities are expressed in terms of these units; thus instead of 1 deciliter, we speak of 100 cubic centimeters, and instead of five hectograms we say either 500 grams or ½ kilo.

For metric prescriptions the use of a decimal line instead of the period is much to be preferred as it prevents possible errors, thus:

℞ Hydrarg. chlorid. corros.......................	0	25	gm.
Potass. iodide.....................................	10		gm.
Aqua...	100		c.c.
Syr. Sarsap. Co....................................	100		c.c.
Mix.			

In order to give a conception of the value of metric terms it is necessary to make comparisons with a system with which we are thoroughly acquainted.

Thus: 1 meter = about 39.37 inches or 1.1 yards.

1 liter = " 34 fl. ozs. or 2½ pints.

1 gram = " 15.5 grs.

For ordinary purposes exact comparisons shoulds not be made as the equivalents so obtained are cumbersome in use and hard to memorize. For instance:

1 meter = 39.370432 inches.

1 liter = 33.81358 fl. ozs.

1 gram = 15.43234874 grs.

1 cubic centimeter = 16.2305 minims.

In writing prescriptions it is sufficiently accurate and safe to consider 1 gram as equal to 15 grains, and to consider 1 cubic centimeter as equal to 15 minims. We accordingly have:

1 gram = 15 grains.

1 grain = ⅟₁₅ gram.

1 cubic centimeter = ¼ fluid dram.

1 fluid dram = 4 cubic centimeters.

Hence—

1. TO CONVERT GRAINS INTO GRAMS, OR MINIMS INTO CUBIC CENTIMETERS:

   a. Divide by 15; or,

   b. Multiply by 2 and divide by 30.

2. TO CONVERT APOTHECARIES' DRAMS INTO GRAMS, OR FLUID DRAMS INTO CUBIC-CENTIMETERS, *multiply by 4.*

To write a metric prescription for 15 doses of any medicine, write it first for *one* dose in *grains* and *minims*, and then rewrite it substituting "grams" and "cubic centimeters" for "grains" and "minims," thus:

℞ Opii..gr. i,

Camphorae.....................................gr. ji.

    Make one pill.

And to get fifteen such doses in metric terms, write:

℞ Opii..1 gm.

Camphorae.....................................2 gms.

    Make 15 pills.

The gram and cubic-centimeter (fluigram), when referring to liquids, may be considered as equal quantities, except the liquids be very heavy (as in the case of chloroform) or very light (as in the case of ether).

Measures may be discarded and weights exclusively employed, if preferred. All quantities in a prescription would then be expressed in grams.

For calculating the number of doses in a certain amount of mixture the following approximate equivalents are useful: The average "drop" (water) may be considered equal to 0.05 c.c. or 0.05 gm., a teaspoonful as 4 c.c. and a tablespoonful as 15 c.c. It must be remembered, however, that teaspoons and tablespoons vary greatly in size and where accuracy is desired a reliable dose measure should be employed.

The above contains all that it is necessary to know or learn of the metric system in order to write metric prescriptions with or without a metric posological table.

To become familiar with the system, the rules given above for the conversion of apothecaries' weights and measures into the corresponding metric quantities, may be used, the result to be varified by comparison with the following table. Just as soon, however, as familiarity with the metric system is established, and a knowledge of doses in metric terms is obtained, it is advisable to drop comparisons and use the system *per se.* Much confusion is thus avoided and time and labor saved.

Table of Equivalents.

APOTHECARIES' WEIGHTS AND MEASURES.	METRIC WEIGHTS AND MEASURES.
Grains or minims.	*Grams or cubic-centimeters.*
$\frac{1}{64}$	$0.001 = (\frac{1}{1000})$
$\frac{1}{32}$	$0.002 = (\frac{1}{500})$
$\frac{1}{16}$	$0.004 = (\frac{1}{250})$
$\frac{1}{8}$	$0.008 = (\frac{1}{125})$
$\frac{1}{4}$	$0.016 = (\frac{1}{60})$
$\frac{1}{2}$	$0.033 = (\frac{1}{30})$
1	$0.066 = (\frac{1}{15})$
2	$0.133 = (\frac{2}{15})$
5	$0.333 = (\frac{1}{3})$
10	$0.666 = (\frac{2}{3})$
15	$1.000 = (1)$
20	$1.333 = (1\frac{1}{3})$
30	$2.000 = (2)$

Drams or fluid drams.	*Grams or cubic-centimeters.*
1	4
2	8
4	16
6	24

Troy ounces or fluid ounces.	*Grams or cubic-centimeters*
1	30
2	60
4	120
6	180
8	240
12	360
16	480

The equivalents given above are approximate only, but they are perfectly safe and are chosen with the view of facilitating calculations.

Rules for Comparing the Centigrade and Fahrenheit Scales.

The Centigrade scale has 100° of temperature between the freezing and boiling points, while the Fahrenheit scale has (212—32) 180°. Hence, 1°C.=1.8° F. or 5° C.=9° F. Therefore, to convert Centigrade into Fahrenheit:

Multiply by 1.8 and add 32; and to convert Fahrenheit into Centigrade:

Subtract 32, divide the remainder by 9 and multiply by 5 (or subtract 32 and divide directly by 1.8).

AN HISTORICAL SKETCH

OF THE INTRODUCTION BY

Dr. J. Marion Sims

OF

SUCCUS ALTERANS

AND ITS SUBSEQUENT USE IN THE

THE TREATMENT OF

SYPHILIS.

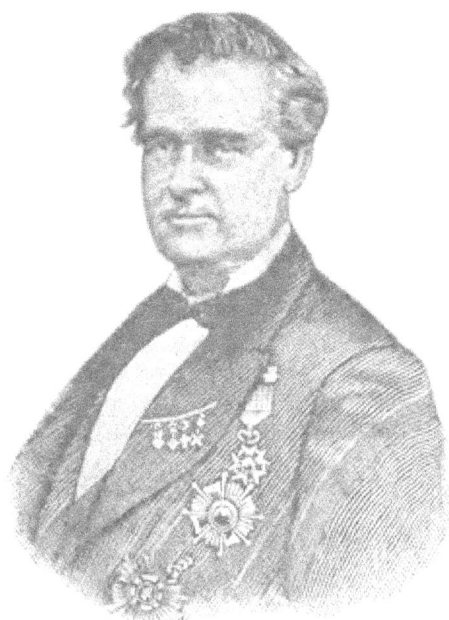

The first article written by DR. J. MARION SIMS for
the medical press was "An Essay on the Pathology and
Treatment of Trismus Nascentium, or Lock Jaw of Infants" published in the *American Journal of Medical
Science*, 1846, a subject which he followed in additional
contributions to the same journal in 1848.   He considered
his treatment of this disease his first great discovery in
medicine.

Previous to this, in 1845, DR. SIMS saw his first case of
Vesicovaginal fistula, and in 1848, through his remarkable operations, his invention of the silver suture and
other appliances, he realized that his efforts had at last
been blessed with success and that he had made one of

the most important discoveries of the age for the relief of suffering humanity.

From this time on his pen was never idle and the records of his wonderful operations fill thousands of pages in medical literature. Of him it is truly said, "Among the galaxy of eminent men of our country in scientific achievements J. MARION SIMS stands forth a great central light illuminating the world of science and fully receiving, not only the due recognition and reverential observation from the *savans* of Europe, but royal homage from crowned heads and grateful tributes from titled peers."

His last article, "The Treatment of Syphilis," was contributed to the British Medical Journal in 1883, when he was in the forty-eight year of his professional career. "This paper," says an eminent New York physician in *Gaillard's Medical Journal*, "shows his character in the lustrous light of a simple, childlike, genuine love of truth, justice and helpfulness to others."

The story in this paper reads like a romance. More than forty years before, DR. SIMS knew that the Creek Indians of Alabama had the reputation of curing syphilis, but supposed when this tribe was removed west of the Mississippi in 1837, that their secret had gone with them. It seems, however, that this was not the case, but that a mulatto slave, named Horace King, who lived among the Creeks had been entrusted with their knowledge. Horace demonstrated his ability to cure the worst cases of syphilis to Dr. Banks and Dr. Freeny who had a number of cases amongst the slaves on the Gibson plantation. These cases were also known to Dr. B. Rush Jones, who was not only DR. SIMS' brotherinlaw, but his bosom friend from youth. Hearing of the cures of the cases at Gibsons', Mr. Nicholas D. Barnett, also a relative of DR. SIMS, sent his servant, Lawson, to learn King's method. The native drugs used in the preparation were shown to Lawson, who was afterwards successful with the remedy at Barnett's plantation, and thus its use became finally known to Dr. George W. McDade, of

whom DR. SIMS speaks as "a very intelligent and ac-
complished physician, whom I have known since boy-
hood."

Dr. McDade, observing the marvelous cures made by
these obscure negroes when the highest representatives
of science had failed, undertook to investigate the remedy
and to reduce it to a scientific basis, which was necessary
for civilized use, as the original decoction was described
as being "so vile that the horrors of syphilis could alone
inspire a man with courage to take it." Learning the
formula from Lawson, he began by eliminating such
articles as he knew to be inert and using the roots and
barks freshly gathered from the woods, combined the
active remedies into a concentrated preparation representing all the valuable constituents. Dr. McDade, Dr.
Rush Jones and many of their medical friends used this
preparation for a number of years with the greatest success, and in 1882 when DR. SIMS was in Montgomery he
learned the facts here stated, which he found abundantly
corroborated on every hand. Shortly DR. SIMS returned
to England, and attended a meeting of the London Medical Society on the 26th of November of the same year,
where papers on the subject of syphilis by Dr. Drysdale
and Dr. Routh were under discussion. DR. SIMS was
greatly impressed with the variance of opinion, and observed that in fifty years there had been no progress in
the treatment of the dread disease. The events at Montgomery were fresh in his mind and he at once wrote to
Dr. Jones and Dr. McDade for a circumstantial account
of the facts which he at once (March 10, 1883) gave to the
world through the *British Medical Journal.* DR. SIMS
had known Dr. Rush Jones all his life and Dr. McDade,
Dr. Freeny and Mr. Nicholas Barnett for over forty years.
He knew their statements to be the truth and without
hesitation announced and endorsed the new treatment.

How many men, having reached the very pinnacle of
professional greatness, would have stood as godfather to
the treatment by vegetable antisyphilitics in opposition
to the ancient and therefore almost sacred methods? His

moral heroism was sublime and his prophetic eye seemed to recognize another great opportunity to bless the age in which he lived. Year after year he had seen the hopeless syphilitic stalk silently through a miserable life to certain death. So it had been for centuries. Here was the demonstrated relief and he said so in a way that no other man in the round world could have said it.

It was nearly six months later that the writer came in contact with Dr. Rush Jones and Dr. McDade personally and Dr. Sims by correspondence, Dr. McDade was overwhelmed with demands for "*his preparation*" which he could not meet. The drug shops were full of inert preparations referred to as McDade's Remedy, inert because the authentic drugs in their recent state had never been obtainable in the markets.

Dr. McDade and Dr. Jones were found at the office of the latter in Montgomery, and as the representatives of Eli Lilly & Company "an alliance, offensive and defensive" was proposed, Dr. McDade to furnish the authoritative green drugs exclusively, Eli Lilly & Company to make and market the preparation under the name of "Succus Alterans." An agreement was speedily reached, and the first order was given on the spot for thirty thousands pounds of drugs. The good doctors were almost paralyzed by the figures, but horses were saddled and the country scoured for diggers. Soon the green roots began to roll northward.

Singularly enough one of the first places visited in search of roots was old Cubahatchie, the early home of J. Marion Sims and the stepping stone to his distinguished career at Montgomery.

Dr. Sims, then in this country, had realized the difficulty encountered by the profession in getting a reliable article and was consequently very much interested in Dr. McDade's arrangements. Writing under date of September 13, 1883, to Eli Lilly & Company, Dr. Sims said "I think you have done wisely to get Dr. McDade to furnish you with the fresh roots. There will always be danger of getting in the market extracts made from roots that have been kept too long and have lost their virtue."

To. Dr. McDade, Oct. 24, 1883, he wrote, "I knew the publication of your experience would create a wide interest, but I had no idea it would have made such a boom. If I had, I would have waited for you to make arrangements for supplying it to the profession." And to ELI LILLY & COMPANY again Oct. 27, 1883, only two weeks before he laid down his earthly labors, he writes, "you have shown a spirit of enterprise and energy and liberality that commands my sympathies. I wish you all the success possible. I get letters daily about it and always answer them promptly."

DR. SIMS seemed to loose no opportunity to direct the attention of his medical friends in New York to SUCCUS ALTERANS, and it rapidly came into use, not only in the active stages of syphilis, where its value met with instant recognition, but in the sequela as well.

Dr. D. H. Goodwillie, Surgeon-in-Chief to the Private Hospital for the treatment of Diseases of the Nose, Mouth and Throat, wrote us in June 1885, "On the recommendation of my lamented friend, J. MARION SIMS, I have been using the SUCCUS ALTERANS in cases of syphilitic disease of the nose, mouth and throat," and a year later Dr. Goodwillie made an elaborate report of a series of cases treated by SUCCUS ALTERANS as a constitutional remedy and support to his surgical treatment. This paper was read before the Medical Society of the State of New York, at Albany, Feb. 3, 1886, and being splendidly illustrated by colored plates was published in the *New York Medical Journal* in June 1886.

Of one of these cases referred to Dr. Goodwillie by Dr. F. N. Otis, of New York, he says: "I put him on full doses of SUCCUS ALTERANS, prepared by ELI LILLY & COMPANY, of Indianapolis, Ind. *A marked improvement commenced at once and in a few days the large ulcerated soft palate and tonsil healed.* The uvula is now of about one-fourth its natural size, and the palate contracted so that the nasopharyngeal space is smaller. *Two years afterward* the voice was normal, the patient's health quite good, and he has *gained twenty pounds in weight*."

Again, Dr. Goodwillie says of a case as reported by Dr. F. E. Miller, House Surgeon St. Frances Hospital, N. Y., "The patient, Mrs. Mary W., entered the hospital and secured treatment by mercury and potas. iod. When all symptoms of the disease had yielded she left the hospital. The following year she returned with sore throat. Both tonsils were found large, ulcerated and accompanied with bronchitis. There was syphilitic wart of the anus. Iodide potassium was administered twice daily in milk. This so distressed her stomach and bowels it was given up and SUCCUS ALTERANS was given in one dram doses twice daily. The large and ulcerated tonsils were amputated by Dr. Goodwilllie. Under the tonic effect of this medicine she regained her health and left the hospital. After a short time she reported as in good health and having *gained twenty-five pounds in weight*." Dr. Goodwillie reports a number of cases coming under his observation quite as important as the above, successfully treated by SUCCUS ALTERANS in connection with surgical attention.

More than twelve years have passed and SUCCUS ALTERANS is professionally known around the globe. The shipments of green roots from about old Cubahatchie have grown steadily with the years and are now running into millions of pounds.

HOW TO USE
SUCCUS ALTERANS.

(JUICES OF THE PLANTS.)

FORMULA ON EVERY LABEL.

IN SYPHILIS.

Begin with teaspoonful doses, either before or after meals and rapidly increase to tablespoonful doses. If slight nausea occurs decrease the dose temporarily. Discontinue the treatment one week in each month. During this period use a tonic such as our Elixir or Pil. Iron and Quinine or Iron, Quinine and Strychnine three times daily and continue the SUCCUS ALTERANS treatment for twelve months.

IN SCROFULA OR OTHER BLOOD OR SKIN DISEASES.

Give from one to two teaspoonfuls three times daily or in severe cases the full doses. For children give from one-half to two teaspoonfuls, according to age and condition, with water or syrup if necessary. SUCCUS ALTERANS is purely vegetable and may be taken any length of time without injury.

AS A GENERAL ALTERATIVE.

Physicians should keep in mind the great value of SUCCUS ALTERANS as a *general* **alterative.** Its use is invaluable in all cases of strumous diathesis, anemia, consumption diagnosed as originating in specific disease, nasal catarrh, rheumatism, eczema, psoriasis, wasting away from general debility, and the whole list of diseases following the train of poisoned and impure, or impoverished blood.

USE SUCCUS ALTERANS pure and simple. It is worse than useless to add mercury or iodides to SUCCUS ALTERANS which is of itself a certain antidote to blood poison and increases red corpuscles in poor blood, while mercury and the iodides produce a condition of the system infinitely worse than the disease it is sought to cure.

The effect of SUCCUS ALTERANS as a constitutional remedy rests, unquestionably, in its power of eliminating specific poison from the blood and its tonic power, increasing the proportion of red corpuscles in impoverished blood, thus enabling the system to throw off disease.

TREATMENT OF SYPHILIS.

By Geo. W. McDade, M. D.

Succus Alterans stimulates the secretions throughout the entire system, acting directly upon the stomach, liver, kidneys and the glandular system. The appetite and digestion are improved, and there is an increased flow of saliva, gastric fluid, bile, urine and perspiration.

Secondary symptoms seldom follow the primary stages if Succus Alterans *is promptly and persistently used on the very first appearance of the chancre. Secondary* cases are usually *discharged* in *from four to eight months.* This is the rule; of course there are exceptions, owing to idiosyncrasies of the patient, amount of constitutional disturbance, condition of patient and the length of time since contracting the disease. Some are cured in less time while others require more. *I have never had to extend the treatment into years.* After all evidences of the disease are subdued, I recommend the patient, as a precautionary measure, to take the medicine every alternate week for several months. No injurious effects are produced even if it should be continued for years.

Patients who have been treated on the old plan usually improve very rapidly after taking Succus Alterans, and soon recover from any bad effects the mixed treatment may have produced. *I think* Succus Alterans *the best remedy for the cure of mercurialism and iodism.*

Succus Alterans sometimes produces temporary nausea; further gastric disturbance I have never witnessed. Almost invariably the appetite and digestion improve after taking the Succus Alterans. There is also abundant evidence of its value in anemia from either syphilitic or other causes.

Unquestionably it eradicates the syphilitic spores from the blood and increases the number of red corpuscles.

Mercury and the iodides, long continued, often produce injurious effects upon the system second only to the disease itself. My mode of administration, as with any other remedy necessary to be continued for any length of time, is to occasionally discontinue it for a few days or a week, alternating with tonics or other medicines, as as are indicated; each return gives renewed benefit.

THE DANGER.

THE DUTY OF THE PHYSICIAN.

In the use of SUCCUS ALTERANS the physician must recognize *his duty* to see that his prescription is filled with the genuine article. It is within our observation that a large amount of spurious stuff is sold as SUCCUS ALTERANS. Cases have even been discovered where imitations have been dispensed from bottles from which the genuine SUCCUS ALTERANS has been removed, thus *selling the imitation under the genuine labels.*

ELI LILLY & COMPANY on their part fill the requirements of DR. J. MARION SIMS and Dr. McDade *to the letter* and it is not their fault if spurious and inferior preparations are used in filling prescriptions when SUCCUS ALTERANS is ordered. *There is absolutely no safety* to the physician or the patient unless the SUCCUS ALTERANS is obtained in the *original, unbroken package.*

ELI LILLY & COMPANY annually receive from the Cubahatchie region of Alabama their supply of the green drugs, native to that country. They are carefully collected at the proper season, shipped in the green state to the laboratory at Indianapolis, the juices extracted and preserved in cool cellars until demanded by the trade. Thus is rendered absolutely certain the utmost uniformity and the greatest activity in the preparation and so we are able to assure the profession that our obligation to furnish the remedy in the highest perfection is honestly fulfilled.

NOTWITHSTANDING ALL THIS we have positive knowledge that thousands of pounds of imitations of SUCCUS ALTERANS are dispensed every year and we can only repeat that SUCCUS ALTERANS should always be obtained in the original pint amber bottles. It is never sold by us in bulk.

THE LABELS IN ENGLISH, SPANISH, GERMAN and French carry the name of ELI LILLY & COMPANY besides their signature in red ink across the front and the certificate of authority of Dr. Geo. W. M. McDade, with *fac simile* of his signature as follows:

WHEN ORDERING OR PRESCRIBING.

322 ELI LILLY & COMPANY

CERTIFICATE OF AUTHORITY.

No. 34 Dexter Ave.,
Montgomery, Ala., December 15, 1884.

This is to certify to the medical profession that ELI LILLY & COMPANY, manufacturing chemists of INDIANAPOLIS, IND., U. S. A., are the only manufactures of "SUCCUS ALTERANS" for blood and skin diseases, and no one has the right to use my name in connection with any other preparation.

That all preparations purporting to be the SAME are wholly unauthorized by me.

That each pint bottle of SUCCUS ALTERANS contains in NATURAL COMBINATION THE UNIMPAIRED VIRTUES OF SIXTEEN TROY OUNCES of the TRUE MEDICINAL PLANTS, STILLINGIA SYLVATICA, SMILAX SARSAPARILLA, PHYTOLACCA DECANDRA, LAPPA MINOR and XANTHOXYLUM CAROLINIANUM, the compound being made in the same proportions as in my original formula.

That I have been impelled to this course solely in answer to the demand upon me personally for a strictly reliable and uniform preparation made only from DRUGS COLLECTED IN PROPER SEASON, and such I guarantee "SUCCUS ALTERANS" to be.

Geo. W. McDade M.D.

PLEASE SPECIFY "LILLY"

SUCCUS ALTERANS;

ALTERATIVE JUICE.

DOSE—One teaspoonful, in water, three **times a day, before meals**, gradually increased to tablespoonful **doses**.

SUCCUS ALTERANS is the preserved fresh juices of the true medicinal plants: *Stillingia sylvatica, Smilax sarsaparilla, Phytolacca decandra, Lappa minor* and *Xanthoxylum Carolinianum;* collected in their native growth under the immediate supervision of DR. G. W. McDADE, of Montgomery County, Alabama, U. S. A., as recommended by DR. J. MARION SIMS, in the *British Medical Journal*, DR. B. RUSH JONES, and many other eminent physicans.

SUCCUS ALTERANS continues to gain favor from its remarkable alterative and tonic properties, *eliminating specific poison from the blood* and *increasing the proportion of red corpuscles in anemic patients* to a wonderful degree; is endorsed by the medical profession and in use by many hospitals of note.

SUCCUS ALTERANS in venereal and cutaneous diseases is fast supplanting Mercury, the Iodides and Arsenic; and is a certain remedy for Mercurialization, Iodism and the dreadful effects often following the use of Arsenic in skin diseases.

SUCCUS ALTERANS is also strongly recommended for its tonic and alterative effects in the myriad forms of scrofulous disease, and in all cases where anemia is a factor. Such patients rapidly develop a good appetite, sleep soundly and gain flesh rapidly. Many cases are on record where patients have increased ten to twenty-five pounds in weight in a few weeks.

SUCCUS ALTERANS is giving satisfactory results in treatment of *Chronic Rheumatism* and can be used with confidence.

SUCCUS ALTERANS may be given for any length of time, without injury to the patient.

SUCCUS ALTERANS is put up in pint, round amber bottles, and *never in bulk.*

ELI LILLY & COMPANY,

PHARMACEUTICAL CHEMISTS,
INDIANAPOLIS, IND., U. S. A.

SUPPLIED BY ALL DRUGGISTS.

LONDON: JOHN M. RICHARDS, 46 Holborn Viaduct, *SOLE AGENT FOR GREAT BRITAIN.*

WHEN ORDERING OR PRESCRIBING.

PIL. APHRODISIACA;

LILLY.

A FOOD AND TONIC FOR THE NERVOUS SYSTEM.

Indicated in Nervousness, Sexual Debility, Mental Overwork, Impotency.

DOSE--ONE TO THREE PILLS AFTER MEALS.

It is necessary that the administration of this pill be continued from three to four weeks, or until the system is thoroughly under the influence of the remedy.

THE GENUINE PILLS

HAVE LILLY ON THE LABEL,

ARE OVAL IN SHAPE,

ARE PINK IN COLOR,

ARE 100 PILLS IN A BOTTLE.

REJECT ALL OTHERS.

Order only original package.   Price $1.00 per bottle by mail.

FOR SALE BY ALL DRUGGISTS.

TWENTY YEARS AGO

ELI LILLY & COMPANY devised the combination of *Damiana, Phosphorus* and *Nux Vomica*, which has since been known as "PIL. APHRODISIACA" and prescribed throughout this country and Great Britain with the greatest success in the treatment of diseases consequent on nervous breakdown from whatever cause, but principally in cases of mental overwork, sexual debility and impotency. It is decidedly beneficial in cases of nocturnal emissions, the result of excesses, mental apathy or indifference, and in an enfeebled condition of the general system, with weakness or dull pain in the lumbosacral region. In diseases of the reproductive organs of the female, and especially of the uterus, it is a most valuable agent, acting as a uterine tonic and gradually removing abnormal conditions, while at the same time, it imparts tone and vigor; hence it is of value in leucorrhea, amenorrhea, dysmenorrhea and to remove the tendency to repeated miscarriages. Careful study of the many reported cases benefited by the remedy leads us to believe the *rationale* of its action upon the nervous system may be considered that of a food and tonic as well as a sedative. In all events it is efficacious as a vitalizing tonic in a way that cannot be claimed for any other remedy or combination in its special sphere, a fact attested by its long and still rapidly increasing use.

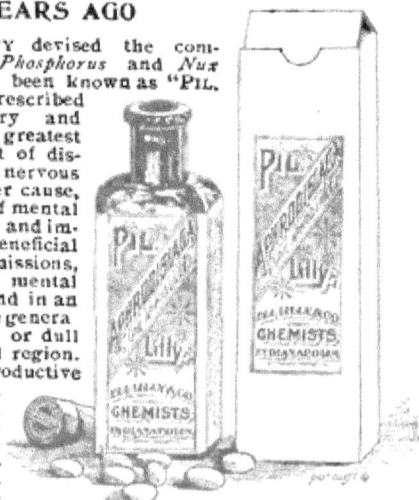

PLEASE SPECIFY "LILLY"

ELIXIR PURGANS;

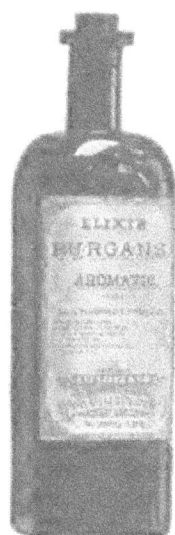

LILLY,

IS NOT ONLY

A Pleasant and Reliable Purgative

AND OF GREAT VALUE IN

Habitual Constipation,

But in every way **Superior to Calomel** in
the treatment of

Chronic Derangements of the Liver,

Malarial Jaundice,

Bilious Remittent Fever

and Duodenal Catarrh.

The popularity of ELIXIR PURGANS; LILLY, with the profession is not surprising, when the formula is considered:

RHAMNUS PURSHIANA. Is tonic, aperient and laxative. Produces large, soft and painless evacuations.

EUONYMUS ATROPURPUREUS. Tonic astringent, mildly cathartic and hepatic stimulant of a high order.

CASSIA ACUTIFOLIA, Purif. Produces copious stools without griping or flatulence.

IRIS VERSICOLOR. Purgative and diuretic. A powerful hepatic stimulant.

HYOSCYAMUS NIGER, in the proportion used, is carminative, laxative and sedative.

AROMATICS are added as correctives and to give palatability.

THIS PREPARATION has been constantly used by many physicians for nearly twenty years, in daily practice, with complete satisfaction.

Physicians in prescribing should be careful to write, "ELIXIR PURGANS; LILLY, that other preparrtions may not be substituted.

Put up in pint Bottles at $1.00 per pint.
SUPPLIED BY THE DRUG TRADE.

ELI LILLY & COMPANY,

PHARMACEUTICAL CHEMISTS,
INDIANAPOLIS, IND.

WHEN ORDERING OR PRESCRIBING.

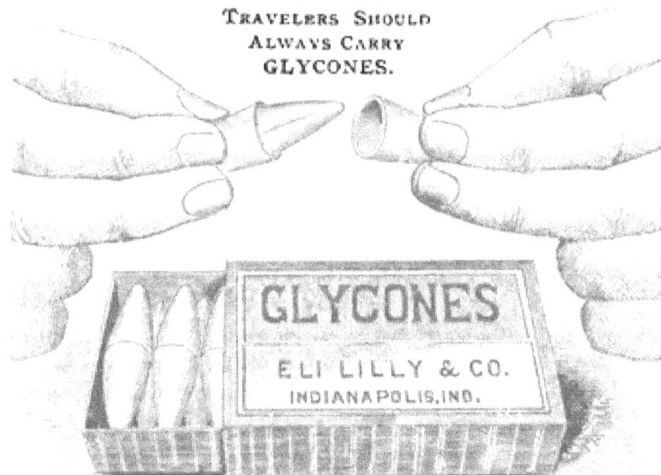

YERBAZIN;

LILLY.

A PERFECT MASK FOR THE BITTERNESS OF QUININE.

We offer this article with the assertion that it is the most perfect liquid vehicle for the administration of Quinine, Cinchonidine, etc., ever produced. It is an elegant, highly flavored preparation, exceedingly agreeable to the taste.

One fluid ounce will PERFECTLY DISGUISE the taste of twenty (20) grains Quinine sulphate.

Full directions for using accompany each package.

A MOST EXCELLENT VEHICLE.

We are using YERBAZIN; Lilly, and think the preparation a most excellent vehicle for masking the taste of Quinine and other bitter medicines.

JAMES R. HEALY, M. D.,
Superintendent Infant's and Children's Hospital, Randall's Island, N. Y.

GEO. H. BOSLEY, M. D.,
Attending physician Out Door Poor, Bellevue Hospital, N. Y.

JOHN A. ARNOLD, M. D.,
Medical Superintendent Kings County Hospital, Flatbush, N. Y.

O. P. HENDRIXSON M. D., Columbus, Ohio, says:
"I have used YERBAZIN; Lilly, for two years, and find it an excellent preparation to disguise the taste of Quinine."

THE KANSAS CITY MEDICAL RECORD, says:
"YERBAZIN; Lilly, is the best preparation we have ever used to mask the taste of Quinine and other bitter medicines. We use the preparation in the proportion of two grains of Quinine to a dram of the Syrup."

FOR SALE BY DRUGGISTS EVERYWHERE.

Please specify LILLY'S in every instance, as there are a large number of inferior preparations in the market.

Pyroferrine;

Lilly.

NUTRITIVE TONIC AND STIMULANT.

Especially Indicated in Nervous Diseases of Women.

FREE FROM CONSTIPATING TENDENCY.

Each fluid dram contains Iron pyrophosphate, 2½ grs.; Strychnine, 1-100 gr.; Phosphoric acid.

Pyroferrine, Lilly, represents the prescription of an eminent specialist in diseases of women, who for many years obtained such uniformly happy results from its use that after his death it was adopted by many of his friends in the profession to whom he had confided the formula. On account of the desire for a preparation which should be always uniform in appearance as well as containing the purest chemicals in strictly accurate proportions, we have been solicited by a prominent physician to supply an article which would fully meet the requirements of the profession. The Iron salt entering into its composition is chemically pure, free from astringency, almost tasteless and does not tend to constipation. It has a tonic influence upon the nerve centers, and improves nutrition principally by its effect upon the circulation; in its combination with Phosphoric acid and Strychnine it presents an elegant preparation, meeting the wants of the practitioner in a wide range of cases where a tonic treatment is indicated. It promotes the appetite, increases digestion, improves the quality of the blood, increasing the number of red corpuscles and exalts the vital powers. Of value in the management of Anemia, Chlorosis and dysmenorrhea. By promoting capillary circulation it is beneficial in cases of habitual coldness of hands and feet; Hysteria, especially when associated with anemia and dysmenorrhea. Certain cerebral disorders which are more or less dependent upon anemia, as some forms of puerperal mania, chronic mania and melancholia, which are not infrequently due to the impoverishment of the blood, are benefited by its use. Pyroferrine is useful with mothers who are anemic and nervous from nursing, and in female debility generally.

Formula is given upon each label.

Dose.—One to two teaspoonfuls three times daily after meals.

```
-----------PYROFERRINE-----------
IS MANUFACTURED ONLY BY
ELI LILLY & COMPANY.
SUPPLIED THROUGH THE DRUG TRADE
AT $1.00 PER PINT.
```

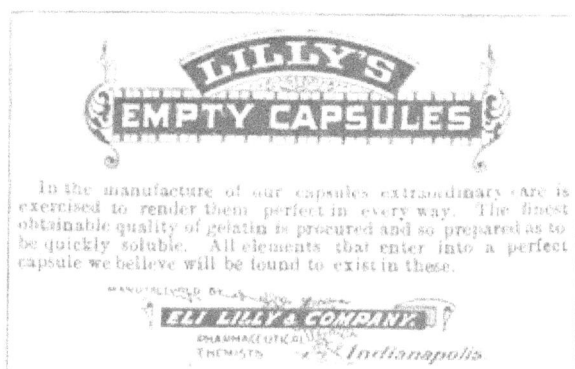

FAC SIMILE OF LABEL

It is with much satisfaction that we announce the completion of a plant devoted to the manufature of highest grade empty gelatin capsules. It is our belief that these products will be found to excel in desirable qualities any heretofore produced in this or any other country. Our aim is to produce the best capsule. With that in view we have constructed a superb plant, which is a monument to mechanical ingenuity, and utilize the best obtainable quality of gelatin. It will give us pleasure to furnish druggists and physicians with samples of these goods.

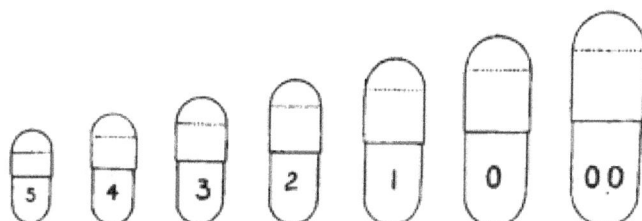

FORMASEPTOL;

LILLY.

To the Physician, Surgeon and Dentist, Formaseptol is a necessity in maintaining the proper sanitary conditions and should be recommended for use in the family as a prophylactic against disease.

For **cleansing the teeth** and as a mouth wash use one to two teaspoonfuls of **Formaseptol** to four fluid ounces of water. One or two tablespoonfuls of the above solution will relieve **fermentive dyspepsia** and **purify the breath.**

As a **gargle for sore throat** equal parts of Formaseptol and water may be used.

As a spray, for treating septic conditions of the mouth, throat and nose, a teaspoonful of Formaseptol may be mixed with four fluid ounces of tepid water may be applied with an atomizer.

For the removal of **dandruff** and **stimulating** the growth of the hair, equal parts of Formaseptol and water should be mixed and rubbed thoroughly into the scalp.

For cleansing and dressing **ulcers, burns and scalds** and relieving itching skin of eruptive diseases, as eczema, etc., **Formaseptol** diluted with an equal part of water should be applied.

For bites and stings of insects apply Formaseptol.

Summer diarrhea of children and adults is relieved by Formaseptol diluted with five to ten parts of water.

For bathing the sick a tablespoonful of Formaseptol to each quart of water purifies and cools the skin, and relieves the odor of perspiration.

As a disinfectant in infectious diseases, as scarlet fever, diphtheria, whooping cough, etc., Formaseptol should be sprayed in the room.

Formaseptol promptly removes odor of excrement and should be used for deodorizing urinals, bed pans, etc. and for sterilizing obstetrical and surgical instruments, for irrigation of catheters, washing the hands before and after surgical operations and for general disinfection.

Formaseptol diluted with an equal part of tepid water should be used for thoroughly cleansing venereal sores and may also be used as a mouth wash and gargle, after which LILLY's Acetanilid powder may be applied to the ulcers. Dr. Thomas S. K. Morton says that upon chancroids the effect of acetanilid is most surprising. He states, "all soft venereal sores have uniformly healed in from one to seven days, with a single exception which one was of a phagadenic nature and required canterization with nitric acid before it would heal under the Acetanilid. He prescribes one drachm of the acetanilid powder." The patient should wash several times a day, using Formaseptol in the water and then rub in the Acetanilid powder. If the sore is beneath the prepuce leave a quantity of the drug which prevents excoriations by urethral discharges. The drug is entirely without odor.

ELI LILLY & COMPANY,

INDIANAPOLIS, IND.

Appendix—Fluid Extracts.

FL. EXT. ALOES, for tincture......................**Dose 10 to 30 m.**
 Standard of strength—One pint represents Purified aloes, 5 troy ounces; Licorice root, 10 troy ounces.
 Action and uses—Purgative, laxative and **emmenagogue.** Used principally for making the official tincture.

PREPARATION.

Tincture Aloes, U. S.—Fl. ext. Aloes, for tincture, Lilly, 4⅞ fl. ozs.; Diluted alcohol, 11⅛ fl. ozs.; Mix—Dose, as a laxative, ½ to 1 fl. dr.; as a purgative, 2 to 4 fl. drs.

FL. EXT. ARBOR VITÆ, Aqueous...................**Dose 30 to 60 m.**
 Thuja occidentalis Linn. **Nat. Ord.**—*Coniferæ.*
 Synonyms—Thuya occidentalis Linn.,—False white cedar.
 Range—New Brunswick to Pennsylvania, along mountains to North Carolina, west to Minnesota.
 Habitat—Swamps and cool rocky banks.
 Part used—Leaves and twigs.
 Standard of strength—That of the U. S. Pharmacopœia, 1890; 1 c. c. representing 1 gram of the drug; or, practically, minim for grain.
 Action and uses—Tonic, stomachic and stimulant. Especially designed for use by inhalation in affections of the lungs and bronchial tubes where the presence of alcohol is objectionable and the antiseptic and stimulant action of the remedy alone desired.

FL EXT. BAYBERRY COMP.....................**Dose 15 to 30 m.**
 Synonym—Fluid composition powder.
 Standard of strength—One pint represents Bayberry bark, 9 troy ounces; Ginger, 4½ troy ounces; Capsicum, Cloves, of each, ¼ troy ounce.
 Note—This formula corresponds to the one given in the National Formulary for compound bayberry powder.
 Action and uses—Aromatic, stimulant and carminative.

FL. EXT. BUCHU COMP., Formula B ....**Dose 30 to 60 m.**
 Standard of strength—One pint represents Buchu, 8 troy ounces; Juniper berries, Cubeb, Uva ursi, of each, 2 troy ounces; Spirit of nitrous ether, 2 fluid ounces.
 Action and uses—Stimulant and diuretic. Valuable in diseases of the urinary organs and the genito-urinary mucous membrane.

FL. EXT. GOLD THREAD......................**Dose 30 to 60 m.**
 Coptis trifolia (Linn.) Salisb. **Nat. Ord.**—*Ranunculaceæ.*
 Synonyms—Helleborus trifolia Linn., Isopyrum trifolium Britton,—Mouth root, Threeleaved gold thread.
 Range—Northeastern United States, south to Maryland, west to Iowa.
 Habitat—Bogs northward, along mountain ranges southward.
 Part used—The entire plant.
 Standard of strength—That of the U. S. Pharmacopœia, 1890; 1 c.c. representing 1 gram of the drug; or, practically, minim for grain.
 Properties and uses—An indigenous bitter tonic, resembling quassia, gentian and columbo, without any astringency. It is beneficial in all cases where a bitter tonic is desired. The infusion is useful as a wash or gargle in ulcerations of the mouth.

FLUID EXTRACTS—Appendix Continued.

PREPARATIONS.

Tincture Gold thread—Fl. ext. Gold thread, Lilly, 2 fl. ozs.; Diluted alcohol, 14 fl. ozs.; Mix—Dose 2 to 4 fl. drs.

Infusion Gold thread—Fl. ext. Gold thread, Lilly, 1 fl. oz.; Hot water, 15 fl. ozs.; Mix—Dose 1 to 2 fl. ozs.

FL. EXT. GRINDELIA Soluble......................Dose 30 to 60 m.

Grindelia robusta Nutt *and G. squarrosa* Dunal.

Nat. Ord.—*Compositæ.*

Synonym—Gum plant.

Range—Western United States, west of the Rocky Mountains.

Habitat—In salt marshes and on alkaline soil.

Part used—The leaves and inflorescence.

Standard of strength—That of the U. S. Pharmacopœia, 1890; 1 c.c. representing 1 gram of the drug; or practically, minim for grain.

Action and uses—Antispasmodic and motor-depressant. Especially efficacious in spasmodic asthma, bronchitis and whooping cough. Useful in dyspnea, hay fever and chronic cystitis. Used as a sedative lotion in poisoning by rhus tox. and for skin diseases in which itching or burning sensations occur.

NOTE—This preparation is made so as to be clearly miscible with aqueous liquids or syrup. The resinous constituents are rendered soluble by combining with a basic salt and are therefore precipitated on the addition of acids.

PREPARATION.

Syrup Grindelia, Soluble—Fl. ext. Grindelia, soluble, Lilly, 4 fl. ozs.; Syrup, 12 fl. ozs.; Mix—Dose 2 to 4 fl. drs.

Infusion Grindelia, Soluble—Fl. ext. Grindelia, soluble, Lilly, 2 fl. ozs.; Hot water, 14 fl. ozs.; Mix—Dose ½ to 1 fl. oz.

FL. EXT. GROUND IVY.............................Dose 30 to 60 m.

Nepeta Glechoma Benth.   **Nat. Ord.**—*Labiatæ.*

Synonyms—N. hederacea B. S. P., Glechoma hederacea Linn.,—Gill-over-the-ground.

Range—Europe, naturalized in the United States; common.

Habitat—Moist shady ground, near dwellings, and in waste places.

Part used—The herb.

Standard of strength—That of the U. S. Pharmacopœia, 1890; 1 c.c. representing 1 gram of the drug, or, practically, minim for grain.

Action and uses—Chiefly used in the treatment of chronic bronchitis with mucopurulent sputa. Also has been found useful in catarrhal affections of the urinary organs and in tonic dyspepsia.

PREPARATION.

Infusion Ground Ivy—Fl. ext. Ground ivy, Lilly, 2 fl. ozs.; Hot water, 14 fl. ozs.; Mix—Dose, ½ to 1 fl. oz.

FL. EXT. LICORICE, for syrup...................Dose 60 to 120 m.

Glycyrrhiza glabra Linn, *and G. glabra var. glandulifera.* (Waldstein et Kittaibel) Regel et Herder. **Nat. Ord.**—*Leguminosæ.*

Synonyms—G. glandulifera Waldstein et Kittaibel.

Range—Southern Europe, Asia Minor and Northern Asia; cultivated in Europe.

Habitat—Moist sandy soil.

Part used—The root.

Standard of strength—That of the U. S. Pharmacopœia, 1890 ; 1 c.c. representing 1 gram of the drug; or, practically, minim for grain.

Action and uses—An excellent demulcent. Useful in catarrhal affections and in diarrhea.

NOTE—This preparation is made from a particularly fine quality of the root, and is intended for use in preparing syrup of licorice. It may also be used for masking the bitterness of quinine.

PREPARATION.

Syrup Licorice—Fl. ext. Licorice, for syrup, Lilly, 4 fl. ozs.; Syrup, 12 fl. ozs.; Mix—Used as a vehicle.

GENERAL INDEX.

GENERAL INDEX—Continued.

GENERAL INDEX—Continued.

www.ingramcontent.com/pod-product-compliance
Lightning Source LLC
Chambersburg PA
CBHW021459210326
41599CB00012B/1053